Critical Topics in an Aging Society

Editorial Advisor, Toni C. Antonucci, PhD

- *Using Technology to Improve Care of Older Adults*
  Diane Chau, MD, FACP, and Thomas F. Osborne, MD, Editors
- *Homeless Older Populations: A Practical Guide for the Interdisciplinary Care Team*
  Diane Chau, MD, FACP, and Arnold P. Gass, MD, FACP, Editors
- *The New Politics of a Majority-Minority Nation: Aging, Diversity, and Immigration*
  Fernando M. Torres-Gil, PhD, and Jacqueline L. Angel, PhD
- *Elder Justice, Ageism, and Elder Abuse*
  Lisa Nerenberg, MSW, MPH
- *Social Isolation in Later Life: Strategies to Bolster Health and Well-Being*
  Lenard W. Kaye, PhD, DWS, and Cliff Singer, MD

Homeless Older Populations

Diane Chau, MD, FACP, is a regional medical director for Molina Healthcare, California, and the director of the San Diego Geriatrics Education Center/Geriatrics Workforce Enhancement Program. She created the University of Nevada School of Medicine Geriatrics, Hospice, & Palliative Medicine fellowship training programs and served as their division chief of geriatric medicine. She has practiced medicine in the field of aging since 1997 as a clinician, educator, and administrator for vulnerable older adults across the care continuum. Her experience in caring for homeless began in 1990 as an Albert Schweitzer Fellow in her work for Boston homeless and Bridge Over Troubled Waters. She has held numerous leadership positions within organizations that offer services to homeless older adults, including the Veterans Affairs, 211 San Diego, San Diego Health Connect (Health Information Exchange), and Molina Healthcare. Throughout her career, she has advocated for systemic change in healthcare services and policies that promote health equity. She is a nationally recognized and grant-funded leader with over $5 million in externally peer-reviewed geriatrics grants. Dr. Chau is an alumna of Boston University and holds an MD from Drexel University College of Medicine. She sits on numerous advisory boards and boards of directors, including the American Geriatrics Society and California Geriatrics Society.

Arnold P. Gass, MD, FACP, an internist and geriatrician, is Health Sciences Clinical Professor of Medicine Emeritus at the University of California, San Diego School of Medicine. Since 1975, he has provided medical care to homeless persons. In 1988 Dr. Gass was the founding medical director of, and continues as senior medical consultant to, Stand Down, a 3-day multi-service reintegration program serving up to 1,000 homeless male and female veterans annually. As a faculty member on a Geriatrics Workforce Enhancement Program (GWEP) grant, Dr. Gass has developed a curriculum focused on geriatric homeless persons.

Homeless Older Populations
A Practical Guide for the Interdisciplinary Care Team

Diane Chau, MD, FACP
Arnold P. Gass, MD, FACP

Editors

SPRINGER **PUBLISHING COMPANY**

Springer Publishing Company, LLC
11 West 42nd Street
New York, NY 10036
www.springerpub.com

Acquisitions Editor: Sheri W. Sussman
Compositor: Exeter Premedia Services Private Ltd.

ISBN: 978-0-8261-7015-6
ebook ISBN: 978-0-8261-7016-3

The author and the publisher of this Work have made every effort to use sources believed to be reliable to provide information that is accurate and compatible with the standards generally accepted at the time of publication. The author and publisher shall not be liable for any special, consequential, or exemplary damages resulting, in whole or in part, from the readers' use of, or reliance on, the information contained in this book. The publisher has no responsibility for the persistence or accuracy of URLs for external or third-party Internet websites referred to in this publication and does not guarantee that any content on such websites is, or will remain, accurate or appropriate.

Library of Congress Cataloging-in-Publication Data

Names: Chau, Diane, editor. | Gass, Arnold P., editor.
Title: Homeless older populations: a practical guide for the
    interdisciplinary care team / Diane Chau and Arnold P. Gass, editors.
Other titles: Critical topics in an aging society.
Description: New York, NY: Springer Publishing Company, LLC, [2018] |
    Series: Critical topics in an aging society
Identifiers: LCCN 2017053220 | ISBN 9780826170156 | ISBN 9780826170163 (e-book)
Subjects: | MESH: Homeless Persons | Aged | Geriatrics
Classification: LCC HV4505 | NLM WT 100 | DDC 362.5/920846—dc23
LC record available at https://lccn.loc.gov/2017053220

Contact us to receive discount rates on bulk purchases.
We can also customize our books to meet your needs.
For more information please contact: sales@springerpub.com

Printed in the United States of America.

Contents

Contributors

Roxana Aminbakhsh, MD, Clinical Assistant Professor, University of California, San Diego, VA San Diego Healthcare System, San Diego, California

Marie Balfour, BA, University of California, Berkeley, Berkeley, California

Kristin Beizai, MD, Clinical Associate Professor, University of California, San Diego, VA San Diego Healthcare System, San Diego, California

Richard Bodor, MD, Faculty Plastic Surgeon, Veterans Affairs Medical Center, San Diego, California

Kevin Broder, MD, Telewound Director, Geriatrics Workforce Enhancement Program, University of California, San Diego; Plastic Surgeon, Veterans Affairs Medical Center, San Diego, California

Diane Chau, MD, FACP, Associate Professor, Health Science Medicine, University of California, San Diego; Project Director, Geriatrics Workforce Enhancement Program; Medical Regional Director, Molina Healthcare, San Diego/Inland Empire, California

Victoria Clark, RD, Dietician, VA San Diego Healthcare System, San Diego, California

Kelly Conright, MD, Clinical Assistant Professor, University of Nevada, Reno, School of Medicine, Reno, Nevada

Elham Faroughi, MD, San Diego, California

Jamie Gannon, PhD, Assistant Clinical Professor, UC San Diego Health Systems, La Jolla, California

Stephanie Diana Garcia, BA, Northridge, California

Arnold P. Gass, MD, FACP, Health Sciences Clinical Professor of Medicine Emeritus, University of California, San Diego School of Medicine; VA San Diego Healthcare System, San Diego, California

Therese Gibson, RN, MSN, FNP-BC, San Diego, California

Veronica Gonzalez, MD, Assistant Clinical Professor of Medicine, UC San Diego Health Systems, La Jolla, California

Helena Harvie, LCSW, VA San Diego Healthcare System, San Diego, California

Rachael Holloway, PsyD, Kaiser Permanente Orange County, Orange, California

Alan Hsu, MD, Assistant Clinical Professor, Veterans Affairs San Diego, UC San Diego Health Systems, La Jolla, California

Alana Iglewicz, MD, University of California, San Diego, San Diego, California

Yash Joshi, MD, PhD, MBE, University of California, San Diego, San Diego, California

Kristoffer Kalisuch, Spatial Design, San Diego, California

Kevin M. Krcmarik, MD, Assistant Professor of Medicine, VA San Diego Healthcare System, San Diego, California

Elizabeth Lake, MS, RD, Escondido, California

Jeanne Maglione, MD, PhD, VA San Diego Healthcare System and University of California, San Diego, San Diego, California

Zack Mahan, BA, University of California, San Diego, San Diego, California

Marlina Mansour, PharmD, Pharmacy Resident, UC San Diego Health Systems, La Jolla, California

Dianne M. McGuirk, ACNS-BC, RN, Case Manager, Homeless Patient Aligned Care, VA San Diego Healthcare System, San Diego, California

Ashlyn Melvin, BA, Care Coordination Administrative Staff, University of Oregon, Eugene, Oregon

Nicola Natsis, BA, Third-Year Medical Student, University of California, San Diego School of Medicine, San Diego, California

Marilee Nebelsick-Tagg, MN, FNP-BC, VA San Diego Healthcare System, San Diego, California

Ian Curtis Neel, MD, Assistant Clinical Professor, UC San Diego Health Systems, La Jolla, California

Beth Palmer, DNP, ACNS-BC, AGPCNP-BC, Primary Care Provider, Homeless Patient Aligned Care Team, VA San Diego Healthcare System, San Diego, California

Jairo Romero, MD, Clinical Professor of Medicine, UC San Diego Health Systems, La Jolla, California

Laura S. Romero, MD, Veterans Administration Medical Center, Associate Professor, Dermatology, University of California, San Diego, San Diego, California

Robert Rumore, MA, New York, New York

Amin Sabet, MD, Riverside Community Hospital, University of California, Riverside, Riverside, California

Ruth Simonis, JD, MSW, LCSW, CCM, Veterans Affairs, Reno, Nevada

Shannon Slama, LVN, VA San Diego Healthcare System, San Diego, California

Roger A. Strong, PhD, ACHPN, FPCN, University of San Diego, San Diego, California

Maria Tiamson-Kassab, MD, DFAPA, FAPM, Director, Psychiatry & Psychosocial Services, UCSD Moores Cancer Center & Jacobs Medical Center, San Diego, California; Clinical Professor, Psychiatry, University of California, San Diego, San Diego, California

Ashkan Vafadaran, MD, Veterans Affairs, Reno, Nevada

Muhammad Atif Waqar, MD, Assistant Professor, Aga Khan University, Karachi, Pakistan

Preface

Homeless Older Populations: A Practical Guide for the Interdisciplinary Care Team began as a solution to a care coordination problem among clinical colleagues who knew their knowledge needed to be shared. These passionate providers have devoted their lives to the service of frail older populations who are increasingly needing care within our complicated healthcare systems. These providers-turned-authors see daily the rise of homeless older populations and want to join to help others improve and provide equitable care for all humans. We as humans must recognize the need to preserve our population and collaborate to solve gaps that contribute to human suffering. This book serves as the pillar for clinical care teams to improve health equity among homeless older adults.

Interdisciplinary care teams are essential in complex homeless older population clinical practice, as all disciplines must work together to address medical, surgical, behavioral, nutritional, and social determinants of health. All clinicians who treat older adults, from the independent to the frail, should approach problem solving via an inclusive approach that includes social work, pharmacy, nursing, rehabilitation, administrative, and medicine inputs. The social determinants of health that contribute to the complexities of clinical care outcomes cannot be addressed within silos. The authors and topics of this book have been assembled to reflect a holistic care model to assist clinicians in the complicated homeless population that is continuing to change in the instability of the homeless environment.

Chapters in this book are organized by problems most commonly faced by clinicians in servicing homeless populations: mental, social, medical, and surgical challenges. We focus on specific conditions and challenges that may benefit the most from the use of interdisciplinary care teams, with special focus on challenges in caring for homeless populations.

Diane Chau, MD, FACP

1

Definition, Background, and Case Studies of Geriatric Homelessness

Arnold P. Gass, Zack Mahan, and Marie Balfour

Geriatric homelessness (GH) is a significant and growing social, political, economic, and humanistic issue throughout the United States. Homeless persons of all ages are obvious to anyone who goes downtown in large as well as in smaller cities and towns. Particularly for GH, one sees scraggly bearded men and gray-haired women of all ethnicities carrying garbage bags stuffed with aluminum cans or bottles, rolling shopping carts containing their worldly goods, or sleeping in doorways. While homelessness has been recognized in all of recorded human history, from the *Book of Ruth* in the Old Testament and Hindu sadhus from South Asia to bums riding the rails during the Depression of the 1930s, current perceptions of homeless persons in our progressive society are that something must be wrong, and that wrong righted, when a person does not have shelter.

But, is that necessarily so? Do homeless persons warrant our concern? If so, why and what can a society or community do to absolve its concern? In particular, does the subset of older homeless persons, geriatric homeless persons (GHPs), have unique vulnerabilities and needs? What if that older homeless person has acute, subacute, or chronic medical and/or psychological problems? What unique challenges do clinicians and an interdisciplinary team face, and what unique skills do they need or they should have in assessing, diagnosing, and ministering to the needs of such persons?

The chapters in this book will address the unique problems of the GHPs, citing case studies as examples and offering possible solutions by clinicians and the interdisciplinary team to the problems raised by the questions listed. The case studies in this chapter will highlight the GH in four urban areas and among veterans.

DEFINITION OF THE HOMELESS AND GERIATRIC HOMELESS

Although the term *geriatric* is used generally in epidemiologic studies to define persons greater than 65 years of age, the Department of Housing and Urban Development (HUD), the agency of the Executive Branch of the Federal Government legislatively tasked by Congress with overseeing programs for all homeless persons, defines a GHP as one who is over 50 years of age and living homelessly. Why is this so? Multiple studies have shown that a 50-year-old person living chronically on the streets has medical and psychological conditions that are usually only seen in persons who are 15 to 20 years older. These conditions include cardiovascular, metabolic, musculoskeletal, and dental conditions, as well as cognitive and psychological ones.

Homelessness itself is defined both temporally and spatially. In terms of time, a person may be homeless temporarily (i.e., for one day, one week, or one month) or chronically (i.e., for three or six months continuously). In terms of space, a homeless person is one who is living in a situation that is not a conventional permanent dwelling. Such a person may be living out of a car, in a tent, or on the streets, or be couch surfing, a situation in which he or she is basically one step from being homeless.

The standard measure of homeless persons in the United States is the Point-in-Time Count (PITC). On the last Friday in January each year, a veritable army of volunteers and paid professionals, using various methods, counts all the persons in demographically selected and diverse locations across the country who are on the streets and in shelters. The count is done in January because it is a winter month; therefore, more homeless persons of all ages are generally in shelters, where they are easier to count. However, the annual PITC only records about one-third of the individuals in the United States who may be homeless during that year.

Other aberrations in the data should make one cautious in viewing any numbers regarding homeless persons as absolutes. It is difficult to obtain population figures for the homeless who, being mobile, may be omitted from measurements if they happen to be away from their usual locale in the United States while any count is being made or, on the local level, moving from city to city within a given county. While data regarding medical and psychological conditions can be collected at clinics and hospitals where the

GH go for medical care, data for those GH who get care in private offices or the Department of Veterans Affairs facilities may be reported using different standards. Finally, advocacy groups may record, calculate, and report data in one manner, while politicians may have motives using these "statistics" in a different manner. Thus, figures used regarding the GH population are open to questions of validity and bias.

As not all studies cited by the authors in this book were stratified using 50 as the definition of GH or use comparable data, the reader should not expect or infer mathematical certainty for every observation or conclusion we have made.

DEMOGRAPHICS

Overall Picture

Is the GH population increasing in absolute or relative numbers, or both? If so, why is it increasing? For one thing, the entire U.S. population is aging. Over the past century, the average age of the entire population of Americans has increased, as has the percentage of those over 65 years. One might expect that, as a population as a whole ages, if there were no reduction in the causes of or solutions addressed to homelessness, the absolute number of homeless persons would also increase. In fact, as of 2017, based on the annual PITC, the absolute number of all homeless unique persons in the United States has been about the same since 2008—about 1.5 million per annum; the number of homeless on the street on any given night has dropped from 647,258 in 2007 to 553,742 in 2017 (U.S. Department of Housing and Urban Development, 2017). Although the absolute number of homeless persons has not increased, the fraction of the homeless of geriatric age, that is, greater than 50 years old, has doubled to about 31% in 2014 (Nagourney, 2016). The percentage increase can be attributed partially to the aging of the overall (housed and nonhoused) U.S. population, as well as to a reduction of younger persons who are homeless. The impact of public policy, public and privately funded programs, and healthcare seems to be affecting the younger homeless, but not the older homeless population.

Factors driving these demographics include (a) loss of employment or bankruptcy among older age groups which, along with a lack of affordable, available housing, is one of the two main reasons for homelessness and (b) the fact that young people who would otherwise be homeless due to unemployment and/or unaffordable housing are moving back into their parents' home, couch surfing with other relatives, or living with friends.

Overall Picture by Locality

GH is a national, state, and local issue. However, the meaning of GH differs depending on the perspective one takes. At the national level, HUD is responsible for producing funding and programs to end, or at least reduce, homelessness.

Overall, HUD policy and grants affect what states and localities can do for their homeless populations. However, individual states add to HUD grants or modify HUD policies as they see fit. For example, programs in Texas and Florida have led to a large decrease in their overall homeless as well as their GH populations. However, the percentage of GH has increased in those states as it has in all other states. Does that mean HUD as well as state and local programs are "failing?"

The aphorism that "all politics is local" is quite applicable to the homelessness issue. Localities take HUD and state money and policies, modify them with local laws and practices, and add the activities of volunteers and private and corporate philanthropy to bring boots-on-the-ground action to the housing, nutritional, and medical needs of the GH population. These programs, significant but as-yet-insufficient remediation to the problems faced by the GH, will be discussed in greater detail in the chapters to follow.

National, Regional, and Local Statistics/ Issues

Does the GH population data represent a crisis, a sort of "silver tsunami" of homelessness? The answer to this question again depends on one's perspective.

As with homelessness (time, space), there are facets to a tsunami; let's say cause and effect. The cause of a tsunami is a perturbation in the undersea environment such as a shift of tectonic plates or an undersea volcanic eruption. The tsunami is the resultant, observed event of the causal trigger. So, we should first ask, what is the cause or causes of the observed GH effect, namely, an increase in their numbers. In the 1930s, there were large numbers of men "riding the rails" looking for work or greener pastures. There were also the certainly homeless Dust Bowl refugee families, memorably depicted in John Steinbeck's *The Grapes of Wrath*. In the mid-1980s, the nightly national news depicted Midwest Rust Belt families emigrating to the Southwest economic meccas of Houston, Denver, and Phoenix. Compared to the 1930s or 1980s, there is currently no tsunami of homelessness, either in absolute or percentage numbers. In June 2017, the overall unemployment in the United States was less than 5%, not the 30% of the depression or the regional 20% or so in the Midwest in the 1980s. However, there is one difference: persons in the homeless population in the 1930s were younger, working-age individuals with or without families.

As previously mentioned, the two main causes of homelessness are loss of employment and the unavailability of affordable housing. While Social Security, which was passed in 1935, and unemployed worker and union benefits helped cushion the economic blows of retirement and loss of employment, respectively, these factors did not affect the other cause of homelessness, namely, available, affordable housing.

As well as approximately 50% of bankruptcy immediately and approximately 75% eventually, medical illness, temporary or permanent, plays a significant causal role in GH, leading to loss of employment in those between 50 and 64 years of age. Bankruptcy, in turn, leads to loss of an owned or mortgaged home, and thus homelessness in this population. Furthermore, those GH on the street experience worsening of these conditions when they cannot get proper treatment for pre-existing conditions or develop new medical and psychological conditions—skin, foot, post-traumatic injury, and depression—as a result of their homelessness.

Among other causes of GH are chronic mental illness and social causes such as family dysfunction. These causes have been present in all societies and at all times in human history. They are only now getting full attention in the United States.

To return to the tsunami metaphor, the effects of a tsunami are modified by multiple factors, such as the elevation of the land where the tidal wave strikes, the structural integrity of the buildings on the land, and the emergency preparedness and response relating to the evacuation and treatment of the population at risk. While some damage to topography and structures cannot be avoided in a tsunami, in theory, not one single life has to be lost if the emergency system works perfectly.

So it is with the effects of job loss, availability and affordability of housing, and medical illness. While a stated goal of mitigating the effect of these causal factors is zero homelessness by politicians and civic leaders, as well as a highly publicized goal of the Department of Veterans Affairs (VA) in 2008, even the VA now admits that zero homelessness among veterans is unattainable. To reduce GH even close to zero, economic, political, social, and medical facets of homelessness have to be addressed both separately and in the aggregate. While this volume will not deal directly with the economic or political effects of GH, these factors must be kept in mind when one reads the chapters on the causes and effects of, as well as the solutions to, the social, medical, and psychological conditions of the GHP with which this volume will deal.

The evidence so far is that only minimal progress is being made toward even a slight reduction in the homeless population and its problems in general while the GH population is increasing. Thus, one can reasonably conclude that there is indeed a silver tsunami in homelessness, the GHP.

A TALE OF FOUR CITIES: CASE STUDIES

New York City

Being the most populous city within the United States, with an estimated population of 8,537,673 people (U.S. Census Bureau, 2017), it is no surprise that New York City (NYC) contains the largest homeless population of any U.S. city. With an astounding 73,523 homeless, this metropolitan jungle contains more dispossessed individuals than the other top five cities combined. Of these 73,523, 70,685 (96.1%) are sheltered, with 2,838 (3.8%) being unsheltered. Based on the annual PITC, compared to the nationwide ratio of sheltered to unsheltered homeless, with 373,571 out of the 549,928 total U.S. homeless being sheltered (67.9%) and 176,357 being unsheltered (32.1%), New York's ratio is truly extraordinary and serves as an example for numerous other cities with exceptionally large homeless populations. This percentage of sheltered homeless is not merely due to coincidence, though; it is probably due to a citywide ordinance designed by New York State Governor Andrew Cuomo to protect the homeless from any extreme cases of weather. According to this act, it is unlawful for the city of New York to leave any individuals without shelter during temperatures of 32°F or below, and thus numerous homeless shelters are constantly established during seasonal periods of cold, such as during the month (January) when the PITC is done.

Additionally, NYC is also one of the largest spenders on homeless care in America. As of 2016, NYC uses a budget of approximately $1.6 billion (Dawsey, 2016) to fight the disenfranchised, a figure that had been rapidly increasing from an already large 2007 budget of $604 million (Fermino, 2015). Despite these massive increases in funding toward homeless shelters/programs, and the admirable ratio of sheltered to unsheltered homeless, the amount of homeless in NYC has been increasing in recent years as opposed to the national trend, which is mostly flat or decreasing slightly. In 2007, 50,372 homeless persons walked the streets of New York; the number was 73,523 in 2016, a 46% increase in disenfranchised individuals, versus the nationwide 11% decrease between the years 2010 to 2015. The reason behind this is unclear, but may be due to the high cost of living and/or the extreme cost of property within the Big Apple.

A majority of the homeless within New York are also part of homeless families, with 44,558 out of 73,523 (60.6%) living alongside of primary relatives; this in itself indicates that most of the homeless within New York have lost their living accommodations due to being unable to afford the cost of housing. The most common occurrence of homelessness within New York is simply unaffordable housing. The hypothesis of excessive costs for living accommodations being correlated with an increased percentage of homeless is further supported by the fact that New York has the most expensive property within America, costing approximately $2,829 per square foot (Elkins, 2015). In recent years, numerous projects designed to supply affordable shelter to all New Yorkers have been established. As of 2014, 62,506 apartments have been financed by Mayor William (Bill) de Blasio's housing plan, enabling numerous families to avoid treating the streets as their home (de Blasio, 2017). With projects such as these, the number of homeless in New York can hopefully begin to decline, and families can be able to afford to live and rear children in a more forgiving environment.

In 2010, the NYC census showed a population of 8,175,133 composed of 3,597,133 (44.0%) Caucasian, 2,088,510 (25.5%) African American, and 2,366,076 (28.6%) Hispanic/Latino. This level of diversity is not seen within the homeless population though; rather, a majority of the financially disenfranchised is of African and/or Hispanic descent. African Americans make up 49,897 out of the 73,523 (67.9%) living on the streets in NYC, and are followed by those of Hispanic/Latino descent, which make up 37,100 (50.4%). Unfortunately, due to the nature of being homeless and the general inability to report crimes committed against oneself upon reaching this level of financial instability, very little is known in regard to the extent of racial crimes against the homeless. From numerous news articles reported with New York though, primarily by sources such as the *New York Times*, it is a fairly common occurrence for those living on the streets to face violence of all kinds. Hopefully, more data will be generated in the years to come regarding abuse of the homeless and the actions of perpetrators will be accounted for. In regard to gender, in NYC, 35,441 (48%) are female, 37,868 (51.5%) are male, and 214 (0.3%) are transgender. All statistics generated were compiled by the HUD 2016 annual report (U.S. Department of Housing and Urban Development, 2016).

According to the NYC Departments of Health and Mental Hygiene and Homeless Services, between the years of 2001 and 2003, 1,170 homeless individuals died on the streets, accounting for 0.7% of all deaths within NYC. In regard to the causes of death, a majority were caused by substance abuse, 151 (16.7%), followed by heart disease, 149 (16.5%), cancer, 137 (15.2%), and HIV/

AIDS, 128 (13.8%) (Barrow, Herman, Córdova, & Struening, 1999). The first three conditions, and increasingly the fourth, are chronic conditions typically seen in the GHP. Thus, as many as 62.5% of the deaths among the homeless in NYC are those of the GHP. Interestingly, the causes of death were affected by shelter use, with frequent shelter users typically dying of cancer and heart disease more often and dying from HIV/AIDS and substance abuse less often. Those using shelters may be older and not actively participating in dangerous drug use and/or harmful sexual activities, behaviors typical of the GHP.

In regard to healthcare within NYC, the homeless make up 48,045 (1.6%) of all hospitalizations despite being only 0.6% of the NYC adult population. Of these hospitalizations, 31% were caused by substance abuse, 24% by alcohol abuse, and 14% by mental health issues, showing an obvious need to establish improved outreach programs regarding substance/alcohol abuse (New York City Departments of Health and Mental Hygiene and Homeless Services, 2005).

In conclusion, with by far the largest absolute number of homeless in the country, NYC demonstrates the causal effect of the unavailability of unaffordable housing on homelessness. However, NYC demonstrates what can be done by political (laws) and fiscal action (monies) to alleviate the human crisis of homelessness. The mortality and hospitalization data show that conditions affecting the GHP are prominent in the population of homeless in NYC.

San Francisco

The City of San Francisco includes about 1.27% of all homeless individuals living in America. This is a surprising fact given its small size (around 47 square miles). A survey performed by the Applied Survey Research in 2015 estimated San Francisco's homeless population to be 6,866, while more recent estimates from HUD's 2016 Annual Homeless Assessment Report claim the number is closer to 6,996 (Applied Survey Research, 2015; Henry, Watt, Rosenthal, & Shivji, 2016). HUD reports San Francisco's homeless population has steadily increased in recent years, including its GHP. As the total homeless population grows, the number of homeless people in San Francisco aged 60 or older has increased by 30% from 2007 to 2015 (Applied Survey Research, 2015).

A 2006 study of 3,534 homeless people surveyed over 14 years in San Francisco showed that, by their mid-forties, many homeless individuals were faced with health problems that are typically associated with senior citizens, highlighting the aging effect of life on the streets, particularly in an urban environment. Over the course of the study, increasing proportions of participants reported spending time ill and experiencing complications with hypertension and diabetes. Additionally, increasing rates of participants reported visiting the emergency department and being hospitalized over the course of the previous year (Hahn, Kushel, Bansberg, Riley, & Moss, 2006). These data indicate that the San Francisco homeless population is encountering more health complications as they age, especially with the effects of chronic conditions.

According to a 2006 study led by Judith Hahn, PhD, the median age of homeless people surveyed increased from 37 years old in the 1990s to 46 years old in 2003, and the median duration of homelessness increased from 12 months to 39.5 months during this period. In the most recent sample of participants, one-third of the population was aged 50 or older. These results led researchers to believe that San Francisco's homeless population is a uniform aging cohort, and homelessness has become more chronic as the years pass. With this information, the authors of the study intimated homeless healthcare providers will experience increased challenges caring for an older homeless population with more chronic conditions, but homeless service programs that combine healthcare and stable housing may provide the key to reducing homeless rates in this static cohort (Hahn et al., 2006).

Another survey reported in 2015 by the Applied Survey Research in San Francisco found that more than two-thirds of the participants reported one or more health conditions, and 37% reported drug or alcohol abuse. In total, 27% reported chronic health problems. The results indicated the surveyed population aged 51 to 60 increased by 8% and the population of respondents aged 61 or older grew by 5% since 2013. Most (61%) respondents first experienced homelessness once past the age of 25 years. In total, 51% of the respondents had been homeless for a year or more, suggesting that San Francisco may have a more long-term homeless group facing an increasing amount of symptoms from chronic conditions and a more complicated healthcare regimen (Applied Survey Research, 2015).

Many attribute San Francisco's sizable homeless population to high housing costs that have increasingly plagued the city and been supported by Northern California's technology boom. In a 2015 survey of homeless individuals in San Francisco, 71% of the respondents said they became homeless while living in the city, up from 61% in 2013. Of those who experienced homeless living first in San Francisco, 49% had lived in San Francisco for 10 or more years. About 37% of the respondents reported staying with friends or family prior to becoming homeless, while 30% lived in a home owned or rented by themselves or their partner immediately before becoming homeless. One-fourth of the participants reported losing their job was their primary cause of homelessness. Almost half (48%) of the participants reported they were unable to obtain permanent housing because they could not afford rent in the city, and 17% reported difficulties with securing permanent housing because of the lack of availability in the area (Applied Survey Research, 2015). The *San Francisco Gate* reports that the shelter system in the city has around 1,200 beds; however, only 39% of homeless individuals reported using an emergency, transitional, or other kind of shelter as their usual accommodations to sleep at night (Applied Survey Research, 2015; Graff, 2016). As San Francisco's shelters fill, their unsheltered population is on the rise, with 57% of unsheltered homeless located in the Tenderloin and South of Market neighborhoods.

Despite these challenges, San Francisco has a relatively strong infrastructure to support homeless services. According to the 2015 San Francisco Homeless Point-in-Time Count and Survey Comprehensive Report, 25% of the homeless participants reported moving to San Francisco to access homeless services or benefits, and 7% reported relocating to the city to access Veterans Affairs services (Applied Survey Research, 2015). Recent Medicaid expansion throughout the city has provided more access to health insurance and primary care clinics for homeless individuals. The *San Francisco Chronicle* estimates that the city spends $241 million each year on homeless services, with an average of $87,480 in medical costs per year for each of the sickest people on the streets and $17,353 per year for each person in city-run supportive housing (Knight & Fagan, 2016). More than half (54%) of the surveyed homeless reported using meal services in the city, and 42% reported using emergency shelter services, up 9% from 2013 data. Also, 72% of San Francisco's homeless also report receiving government assistance outside of the city's homeless services (Applied Survey Research, 2015). Notwithstanding all of these resources and programs, the homeless population in San Francisco continues to climb every year.

A specifically geriatric program comes in the form of the San Francisco Medical Respite Center, which provides specialized healthcare to homeless individuals with a focus on those over the age of 50. The facility serves as a discharge point for many San Francisco hospitals and a drop-off facility for individuals in need of chronic alcoholism stabilization services, which help to offset expensive emergency department use by homeless individuals. In addition to medical care, the program facility offers transportation to medical and social service appointments, links to benefits and housing, after care and support from an alumni network, social services, case management, and three meals a day. This integrative approach may be an important case study in expanding services offered to the GH, as the center offers 60 medical respite beds and includes a 12-bed sobering center on-site. However, because of the toll of living on the streets, staff members report that the center's average patient stay has been growing since their client population has aged (Liss-Schultz, 2016).

If San Francisco has so many resources available to their homeless population, why is the population of older homeless individuals increasing? The answer may be that the city has just begun to focus homeless services programs on its aging population since the most recent tallies of elderly homeless individuals were released from point-in-time (PIT) counts in 2015 and 2016. Additionally, the results of 2015 PITC data show that only 17% of homeless respondents reported using health services, suggesting that the city may have to develop healthcare programs that are more accessible to their homeless population. Because data show that chronic health conditions are on the rise in the San Francisco population, healthcare development is an important step in improving the quality of life for homeless individuals in the area. Research shows that geriatric individuals in San Francisco are facing different and more complex conditions than their nonhomeless counterparts, implying the need for a more specialized healthcare approach for these individuals. There is, however, a silver lining to San Francisco's situation. A 2017 donation from the Tipping Point Community charitable organization pledged $100 million to try and cut the chronically homeless population in San Francisco (Fagan, 2017). Although plans for allocating this donation have not yet been released, it provides a promising option for the city to alleviate the struggles of the elderly homeless of San Francisco.

Oakland

Oakland, California, is a city with an ever-increasing homeless population. However, recent in-depth studies of the local subset of the GH combined with PITC data for the overall homeless population have provided insights into potential avenues to decrease the total homelessness rate. The City of Oakland officially declared a homeless crisis in 2016, and data from PIT counts show the overall homeless population has increased 25% from 2015 to 2017 (EveryOneHome, 2017; Hedin, 2017). The current total population based on 2017 tallies by EveryOne Home, a nonprofit based in Alameda County, has reached 2,761 individuals. In 2017, EveryOne Home utilized homeless "guides" to identify where homeless people congregate, which may provide a more accurate tally for 2017 than previous years.

Oakland's rising homeless tally may take root in increased growth of the city in recent years. Although there has been a rapid job growth within the city, income inequality and the lack of recent housing development may have caused more people with limited options to turn to the streets. Additionally, with the rising housing demand, the *East Bay Times* reports that fewer land-lords are willing to accept Section 8 housing vouchers that many low-income individuals have relied on in past years to subsidize their rent (Hedin, 2017). In total, 82% of homeless individuals surveyed by EveryOne Home reported they lived in Alameda County before becoming homeless. By the most recent 2017 tallies, over 68% of the homeless population in Oakland is unsheltered, living in homeless encampments, overpasses, and parks, emphasizing the overcrowding of shelters and housing programs in the city's current state (Applied Survey Research, 2017).

Although there has been a growth in homeless services offered by the city over the years, there are only a few programs related directly to the older homeless population. Oakland has established Coordinated Entry, a pro-gram to connect people at risk for homelessness with resources and leads to acquire long-term supportive housing, but this program is currently only available to families. The main geriatric housing program is St. Mary's Center, which receives 60% of its funding from the government and got its start as a center for the elderly and a preschool in 1973. The program expanded in 1979 to a secondary facility that provides low-income seniors with one-bed-room apartments, and the current facility includes the Recovery 55 program, which educates homeless seniors on strategies to cope with mental health issues and drug and alcohol addictions. The facility also sponsors money management programs and has social workers, case managers, and senior advocates on site. St. Mary's Center also provides emergency winter shelter for 25 individuals who become connected with a social worker after staying in the shelter for more than two nights. The program continues to expand its reach, having purchased and renovated new properties for senior living in 2005, 2008, and 2014. The facility reports that most of its senior participants receive a Supplemental Security Income (SSI), which provides a maximum stipend of $10,500 each year. The center estimates that the average cost of a small studio apartment in West Oakland is around $1,200 per month, while most of the seniors in their facilities receive only $877 a month in SSI sup-port (St. Mary's Center, n.d.). St. Mary's Center currently has two operating housing facilities that utilize a common living space connected to private rooms, but their homes can only house around six seniors at a time (20–24 are reported to be helped each year as they are transitioned into permanent housing options), suggesting that expansion is needed in order to combat the rising tide of the older homeless population in Oakland.

The main GH statistics coming out of Oakland in recent years are a product of the Health Outcomes in People Experiencing Homelessness in Older Middle Age (HOPE HOME) study published in 2016. In this study, researchers interviewed 350 homeless adults aged 50 and older enrolled through population-based sampling in Oakland for a prospective cohort study. The results of these interviews indicated that more than 40% of the participants became homeless for the first time after age 50. The group of participants that had experienced homelessness for the first time after age 50 reported a higher prevalence of several mental health issues, positive screens for PTSD, hallucinations in the past six months, and hospitalization for mental health reasons in the past six months than their counterparts who had experienced homelessness before age 50. The participants who reported becoming homeless for the first time before age 50 had a higher chance of adverse life experiences and a lower chance of meeting typical milestones of young adulthood, such as marriage. Researchers also found that those who had experienced homeless living before 50 years had more current mental and physical vulnerabilities than their counterparts who experienced homelessness after 50 years (Brown et al., 2016). These results imply that those who have spent more time on the streets have more health difficulties (which is not surprising), but those who became homeless later may be experiencing a different set of health conditions that service programs can aid with more focus on this subset of Oakland's homeless population.

In addition to investigating the causes of homeless living in Oakland, the HOPE HOME study also investigated smoking behaviors, mental health outcomes, substance abuse, residential behaviors, and emergency department use in this older homeless cohort. According to the results, rates of quit attempts for tobacco smoking were similar to rates in the nonhomeless population, but homeless individuals had lower rates of successful quitting (Vijayaraghavan, Tieu, Ponath, Guzman, & Kushel, 2016). The participants with experience with one childhood adversity (i.e., the death of a parent) had higher chances of reporting moderate to severe depressive symptoms and a lifetime history of suicide attempt (Lee et al., 2017). Three-quarters (75.3%) of the participants reported a personal history of abuse. The participants with a history of PTSD and abuse had higher chances of chronic moderate to severe pain (Landefeld et al., 2017). Over 64% of those surveyed had moderate or greater severity systems for at least one illicit drug (Spinelli et al., 2017). About 46% of the participants were unsheltered, while 25% resided in multiple institutional settings such as jails, shelters, or transitional housing (Lee et al., 2016). The participants who used multiple institutions for housing and who were unsheltered had higher rates of emergency department use than participants who had access to housing in the six months prior to the interviews (Raven et al., 2017). These statistics help to paint a more accurate picture of the kinds of health conditions that the aging homeless population is facing and provides the framework for healthcare services and integrative transitional housing services to better serve the older homeless cohort.

These results suggest a specific action plan that Oakland could adopt in order to decrease its older homeless population and avert a continued homelessness crisis. The HOPE HOME study is amongf the first of its kind to thoroughly analyze the multiple facets of homelessness in older populations and provide a detailed account of the many ways a specific city can intervene in an individual's life, even before he or she becomes homeless. Although the recent state of crisis declared by the city has caused local politicians to promote increased homeless services (such as city-funded transitional housing), Oakland does not currently have the pre-existing integrative infrastructure that some other cities have to combat rising homeless statistics, which may explain their rapidly increasing homeless population.

San Diego

San Diego County has a population of approximately 2.6 million, half of which, approximately 1.3 million, live in the city of San Diego, the eighth largest city in the United States. San Diego is generally within the top five in the absolute number of homeless individuals. Homeless persons, seemingly all of them GH, are readily visible in the downtown area. The 2016 PITC administered by the Regional Task Force (HUD) found 8,669 homeless within San Diego County, slightly over half in the city of San Diego itself. Of these homeless, 3,729 (43.0%) were found to be using government-funded shelters, such as emergency shelters and/or transitional housing, and 4,940 (57.0%) were left unsheltered (Warth, 2016). The number of homeless within San Diego has been increasing in recent years, counter to the national trend. Despite a national 11% decrease in homelessness between the years 2010 and 2015, San Diego's homeless have been seen to increase by 4% between the years 2010 and 2015. Although all the reasons behind the increase in homelessness compared to the nationwide figures are not entirely known, at play may be a plethora of factors ranging from availability of healthcare, general living conditions for homeless individuals in San Diego, particularly its year-round moderate climate, or simply the geographical location.

San Diego's proximity to Tijuana, Mexico, the sixth largest city within Mexico with the busiest land border crossing in the western hemisphere, with over 30 million people crossing in 2016 alone (Bureau of Transportation Statistics, 2016), makes for a culturally unique and diverse distribution of its homeless population—2,469 (28.5%) of San Diegan homeless ethnically identify as Hispanic/Latino (compared to the national percentage of Hispanic homeless, 11%) and 1,836 (21.2%) as Black (compared to the national percentage of Black homeless, 40%). Additionally, of the 8,669 homeless accounted for within San Diego County, 2,953 (34.1%) were found to be female, 5,674 (65.4%) were found to be male, and 42 (0.5%) were found to be transgender. All statistical summaries involving homeless individuals were found by a 2016 HUD consensus and from the National Coalition for the Homeless published in July 2009.

San Diego has a massive military presence, with over 100,000 individuals being active duty personnel and seven military bases being located within the county (U.S. Navy Dispatch Newspaper, 2017). Possibly due to this presence, San Diego has the third largest homeless veteran population, with 1,156 homeless individuals being veterans (13.3%). This quantity of homeless veterans has led to an extensive amount of federal aid to care for such individuals, such as housing assistance, employment assistance, and healthcare, all specifically designed for ex-military personnel. In terms of healthcare, programs aiding in everything from medical assistance, dental maintenance, and mental health evaluations have become a staple within many San Diego healthcare facilities. Possibly due to these benefits, the quantity of homeless veterans within San Diego County has steadily declined, despite the general rise in homeless individuals of all backgrounds. This decrease in a specific portion of homeless individuals due to increased access to healthcare and federal aid may directly reveal a correlation between homeless population and increased federal spending, but unfortunately no such study analyzing this correlation within San Diego homeless exists.

Unlike San Francisco, Los Angeles, and Boston in terms of clinical or research papers on medical and psychological conditions related to homelessness, not much work has been done within San Diego analyzing either on the general homeless or the GHPs. What few reports there are, though, such as "An Assessment of Homeless Individuals; Perceptions of Service Accessibility in Downtown San Diego" (Welsh & Abdel-Samad, 2016), are incredibly valuable in both assessing a homeless perspective on the necessities required to live within San Diego and how safe living on said streets truly is. With that being said, though, much raw data containing information on the background of most homeless individuals, their respective health/medical issues, and other possibly valuable pieces of information is not truly utilized. Much of this information can simply be found within the databases of the 29 nonprofit institutions scattered across San Diego County (www.homelesss-helterdirectory.org/cgi-bin/id/city.cgi?city=San Diego&state=CA). Some of these homeless shelters, such as the most prominent, Father Joe's Villages, conduct their own data gathering for grant and fund-raising purposes. While not empirically based epidemiologically, these reports are informative and reveal insights into interpretation of the raw homeless population data presented by the annual HUD assessments (DeLessio, n.d.). They do not contain much medical information, however. Therefore, although much information behind homelessness is readily available and easily accessible within San Diego, for unknown reasons few formal medical studies have been conducted for academic publication by the scientific community.

San Diego, one of the most expensive and most limited housing markets in the country, has focused mainly on increasing the availability of and affordability of housing. However, despite San Diego being home to the fourth largest homeless population in the United States in 2015, it placed only 22nd in the amount of HUD funding it receives according to the 2015 Annual Homeless Assessment Report to Congress. For many, this is not surprising due to San Diego's long-standing practice of spending little public money on the financially disenfranchised. This practice has recently changed, though. As of July 5, 2017, city officials led by Mayor Kevin Faulconer announced an $80 million homeless plan designed to greatly diminish the size of San Diego's unsheltered homeless (Warth, 2017). With a goal of housing 3,000 in the course of three years, this federally, state, locally, philanthropic, and NGO-funded initiative involves a plethora of projects ranging from permanent supportive housing to homeless prevention projects focused around keeping families off of the streets. This massive project designed by the city of San Diego is not alone, though, with numerous other private shelters announcing plans to better assist the homeless in the years to come. The best example of this is the upcoming Father Joe's Village project, which involves a $531 million plan to create 2,000 housing units in the next five years, a charity project that is potentially the largest in county history. With these projects, and many others like them, San Diego's homeless projects may finally become comparable to those of the rest of the nation, and their homeless population will receive the help it so desperately needs.

HOMELESS VETERANS: CASE STUDY

Overview

Approximately 9% of chronically homeless persons are veterans, a percentage that exceeds the proportion of veterans in the U.S. population as a whole and even among men. Since, prior to the Gulf War in 1990, over 90% of the American veterans were men, the proper denominator for the comparison is males in the population. However, even this denominator is not fully accurate as, in order to be accepted into military service, both men and women have to be more than adequately physically and psychologically fit for service.

Thus, as homeless risks include chronic physical and/or psychological factors, one would expect less homelessness among the nonveteran than the veteran population. Therefore, one might reasonably ask why veterans are disproportionately represented among the homeless, particularly the chronically homeless. Similarly, are there similar demographics and demographic trends for veteran homeless persons as for nonveterans?

As veteran homelessness seems like a particular social blight, the public in general and the VA in particular are very concerned about the issue of veteran homelessness. In fact, the focus on veteran homelessness dates back to the Revolutionary War. Veteran homelessness was experienced by and commented on by the Civil War generation of veterans. The issue became particularly prominent immediately after World War I and during the Great Depression (Coxie's Army and the veteran encampment in the Anacostia area of Washington, DC). Finally, along with nonveteran homelessness, the issue resurfaced after the Vietnam War in large part because of the political tensions during and after Vietnam and economic conditions in the early and mid-1980s. A unique aspect of this tension related to Vietnam was a divided public during the war and a decidedly ambivalent feeling regarding returning veterans. Also, the Vietnam veteran cohort was particularly vocal and politically active, a trait congruent with attitudes of the generation, which came of age in the 1960s and 1970s.

Therefore, there is a particularly rich database regarding veteran homelessness, particularly veterans from Vietnam, whose youngest members are now 59 (i.e., GH), and the Gulf War in 1990 (GW 1), whose youngest members are now 44, approaching the GH age. However, as both Reserves and National Guard Units were mobilized in 1990, many GW 1 veterans are, in fact, GHP age.

Can the data on homeless veterans and the responses the VA has made to veteran homeless instruct the way we approach other homeless populations? While it is beyond this introductory chapter to explore all the pros and cons of the answer to these questions, the answers are "Yes" and "No."

While sociologic, demographic, and epidemiologic studies can shed light on populations and even subpopulations of the homeless, it is important to recognize that every homeless person is an individual. Thus, for both veteran and nonveteran homeless populations, individuals within the population have unique characteristics, including family background, social class, ethnicity, environmental effects during childhood (e.g., orphan status, substance abuse by parents, physical and psychological abuse), and education. For veterans, living in regimented conditions and being in combat are unique stressors. Some of the aforementioned factors, in fact, lead both men and women to enter military service, perhaps skewing the risk factors toward homelessness and predisposing veterans toward homelessness. Thus, while there is a considerable overlap between veteran and nonveteran homeless populations, they are not similar populations. What works for veterans may or may not work for some or all of the nonveteran homeless population.

On the positive side, the selective factors, which allow men and women to be accepted for military service, give them strengths that they may draw on in an attempt to end their homelessness. Among these strengths are the experience of group living and the camaraderie of having "buddies," watching out for one another in combat situations, learning survival skills, and receiving education on recognizing and coping with stress of all kinds. Veterans often regard themselves as a community, and, as such, often offer to help one another.

Department of Veterans Affairs Efforts

The Department of Veterans Affairs, formerly the Veterans Administration, which became a cabinet-level federal agency in 1984, is responsible for many aspects of veteran life, including housing loans, education, healthcare, and burial and survivor benefits. The VA has been concerned and continuously proactive with and responsive to veteran homelessness since the mid-1980s, particularly with the post-Vietnam War veteran population.

The VA's programs include housing, detoxification and medical care, employment, and outreach. Some of its programs are direct, and others are partnered ventures with other organizations such as the Urban League; local governments such as in NYC, San Francisco, and San Diego; and local housing commissions.

While the stated goal of the VA is to end veteran homelessness entirely, it has recognized that such a goal is likely not achievable. However, that goal has led to comprehensive programs, not just shelter, which, with the type of fiscal and staff support the VA can muster, could be models for homeless programs in general. For example, while nonveteran GHPs have chronic medical conditions and may only have fragmented, noncontinuous care, the VA has provided outreach teams that treat homeless veterans where they are located and/or provide transportation to local VA clinics or hospitals. This care is all documented in a single electronic health record allowing for continuity of care without reduplication of history-taking, testing, or provision of medication.

Regarding housing, VA-sponsored housing (VASH) is available both as transitional and long-term residences for selected veterans and their families.

Stand Down

Stand Down is a military term that refers to a soldier in a combat zone being brought "inside the wire" into a relatively safe haven in which his or her fellow soldiers stand guard while the soldier recoups both physical and psychological resources prior to going back on patrol or into battle.

In the San Diego Stand Down community model, homeless veterans were brought off the street into a tent city for 54 hours during which time they received food; clothing; medical care, including detoxification; and protection from life on the streets. Uniquely, the residents of Stand Down were grouped into 30-person tents with two to three tent leaders, one of whom was experienced in mental health techniques to foster the recreation of the military unit *esprit de corps* wherein the individual homeless veteran could "connect" with his or her fellows and become activated and empowered to begin to cope with the factors keeping him or her homeless. Transitional and safe haven housing and extended services leading to more permanent housing and jobs were made available to those men and women interested in such opportunities. Eventually, a cadre of former homeless persons, alumni of Stand Down, became peer counselors in the residential tent.

The Stand Down idea has been duplicated in many cities and communities around the United States, although not all Stand Down programs have employed the core concept of the veteran community unit. It is important to realize that Stand Down, which, from its inception had the support of the VA, was generated by an NGO, the VVSD, now called the Veterans Village of San Diego.

CONCLUSION

We have tried in this chapter to define geriatric homelessness, outline its general dimensions, explicate its two primary etiologies (loss of employment and the lack of affordable housing in the areas where most homeless persons are located), and give examples of the diversity of the problem and attempts at solutions in four cities and among veterans. While other chapters in this volume describe the medical and psychological conditions relating to the GHP, the case examples in this chapter, including the VA, show that the solution to the medical and psychological issues in the GHP involves much more than traditional medical practices and therapies. The solutions, involving among others politics, economics, and housing, are those of communities and localities acting to positively affect the lives of individuals and families of all ages, particularly the growing population of GHPs in the United States.

REFERENCES

Applied Survey Research. (2015). San Francisco point-in-time count & survey comprehensive report 2015. Retrieved from https://sfgov.org/lhcb/sites/default/files/2015%20San%20Francisco%20Homeless%20Count%20%20Report_0.pdf

Applied Survey Research. (2017). Alameda County homeless census & survey comprehensive report 2017. Retrieved from http://everyonehome.org/everyone-counts

Barrow, S. M., Herman, D. B., Córdova, P., & Struening, E. L. (1999). Mortality among homeless shelter residents in New York City. *American Journal of Public Health, 89*(4), 529–534. Retrieved from http://ajph.aphapublications.org/doi/pdf/10.2105/AJPH.89.4.529

Brown, R. T., Goodman, L., Guzman, D., Tieu, L., Ponath, C., & Kushel, M. B. (2016). Pathways to homelessness among older homeless adults: Results from the HOPE HOME Study. *PLOS ONE, 11*(5). doi:10.1371/journal.pone.0155065

Bureau of Transportation Statistics. (2016). Border crossing/entry data. Retrieved from https://transborder.bts.gov/programs/international/transborder/TBDR_BC/TBDR_BCQ.html

City of New York. (2017). Retrieved from http://www1.nyc.gov

Dawsey, J. (2016, November 20). NYC's homeless spending surges to $1.6 bBillion. Retrieved from https://www.wsj.com/articles/nycs-homeless-spending-surges-to-1-6-billion-1479676408

de Blasio, B. (2017). Transcript: Mayor de Blasio announces major progress helping New Yorkers afford their homes and neighborhoods. Retrieved from http://www1.nyc.gov/office-of-the-mayor/news/016-17/-still-your-city-mayor-de-blasio-major-progress-helping-new-yorkers-afford-their-homes#/0

DeLessio, P. (n.d.). By the numbers: Deciphering We All Count. Retrieved from http://my.neighbor.org/deciphering-homelessness-count

Elkins, K. (2015, October 4). The most expensive zip codes in 15 major US cities. Retrieved from http://www.businessinsider.com/the-most-expensive-neighborhoods-in-major-us-cities-2015-9

EveryOneHome. (2017). EveryOne Counts! 2017: Alameda County's homeless person point-in-time count. Retrieved from http://everyonehome.org/wp-content/uploads/2016/02/Homeless-Count-Notes-5-22-17-w-EdC-edits-1.pdf

Fagan, K. (2017, May 8). Nonprofit pledges $100 million to aid SF's chronically homeless. *San Francisco Chronicle.* Retrieved from http://www.sfchronicle.com/bayarea/article/Nonprofit-pledges-100-million-to-aid-SF-s-11126953.php

Fermino, J. (2015, October 16). Spending on homeless to reach close to $1B in 2015: Study. Retrieved from http://www.nydailynews.com/new-york/spending-homeless-reach-close-1b-2015-study-article-1.2399388

Graff, A. (2016, June 28). San Francisco homelessness Q&A: Frequently asked questions, answers. *San Francisco Gate.* Retrieved from http://www.sfgate.com/news/article/Questions-about-San-Francisco-s-homeless-answered-8323297.php

Hahn, J. A., Kushel, M. B., Bansberg, D. R., Riley, E., & Moss, A. R. (2006). Brief report: The aging of the homeless population: Fourteen-year trends in San Francisco. *Journal of General Internal Medicine, 21*(7). doi:10.1111/j.1525-1497.2006.00493.x

Hedin, M. (2017, June 5). Survey confirms Oakland homeless crisis growing worse. *East Bay Times*. Retrieved from http://www.eastbaytimes.com/2017/06/02/survey-confirms-oakland-homeless-crisis-growing-worse

Henry, M., Watt, R., Rosenthal, L., & Shivji, A. (2016, November). *The 2016 Annual Homeless Assessment Report (AHAR) to Congress*. Retrieved from https://www.hudexchange.info/resources/documents/2016-AHAR-Part-1.pdf

Holland, G., & Smith, D. (2017, June 2). L.A. leaders promised to spend $138 million on homelessness this year. Then reality hit. Retrieved from http://www.latimes.com/local/lanow/la-me-ln-city-homeless-budget-20170602-story.html

Knight, H., & Fagan, K. (2016, February 5). S.F. spends record $241 million on homeless, can't track results. *San Francisco Chronicle*. Retrieved from http://www.sfchronicle.com/bayarea/article/S-F-spends-record-241-million-on-homeless-6808319.php

Landefeld, J. C., Miaskowski, C., Tieu, L., Ponath, C., Lee, C. T., Guzman, D., & Kushel, M. (2017). Characteristics and factors associated with pain in older homeless individuals: Results from the Health Outcomes in People Experiencing Homelessness in Older Middle Age (HOPE HOME) Study. *Journal of Pain, 18*(9), 1036–1045. doi:10.1016/j.jpain.2017.03.011

Lee, C. M., Mangurian, C., Tieu, L., Ponath, C., Guzman, D., & Kushel, M. (2017). Childhood adversities associated with poor adult mental health outcomes in older homeless adults: Results from the HOPE HOME Study. *American Journal of Geriatric Psychiatry, 25*(2), 107–117. doi:10.1016/j.jagp.2016.07.019

Lee, C. T., Guzman, D., Ponath, C., Tieu, L., Riley, E., & Kushel, M. (2016). Residential patterns in older homeless adults: Results of cluster analysis. *Social Science & Medicine, 153*, 131–140. doi:10.1016/j.socscimed.2016.02.004

Liss-Schultz, N. (2016, June 30). Homeless people are older and sicker than ever before. Here's one way to help. Retrieved from http://www.motherjones.com/politics/2016/06/homeless-san-francisco-medical-respite-health-care-aging

Nagourney, A. (2016, May 31). Old and on the street: The graying of America's homeless. *International New York Times*. Retrieved from http://nyti.ms/1WVQRYp

New York City Departments of Health and Mental Hygiene and Homeless Services. (2005, December). The health of homeless adults in New York City. Retrieved from https://www1.nyc.gov/assets/doh/downloads/pdf/epi/epi-homeless-200512.pdf

Raven, M. C., Tieu, L., Lee, C. T., Ponath, C., Guzman, D., & Kushel, M. (2017). Emergency department use in a cohort of older homeless adults: Results from the HOPE HOME Study. *Academic Emergency Medicine, 24*(1), 63–74. doi:10.1111/acem.13070

Spinelli, M. A., Ponath, C., Tieu, L., Hurstak, E. E., Guzman, D., & Kushel, M. (2017). Factors associated with substance abuse use in older homeless adults: Results from the HOPE HOME Study. *Substance Abuse, 38*(1), 88–94. doi:10.1080/08897077.2016.1264534

St. Mary's Center. (n.d.). Housing. Retrieved from http://stmaryscenter.org/housing

U.S. Census Bureau. (2017). Census.gov. Retrieved from https://www.census.gov

U.S. Department of Housing and Urban Development. (2016, November). The 2016 Annual Homeless Assessment Report (AHAR) to Congress: Part 1: Point-in-time estimates of homelessness. Retrieved from https://www.hudexchange.info/resources/documents/2016-AHAR-Part-1.pdf

U.S. Department of Housing and Urban Development. (2017, December). The 2017 Annual Homeless Assessment Report (AHAR) to Congress. Exhibit 1.1. Retrieved from https://www.hudexchange.info/resources/documents/2017-AHAR-Part-1.pdf

U.S. Navy Dispatch Newspaper. (2017). San Diego military facts. Retrieved from http://www.navydispatch.com/military.htm

Vijayaraghavan, M., Tieu, L., Ponath, C., Guzman, D., & Kushel, M. (2016). Tobacco cessation behaviors among older homeless adults: Results from the HOPE HOME Study. *Nicotine & Tobacco Research, 18*(8), 1733–1739. doi:10.1093/ntr/ntw040

Warth, G. (2016, August 24). Who are the homeless? Retrieved from http://www.sandiegouniontribune.com/sdut-who-are-the-homeless-2016aug24-htmlstory.html

Warth, G. (2017, April 20). Homeless up 5 percent in the county, skyrockets downtown. Retrieved from http://www.sandiegouniontribune.com/news/homelessness/sd-me-homeless-count-20170419-story.html

Welsh, M., & Abdel-Samad, M. (2016). An assessment of homeless individuals' perception of service accessibility in downtown San Diego. Retrieved from http://sdsu-dspace.calstate.edu/bitstream/handle/10211.3/183014/SD001%20PA497_CJ540_Sp16%20An%20Assessment%20of%20Homeless%20Individuals%27%20Perceptions%20of%20Service%20Accessibility%20in%20Downtown%20SD.pdf?sequence=1

2

Chronic Mental Health Issues (Psychosis) in the Geriatric Homeless

Jamie Gannon and Alan Hsu

The population of geriatric homeless individuals diagnosed with serious mental illness is a largely underrepresented subpopulation in the research literature despite the notion that this population is one of the most vulnerable to negative outcomes due to physical, mental, and psychosocial factors. This subgroup is a vulnerable population because each of these factors (being homeless, being diagnosed with a serious mental illness, and being in the geriatric population) has an impact on the quality of life and functional status of these identified individuals (Lam & Rosenheck, 2000; Sullivan, Burnam, Koegel, & Hollenberg, 2000). Research and healthcare data in each of these areas highlight the challenges with resources and accessibility of care for the individual factors, but there have not yet been studies looking at these three factors combined. More research needs to be done for specific subgroup populations for needs assessment and clinically indicated treatment options.

Therefore, this chapter will briefly summarize the separate impact of each of these three factors:

- Being homeless
- Being in the geriatric population
- Being diagnosed with a serious mental illness (SMI)

In addition, this chapter will illustrate how these three factors combined impact overall subjective quality of life and poor outcomes for mental health through the use of a case vignette of a homeless, geriatric individual with a severe mental illness.

FACTOR I: BEING HOMELESS

The prevalence rate of homelessness varies across sampling studies due to differences in methodology and in the definition of homelessness. In addition, most of these studies are cross-sectional, which means changes across time cannot be examined for this population. It has been suggested that specific variables may contribute to continued homelessness, such as economics and federal and state policies (Aviram, 1990), the closing of large psychiatric institutions (Appleby & Desai, 1985), a decrease in low-income housing or increased rent (Quigley, Raphael, & Smolensky, 2001), and the lack of community services (Kushel, Vittinghoff, & Haas, 2001).

Identifying the priorities of this population can help health service agencies tailor the most helpful interventions. Homeless persons face a variety of day-to-day problems, including physical and mental health issues; victimization as a result of physical, sexual, or emotional abuse; social isolation; competing needs with others; and insufficient, safe housing options (Gelberg, Andersen, & Leake, 2000). Practical concerns such as obtaining food and shelter often take priority over the treatment of chronic mental and physical health issues (Dennis, Buckner, Lipton, & Levine, 1991). In addition, these individuals' poor living conditions themselves can lead to the development of psychiatric conditions, such as depressive or other severe affective disorders. Homeless individuals are at higher risk of traumatization (Lee & Schreck, 2005), including sexual or emotional abuse, and as a result may also develop traumatic sequalae such as post-traumatic stress disorder or worsening in pre-existing psychiatric disorders (Goodman, Saxe, & Harvey, 1991; Lee & Schreck, 2005). If they are forced to return to the same environment, this can lead to severe physical endangerment, psychological decompensation, or use of substances to avoid or numb these difficult emotional reactions.

Although homeless individuals tend to have poorer overall physical health status and are less likely than comparison cohorts to utilize outpatient medical services, a concern important enough to an individual will lead to the individual seeking appropriate medical care (Gelberg et al., 2000). Generally speaking, homeless individuals tend to seek treatment for immediate concerns causing noticeable symptoms, rather than interventions targeted for long-term health ailments (Gelberg et al., 2000). Healthcare data suggests that, for homeless patients, there is a higher utilization of emergency care and inpatient hospitalization than for preventive or outpatient care (Folsom et al., 2005). There appears to be an association between high insurance rates with homeless and housed individuals more frequently utilizing acute care services (through ED visits and hospitalizations), as opposed to ambulatory care or outpatient clinics (Brown et al., 2016). Homelessness is negatively associated with medication adherence, including adherence to psychotropic medications. A study in 2006 found that only 9.5% of homeless veterans were fully adherent with antipsychotic medications prescribed for bipolar disorder, compared with 90.5% of nonhomeless veterans (Sajatovic, Valenstein, Blow, Ganoczy, & Ignacio, 2006).

Interventions targeting improvement in the quality of life of homeless individuals include securing stable housing, accessing clothing and food, addressing physical health problems, and teaching individuals how to decrease their risk of victimization (Sullivan et al., 2000). Alongside interventions for practical matters, addressing depression and other mental disorders can also have an important role in improving the quality of life for these individuals.

Involuntary commitment statutes vary from state to state, ranging from Georgia, which allows involuntary hospitalization for any individual who has a mental illness in need of treatment, to states such as New York or Maryland that require one to be a danger to himself/herself or others, or, most commonly, that one poses a danger to himself/herself or others *due to mental illness.* Some states also specify grave disability or inability to meet basic needs (including the ability to meet the need for food, shelter, and basic self-care) as criteria allowing for involuntary hospitalization (Hedman et al., 2016). For homeless individuals, the ability to meet these basic needs can be quite broadly defined. Shelter can mean sleeping in their automobile or "couch surfing" at a peer's residence, and obtaining food or clothing can mean searching for usable or edible items that have been discarded by others. Interventions addressing concerns that fall under the category of grave disability may call upon a psychiatrist, psychologist, or licensed clinical social worker (LCSW) to describe and make recommendations to remover patients' psychological barriers to their providing these basic needs to themselves. Social workers can also be instrumental in utilizing federal, state, or local resources to help secure housing, food stamps, volunteer donations of clean clothing, and other practical supports.

FACTOR 2: BEING IN THE GERIATRIC POPULATION

The U.S. Census Bureau projected that, by 2050, there will be 89 million people over the age of 65, which translates to double the current elderly population (Sermons & Henry, 2010). This projection means that we will overall have an older nation accessing healthcare services and agencies, such as Social Security and Medicare. Researchers have hypothesized that, if the rates of geriatric homelessness are due to the fact that the chronically homeless population is aging, greater economic hardship due to rise in housing costs or untreated mental health conditions may impact the ability for homeless persons to maintain stable housing.

The geriatric population in general has more medical comorbidities (cognitive issues, overall health risk increases for certain conditions) than younger individuals due to the general decrease in physical functioning that occurs as a part of the natural aging process. As a person ages, his or her general faculties start to decline, which places the person at greater risk for falls, adverse health events, and/or needed greater assistance from others to perform general activities of daily living. Collateral information from friends and family about a person's day-to-day functioning across a period of time can help providers assess a pattern of decline to be used for diagnostic and treatment interventions.

As covered more extensively in the chapter on cognitive disorders within the homeless population, interventions for a geriatric population include receiving a full workup by health providers for possible neurocognitive disorders versus deliriums versus severe mood disorder causing cognitive deficits.

FACTOR 3: BEING DIAGNOSED WITH A SERIOUS MENTAL ILLNESS

An estimated one-fourth to one-third of the homeless population has an SMI, including schizophrenia, severe and recurrent major depression, and bipolar disorder (Folsom et al., 2005; Sullivan et al., 2000), and an estimated 15% of all patients treated for these serious mental illnesses are homeless (Folsom et al., 2005).

SMIs have an adverse effect on health outcomes. Having a diagnosis of schizophrenia has been associated with a 20% reduced life span due to unhealthy lifestyle factors, such as an unhealthy diet, sedentary behavior, smoking, alcohol use, and unsafe sexual practices. Metabolic and neurologic side effects of psychiatric medications can also adversely affect health (Bartels, 2004). The cornerstone of treatment of schizophrenia is antipsychotic medications, which have been associated with metabolic side effects, including insulin resistance, hyperglycemia, weight gain, and dyslipidemia. Antipsychotics are also commonly used in bipolar disorder, as well as more severe forms of major depressive disorder, and given the chronic, recurrent nature of all of these disorders, lifelong treatment is generally recommended (Miyamoto, Duncan, Marx, & Lieberman, 2005). Best practices for treatment of an SMI include a combination of psychiatric medications with psychotherapy interventions, such as cognitive behavioral therapy (Miyamoto et al., 2005). Poor medication compliance with individuals with an SMI is associated with clinical patient factors of poor insight into their mental health condition, forgetfulness, or poor organizational skills associated with many chronic mental health conditions, such as psychosis, difficulty following complex medication regimes, personal health beliefs about what it means to take medications, family or cultural beliefs about medications, substance-abuse difficulties, experiencing negative medication side effects, or increased symptom severity (Nageotte, Sullivan, Duan, & Camp, 1997). Assessment of a patient's personal health beliefs can allow providers to learn of potential barriers, including poor health literacy, which may contribute to nonadherence to psychiatric medications or regular mental health follow-up. Improved medication adherence is associated with increased awareness and understanding about one's mental health condition and the need for continued treatment (Nageotte et al., 1997).

Some individuals who are part of a specialized mental health treatment program or intensive case management system designed for individuals with an SMI can be assigned a mental health-intensive case manager, who assists patients with coordinating their appointments, creating appointment reminders, assisting with travel, and maintaining ongoing contact with the patients to proactively monitor risk or adverse events. However, for other individuals, this level of care is not sufficient and may warrant the use of involuntary commitment, public guardianship, or conservatorship. As with involuntary hospitalization, laws differ by state for public guardianship and conservatorship. Health data has shown that, for some individuals, conservatorship may improve conditions and create an option that can increase engagement in routine care (Richard, Lamb, & Weinberger, 1992).

Individuals with an SMI frequently have difficulty sustaining employment and rely on federal, state, or government assistance for funds or resources to access safe food, shelter, and clothing necessities at higher rates than the general population (Wilton, 2004). Interventions for this population include recovery-oriented programs with the goal of improving overall health by teaching skills-based interventions in programs specifically designed for individuals with serious mental illness, such as the Psychosocial Recovery and Rehabilitation Center (PRRC) or the Center of Recovery Education (CORE) at the Veterans Mental Health Administration. These programs teach individuals with an SMI life skills, such as money management, food preparation, and medication organization. Social skills training has also shown an increase in individuals with an SMI to establish and maintain interpersonal relationships for both peer and family relationships, which is also helpful for those seeking employment or who are gainfully employed. Furthermore, the psychotherapies for those with an SMI teach patients life skills that target increasing their level of functioning and involvement in their own personal health, which can include vocational rehabilitation to obtain employment or participate in volunteer services.

As is true in the treatment of other conditions, geriatric adults can be more vulnerable to adverse effects of medications due to age-related pharmacokinetic and pharmacodynamic changes, which impact effective treatment of an SMI (Hajjar, Cafiero, & Hanlon, 2007). Selective serotonin reuptake inhibitors (SSRIs) are associated with higher risk of hyponatremia in the elderly, which can lead to life-threatening complications, including seizures, coma, and death (Liu, Mittmann, Knowles, & Shear, 1996). Benzodiazepines are associated with increased risk of falls, cognitive impairment, sedation, delirium, and impairment of driving skills, all of which may lead to increased morbidity and mortality (Olfson, King, & Schoenbaum, 2015).

Especially difficult are decisions regarding the use of antipsychotics in this population, given the findings of increased risk of death and cerebrovascular events in elderly patients prescribed either conventional or atypical antipsychotic medications (Wang et al., 2005). While the Food and Drug Administration (FDA) black box warning pertains specifically to elderly patients treated for dementia-related psychosis, antipsychotics are associated with a variety of adverse physiological effects, including orthostatic hypotension, QTc prolongation and increased risk of life-threatening arrhythmias, insulin resistance, and the metabolic syndrome. Other serious side effects seen in the elderly include a higher risk of pneumonia and higher risk of deep venous thrombosis (Gareri et al., 2014). However, effective treatment of SMIs, including schizophrenia, schizoaffective disorder, and bipolar disorder, often does require use of antipsychotic medications. The Expert Consensus Guidelines recommend risperidone 1.25–3.25 mg/day as the first-choice treatment for late-onset schizophrenia, with quetiapine 100–300 mg/day, olanzapine 7.5–15 mg/day, and aripiprazole 15–30 mg/day as second-line choices (Alexopoulos, Streim, Carpenter, & Docherty, 2003). Late-onset bipolar disorder often presents with less severe mania and higher incidence of neurological and medical conditions, but treatment strategy frequently follows guidelines established for younger patients (Gareri et al., 2014). For patients with chronic but well managed mental illness, generally, it is recommended that they remain on the medications that have been effective for them in the past.

THE BIG 3 COMBINED

In Western countries, there is an increased rate of individuals with alcohol and drug-use disorders, as well as psychotic illnesses and personality disorders, among the homeless population compared to nonhomeless individuals of similar age (Fazel, Khosla, Doll, & Geddes, 2008). In addition, there is evidence with the aging of the baby boomers that the prevalence rates of geriatric homeless individuals with serious mental illness is expected to significantly increase in number. In the past two decades, the overall rates of geriatric homeless have been lower or more infrequent than the younger adults over 18 years of age who are homeless. The national data has shown the prevalence rates for geriatric homelessness is "modestly increasing"; over the course of a three-month period in 2005, there was an estimated 2.4% of sheltered homeless adults aged 62 years of age or older (Sermons & Henry, 2010).

The interplay of these three factors puts these identified individuals at risk for substantially decreased life expectancy, poor physical and mental health issues, and poor overall quality of life. However, there is limited research that defines needs for this subgroup. Health service agencies are learning how to integrate treatments to meet the needs of this group. What is known is that, by not prioritizing healthcare, we are left with very medically ill individuals who are not getting appropriate care and are suffering more morbidity and mortality at a younger age. Therefore, different interventions need to be tailored to meet the unique needs of this subgroup to address the impact of each factor on an individual's overall health status and quality of life.

CASE EXAMPLE PART I

The patient is a 69-year-old, never married, homeless male with alcohol abuse, schizophrenia disorder, unspecified neurocognitive disorder, diabetes mellitus type 2, chronic osteomyelitis of right hip, iron deficiency anemia syndrome, and hypertension, wheelchair bound due to unknown reasons who first presented to the emergency department (ED) after having a fall and sustaining a forehead laceration while intoxicated. He reported that he recently moved to California from another state via Greyhound bus.

Upon initial evaluation in the ED, he was found to be sitting in his own bodily wastes and to have pressure ulcers on his buttocks, sacrum, and right hip. His unstageable sacral ulcer had been exacerbated by fecal and urinary incontinence, and was treated. He received a CT scan, which revealed right testicular versus infratesticular abscess, possible right femoral head osteomyelitis (OM) versus septic arthritis, and, finally, sacral abscesses, which were treated with ceftriaxone. While his right hip lesions were being examined, he batted the doctor's hand away and shouted verbal profanities. His mental status was observed to be altered with poor insight and impaired judgment, with irritability, disruption, and yelling toward staff members, paranoia, and mood dyscontrol.

Although the patient was presenting with probable delirium or dementia, he always refused to be examined for cognitive deficits; therefore, providers had to rely primarily on mental status exams, collateral information, and medical lab results to help with diagnostic clarification. Lab results were positive for urinary tract infection, which could have been causing his delirium; however, the question still remained whether the patient had an underlying progressive neurocognitive disorder. Generally, patients are reassessed regularly for the presence and persistence of cognitive deficits as etiologies for delirium are addressed and resolve. As previously mentioned, this patient refused to answer questions from cognitive screening tools and also refused to answer informal attempts to test cognition.

For homeless individuals, who may move frequently between different geographical locations to find safe shelter or better access to community resources, providers must search broadly for records from hospital admissions or care at multiple inpatient and outpatient facilities to collect collateral information to inform their diagnostic and treatment plans. Patient mobility also creates particular difficulty in setting up ongoing outpatient care to manage their conditions, as the patient cannot be relied on to be in the same area for any length of time.

The patient was subsequently admitted to the inpatient medical unit for treatment of these conditions. In the ED, he reported smoking two packs of cigarettes per day and drinking a liter of vodka, but denied any history of withdrawal. He denied illicit or prescription drug abuse. In the ED, he was given thiamine, folate, and multivitamins, which he continued throughout his inpatient hospitalization.

This course of proactive vitamin supplements while on inpatient hospitalization is used to prevent Wernicke encephalopathy (WE) and Korsakoff syndrome, which results from deficiency of thiamine arising from malnutrition and is often seen in severe, chronic alcohol-use disorders. The European Federation of Neurological Sciences (EFNS) guidelines for the diagnosis, management, and treatment of WE suggest that the clinical diagnosis requires two of the following four signs: (a) dietary deficiencies (which are frequently presumed to be present in individuals with chronic alcohol use disorders), (b) eye signs, (c) cerebellar dysfunction, and (d) either an altered mental status or mild memory impairment (Galvin et al., 2010). Treatment of WE, in contrast to prevention, requires the use of high dose, parenteral thiamine, which must be given before any carbohydrate, which can lead to rapid depletion of existing thiamine stores. Oral thiamine supplementation is often recommended following hospital discharge; however, once individuals are discharged from the hospital, they typically display poor adherence to continued nutritional and supplement recommendations due to continued drinking of excessive amounts of alcohol and limited access to healthy food options that could lead to improved overall health.

Throughout his hospitalization, the patient was often agitated and not cooperative with staff for the interview, refused physical examination, and declined medical treatment or care. At times, he would refuse to participate in a productive conversation about his medical conditions and would resort to scolding the staff. By leveraging contingencies the patient deemed as rewarding, he agreed to be treated by wound care and was noted to have significant improvement in wound healing.

Despite multiple attempts by providers, the patient declined engaging in mental health or alcohol/drug treatment. Although the patient had a psychiatric diagnosis of schizophrenia, the course of this disorder for him as he aged had been marked by a decrease in the frequency and intensity of positive symptoms, that is, hallucinations or florid delusions, and instead was characterized predominantly by pervasive paranoia and negative symptoms such as avolition. Because the patient refused his oral medications, and there was no injectable form of his current antipsychotic medication, quetiapine, the consulting psychiatrist recommended switching him to a different antipsychotic medication, haloperidol, which was available in a long-term injectable form. Because he continued to demonstrate belligerent abusive behavior and language toward staff, the medical team was given recommendations from psychiatry to use "as needed" or PRN doses of haloperidol to manage agitation. The patient was provided psychoeducation about the importance of engagement in mental health services for improvement in general functioning, adherence to the medical team's recommendations, and to his overall quality of life.

Following medical treatment, social work was able to obtain funding to qualify for multiple skilled nursing facilities (SNFs). However, the patient adamantly refused placement to an SNF and stated that he preferred to be discharged to the streets. The medical team made numerous attempts to provide psychoeducation about the risks of living on the streets, highlighting his mental and physical health conditions that could be worsened. Because at this time the patient had been deemed by psychiatry to have capacity to leave against medical advice and to determine his own disposition upon discharge and he continued to refuse SNF placement, he was discharged to the streets.

CASE EXAMPLE PART II

Over the subsequent year, the patient was hospitalized multiple times for chronic wounds and sepsis, living on the streets when an outpatient with a span of one month or less between inpatient stays. The patient did not follow the interdisciplinary team's recommendations for either mental or physical health conditions, including not pursuing outpatient medical care or mental health follow-up. In addition, his inability to follow-up routinely with continued wound care to ensure healing of his ulcer once discharged from inpatient medical level of care complicated the typical progression and recovery time. This pattern led to permanent conservatorship paperwork to be sent for approval during one of his inpatient stays. Now, one month after his last discharge, he was hospitalized again with a similar presentation of intoxication, poor compliance with health regimes, and continued daily use of alcohol.

During the court date, the judge questioned the psychiatrist about the patient's diagnostic and treatment history, including a summary of his recent behavior on the unit and adherence to medical treatment recommendations. The judge ruled that this patient met the standards for incompetency, finding that the patient was unable to clearly verbalize a safe plan for finding food, clothing, and shelter. Consequently, once he was stabilized medically, he was discharged to an SNF. The patient continued to have frequent inpatient medical admissions to help manage agitation and refusal of care at his SNF; with each admission, it became clear to the treating teams that the patient's presentations reflected a baseline of a major neurocognitive disorder, as well as chronic schizophrenia. Frequently, at the beginning of each admission, he was suffering from delirium secondary to various causes, most frequently an infectious or metabolic etiology that could be traced to nonadherence with medical care. Once conservatorized, however, the patient was continued on an injectable antipsychotic medication to manage his mood symptoms from his diagnosis of schizophrenia disorder. He continued with occasional irritability and poverty of thought content, but otherwise denied active hallucinations or expressed emotions.

Based on the paucity of literature on the clinical management of geriatric homeless individuals with serious mental illness, we have provided a clinical vignette of a clinical case that depicts how these factors interact. This case highlights how psychiatry and psychology helped make recommendations for the interdisciplinary team members on how to take care of this patient, including creating parameters, such as using involuntary commitment when necessary to be able to get him treated for his complex conditions, as well as strategies for behavioral management of disruptive behaviors toward nursing while an inpatient. Providers illustrated the need for involuntary commitment to the patient by summarizing that, at every admission, he returned with his severe wounds worsened by lack of following treatment recommendations. Patients who fall under this subgroup of being a geriatric homeless individual with a serious mental illness are at risk for decision-making difficulties during an acute medical or psychiatric event. The medical conditions may result in the development of delirium, which can then exacerbate neurological, metabolic, or psychiatric conditions.

Our case illustrates that high comorbid substance abuse along with an SMI (i.e., dual diagnosis) associated with complex medical conditions create seemingly insurmountable challenges for the interdisciplinary care team. Assessment and treatment of patients with comorbid psychiatric and medical illness can be complex, especially when patients are non-cooperative with staff or are refusing care altogether. Ultimately, after a series of interventions—psychoeducation and encouragement of patient involvement and engagement in care—failed to achieve optimal outcomes, the team pursued involuntary commitment and, eventually, conservatorization. The laudatory outcome of this patient's beneficent care was the prevention of further decompensation of both his medical and psychiatric conditions, thus resulting in better overall health and a better quality of function and life for this man.

REFERENCES

Alexopoulos, G. S., Streim, J., Carpenter, D., & Docherty, J. P. (2003). Using antipsychotic agents in older patients. *The Journal of Clinical Psychiatry, 65,* 5–99. Retrieved from https://www.ncbi.nlm.nih.gov/pubmed/14994733

Appleby, L., & Desai, P. N. (1985). Documenting the relationship between homelessness and psychiatric hospitalization. *Psychiatric Services, 36*(7), 732–737. doi:10.1176/ps.36.7.732

Aviram, U. (1990). Community care of the seriously mentally ill: Continuing problems and current issues. *Community Mental Health Journal, 26*(1), 69–88. doi:10.1007/BF00752677

Bartels, S. J. (2004). Caring for the whole person: Integrated health care for older adults with severe mental illness and medical comorbidity. *Journal of the American Geriatrics Society, 52,* S249–S257. doi:10.1111/j.1532-5415.2004.52601.x

Brown, R. T., Hemati, K., Riley, E. D., Lee, C. T., Ponath, C., Tieu, L., . . . & Kushel, M. B. (2016). Geriatric conditions in a population-based sample of older homeless adults. *The Gerontologist, 57*(4), 757–766. doi:10.1093/geront/gnw011

Dennis, D. L., Buckner, J. C., Lipton, F. R., & Levine, I. S. (1991). A decade of research and services for homeless mentally ill persons: Where do we stand? *American Psychologist, 46*(11), 1129–1138. Retrieved from https://www.researchgate.net/publication/21383941

Fazel, S., Khosla, V., Doll, H., & Geddes, J. (2008). The prevalence of mental disorders among the homeless in Western countries: Systematic review and metaregression analysis. *PLoS Med, 5*(12), e225. doi:10.1371/journal.pmed.0050225.

Folsom, D. P., Hawthorne, W., Lindamer, L., Gilmer, T., Bailey, A., Golshan, S., . . . & Jeste, D. V. (2005). Prevalence and risk factors for homelessness and utilization of mental health services among 10,340 patients with serious mental illness in a large public mental health system. *American Journal of Psychiatry, 162*(2), 370–376. doi:10.1176/appi.ajp.162.2.370

Galvin, R., Bråthen, G., Ivashynka, A., Hillborn, M., Tanasescu, R., & Leone, M. A. (2010). EFNS guidelines for diagnosis, therapy and prevention of Wernicke encephalopathy. *European Journal of Neurology, 17*(2), 1408–1418. doi:10.1111/j.1468-1331.2010.03153.x

Gareri, P., Segura-García, C., Manfredi, V. G. L., Bruni, A., Ciambrone, P., Cerminara, G., . . . & De Fazio, P. (2014). Use of atypical antipsychotics in the elderly: A clinical review. *Clinical Interventions in Aging, 9,* 1363–1373. doi:10.2147/CIA.S63942

Gelberg, L., Andersen, R. M., & Leake, B. D. (2000). The behavioral model for vulnerable populations: Application to medical care use and outcomes for homeless people. *Health Services Research, 34*(6), 1273–1302. Retrieved from https://www.ncbi.nlm.nih.gov/pmc/articles/PMC1089079

Goodman, L., Saxe, L., & Harvey, M. (1991). Homelessness as psychological trauma: Broadening perspectives. *American Psychologist, 46*(11), 1219–1225. Retrieved from http://www.academia.edu/26235515/Homelessness_as_psychological_trauma_Broadening_perspectives

Hajjar, E. R., Cafiero, A. C., & Hanlon, J. T. (2007). Polypharmacy in elderly patients. *The American Journal of Geriatric Pharmacotherapy, 5*(4), 345–351. doi:10.1016/j.amjopharm.2007.12.002

Hedman, L. C., Petrila, J., Fisher, W. H., Swanson, J. W., Dingman, D. A., & Burris, S. (2016). State laws on emergency holds for mental health stabilization. *Psychiatric Services, 67*(5), 529–535. doi:10.1176/appi.ps.201500205

Kushel, M. B., Vittinghoff, E., & Haas, J. S. (2001). Factors associated with the health care utilization of homeless persons. *Journal of the American Medical Association, 285*(2), 200–206. doi:10.1001/jama.285.2.200

Lam, J. A., & Rosenheck, R. A. (2000). Correlates of improvement in quality of life among homeless persons with serious mental illness. *Psychiatric Services, 51*(1), 116–118. Retrieved from https://ps.psychiatryonline.org/doi/pdf/10.1176/ps.51.1.116

Lee, B. A., & Schreck, C. J. (2005). Danger on the streets: Marginality and victimization among homeless people. *American Behavioral Scientist, 48*(8), 1055–1081. doi:10.1177/0002764204274200

Liu, B. A., Mittmann, N., Knowles, S. R., & Shear, N. H. (1996). Hyponatremia and the syndrome of inappropriate secretion of antidiuretic hormone associated with the use of selective serotonin reuptake inhibitors: A review of spontaneous reports. *CMAJ: Canadian Medical Association Journal, 155*(5), 519–527. Retrieved from http://www.cmaj.ca/content/155/5/519

Miyamoto, S., Duncan, G. E., Marx, C. E., & Lieberman, J. A. (2005). Treatments for schizophrenia: A critical review of pharmacology and mechanisms of action of antipsychotic drugs. *Molecular Psychiatry, 10*(1), 79–104. doi:10.1038/sj.mp.4001556

Nageotte, C., Sullivan, G., Duan, N., & Camp, P. L. (1997). Medication compliance among the seriously mentally ill in a public mental health system. *Social Psychiatry and Psychiatric Epidemiology, 32*(2), 49–56. doi:10.1007/BF00788920

Olfson, M., King, M., & Schoenbaum, M. (2015). Benzodiazepine use in the United States. *JAMA Psychiatry, 72*(2), 136–142. doi:10.1001/jamapsychiatry.2014.1763

Quigley, J. M., Raphael, S., & Smolensky, E. (2001). Homeless in America, homeless in California. *The Review of Economics and Statistics, 83*(1), 37–51. Retrieved from https://escholarship.org/content/qt4v61c0ws/qt4v61c0ws.pdf?nosplash=68059928cfac-72d2abb98f4548341f16

Richard, H., Lamb, M. D., & Weinberger, L. E. (1992). Conservatorship for gravely disabled psychiatric patients: A four-year follow-up study. *American Journal of Psychiatry, 149,* 909–913.

Sajatovic, M., Valenstein, M., Blow, F. C., Ganoczy, D., & Ignacio, R. V. (2006). Treatment adherence with antipsychotic medications in bipolar disorder. *Bipolar Disorders, 8,* 232–241. doi:10.1111/j.1399-5618.2006.00314.x.

Sermons, M. W., & Henry, M. (2010). *Demographics of Homelessness Series: The rising elderly population*. Washington, DC: National Alliance to End Homelessness.

Sullivan, G., Burnam, A., Koegel, P., & Hollenberg, J. (2000). Quality of life of homeless persons with mental illness: Results from the Course-of-Homelessness Study. *Psychiatric Services, 51*(9), 1135–1141. doi:10.1176/appi.ps.51.9.1135

Wang, P. S., Schneeweiss, S., Avorn, J., Fischer, M. A., Mogun, H., Solomon, D. H., & Brookhart, M. A. (2005). Risk of death in elderly users of conventional vs. atypical antipsychotic medications. *New England Journal of Medicine, 353*(22), 2335–2341. doi:10.1056/NEJMoa052827

Wilton, R. (2004). Putting policy into practice? Poverty and people with serious mental illness. *Social Science & Medicine, 58*(1), 25–39. doi:10.1016/S0277-9536(03)00148-5

3

Neurocognitive Disorders in the Geriatric Homeless Population

Rachael Holloway and Maria Tiamson-Kassab

Neurocognitive disorders are life-disrupting disorders that complicate the lives of those who have them, as well as those who care for them. As the homeless population ages and is increasingly comprised of geriatric individuals, it will become more common for homeless older adults with neurocognitive disorders to present for medical care, social services, and other services. The aging of the homeless population is a relatively recent phenomenon, which is reflected in the relative paucity of research at present. However, a cohesive understanding of the current state of the literature and related literature, as well as how to apply that to practice, is necessary when working with this population moving forward.

Any discussion of neurocognitive disorders within the homeless population must be prefaced by the fact that accurate and full assessment of these disorders is difficult in this population, practically speaking. Full neuropsychological batteries that would provide a detailed and clear picture of the characteristics of neurocognitive disorders within the population are rare, as are detailed medical records that would accurately document diagnosed neurocognitive disorders. As such, the research that exists varies widely among brief cognitive screeners, more detailed measures of specific cognitive domains, and full diagnoses of neurocognitive disorders. The state of this research is not conducive to speaking extensively about specific diagnoses of neurocognitive disorders. However, despite these inconsistencies in research measures and gaps in knowledge, there has emerged a clear evidence that neurocognitive deficits are prevalent among the homeless adult population in general, and also specifically in the geriatric homeless population.

Speaking about neurocognitive disorders among the geriatric homeless populations is further complicated by the fact that not only is the existing research inconsistent, research on this topic in general is relatively sparse. Much of the research that exists in this area examines homeless populations in general, rather than geriatric homeless populations specifically, but examining this research is still useful for the purposes of better understanding this issue within the geriatric homeless population. This chapter endeavors to do so in order to highlight relevant research and clinical issues.

NEUROCOGNITIVE DISORDERS IN GERIATRIC HOMELESS ADULTS

With these caveats in mind, shifting to the existing research can help illuminate what is currently known about neurocognitive disorders in the geriatric homeless population. Much of the research into this population in general has found that homeless adults tend to age more quickly, both physically and cognitively. For instance, neurocognitive impairments are common among homeless adults, even when there are very few individuals over age 65 in the research samples (Buhrich, Hodder, & Teesson, 2000). As such, researchers have generally defined *geriatric* differently among homeless adults compared to the general population. Although various ages have been proposed as being used to define *geriatric* among homeless adults throughout the years, the common consensus is that age 50 is considered geriatric, rather than the cutoff of aged 65 or older that is used in the general population (Cohen, 1999). This cutoff has been affirmed with recent research as well. For instance, researchers have found that the mean age of death is 10 to 15 years younger among homeless individuals than their housed counterparts (Baggett et al., 2013). Based on this research, chronically homeless individuals aged 50 or older can generally be considered geriatric.

With this research in mind, it can be helpful to be especially mindful of a homeless adult's age when providing medical, social, or other services to them. Common age-related conditions, including neurocognitive disorders, are more likely to occur at even younger ages when someone is homeless, so being watchful and aware of this may help providers tailor care to be more appropriate.

Understanding more specifics about neurocognitive disorders among homeless geriatric adults can help guide care of this population. Although the research looking specifically at cognitive deficits in geriatric homeless individuals is sparser than that examining adults in general, there does exist research that establishes evidence for the high prevalence of cognitive deficits in the homeless geriatric population. For instance, research by Buhrich et al. (2000) found that cognitive impairment was prevalent among their sample in Sydney, Australia, and that those with cognitive deficits were significantly older than those without. Specifically, 10% of their sample screened positive for cognitive impairments as measured by the Mini Mental Status Examination (MMSE), and those with cognitive impairments tended to be significantly older than those without (Buhrich et al., 2000). This research established that cognitive disorders were common among homeless adults, but particularly among older homeless adults. However, because it used the MMSE, the study was not able to establish any data about specific cognitive deficits, disorders, or specific domains affected.

Other research has also confirmed the prevalence of neurocognitive impairments in the geriatric homeless population. Hategan, Tisi, Abdurrahman, and Bourgeois (2016) examined how the geriatric homeless population utilizes emergency services. The researchers examined electronic medical records (EMRs) and found that 28% of those in the study had psychiatric disorders, including neurocognitive disorders (Hategan et al., 2016). Although this study does not distinguish between neurocognitive disorders and other psychiatric disorders, the fact that it uses EMR data rather than cognitive screeners such as the MMSE indicates more restrictive criteria. This suggests that actual diagnoses of neurocognitive disorders, rather than positive screeners of neurocognitive impairments, are likely common among this population.

Despite the lack of specificity about type of cognitive deficits and somewhat unclear information about diagnoses of neurocognitive disorders, this information is still useful in guiding care. Cognitive screening measures such as the MMSE provide information about gross cognitive deficits, which may give information about how well patients understand medical diagnoses and advice, how well they will be able to remember to take medications, or how well they will be able to navigate complex systems to access social services. Medication adherence is a particularly difficult issue for homeless adults in general, as certain medications are prone to being stolen by other homeless individuals either on the streets or in shelters. Lack of secure locations to store vital medications is often compounded by inconsistent routines and regular environmental cues, resulting in it being particularly difficult for homeless adults with neurocognitive deficits to adhere to medical advice or successfully take advantage of other services provided. The types of cognitive deficits that would result in such real-world difficulties are detectable via measures such as the MMSE and other measures of gross cognitive deficits. As a result, research demonstrates that, while brief cognitive screeners like the MMSE are imprecise, a poorer MMSE score is still useful information when working with this population.

There does exist research that looks more thoroughly at specific neurocognitive impairments in the geriatric homeless population, which provides supporting evidence for the high prevalence of these disorders in this population and also provides more information about specific deficits and functional impairments. For instance, Brown, Kiely, Bharel, and Mitchell (2012) found evidence of prevalent cognitive impairments, as well as associated functional impairments. The researchers looked at global cognitive impairments with the MMSE, and also looked at more specific deficits. Nearly one-quarter of the participants experienced deficits as measured by the MMSE, and 28.3% demonstrated impaired executive functioning. The researchers also found that more than half of participants had experienced a fall in the past year, and that self-reported hearing and vision impairment were relatively common as well. They concluded that geriatric syndromes such as cognitive impairment occur at a significantly younger age among homeless older adults than their housed counterparts (Brown, Kiely, et al., 2012).

Furthering this research, Brown, Hemati, et al. (2017) interviewed 350 geriatric homeless individuals, which they defined as those aged 50 and older. They assessed activities of daily living (ADLs), such as eating, bathing, dressing oneself, and toileting, as well as instrumental activities of daily living (IADLs), such as managing one's own medications, managing finances, taking transportation, completing job applications, and scheduling a job interview. Other outcome variables measured include mobility impairments, cognitive impairments as assessed with the MMSE, and vision and hearing impairments. Consistent with research finding that homeless adults tend to age more quickly, the researchers found that geriatric conditions were common in the study sample. For instance, they found that 25.8% of participants had cognitive impairments. Functional impairments were also common; the researchers found that 38.9% of the geriatric homeless in their sample experienced difficulty with ADLs, and 49.4% experienced difficulty with IADLs (Brown, Hemati, et al., 2017).

Overall, this research found not only that general geriatric conditions were common among homeless adults aged 50 and over, but they also found evidence that cognitive impairment, specifically, was prevalent. Furthermore, functional impairments frequently associated with neurocognitive disorders were common. Nearly 40% experienced ADL deficits, and half of the participants experienced difficulty with one or more IADL (Brown, Hemati, et al., 2017), which underscores the practical implications of such prevalent neurocognitive impairments in this population. Not only are geriatric homeless more likely to screen positive for neurocognitive impairments on brief screeners, but it is also common for them to struggle with basic functional tasks.

Although this research established both high prevalence of neurocognitive impairments and functional deficits, it is somewhat limited. Because the researchers used the MMSE to study cognitive impairments, it was not possible to make more specific conclusions about types of cognitive impairments, or the cognitive domains that were commonly affected. However, this research does provide evidence for what was previously discussed, that even the MMSE can provide useful information about someone's functional level. As the research of Brown, Hemati, et al. (2017) shows, difficulty performing basic daily tasks is common in this population, and this can change the type of care that is necessary when working with older homeless adults. For instance, it may be necessary to place referrals to additional services and specialists who can assist homeless adults to adhere to medical advice, complete complex tasks, or otherwise assist them so that they can better take advantage of services.

Some research does provide more information about specific cognitive deficits in this population. For instance, in a recent study, Rogoz and Burke (2016) looked at more specific cognitive deficits in older homeless adults by looking at the characteristics of homeless older adults in Sydney, Australia. The researchers collected cognitive data on general neurocognitive deficits, as well as specific frontal lobe deficits. They gave all participants the MMSE to check for gross cognitive deficits, and gave 150 out of 171 participants frontal lobe assessments. Frontal lobe assessments included a clock drawing test, the FAS verbal fluency test, and the trail-making test (part B). They found that 78.4% of the sample screened positive for cognitive impairment on the MMSE, and that of those who took the frontal lobe testing, 33.3% demonstrated deficits on clock drawing, 62.7% demonstrated deficits on verbal fluency, and 75.3% demonstrated deficits on trail-making (Rogoz & Burke, 2016).

Based on this research, it is clear that cognitive deficits, and specifically frontal lobe deficits, are likely common among the geriatric homeless population. The measures administered are not sufficient to make any conclusions about specific diagnoses, but they do offer a clearer picture of some of the specific impairments that are common in this population. The prevalence of frontal lobe deficits is also consistent with the research by Brown, Hemati, et al. (2017), which found that IADL deficits were common. Although more research is needed before making any definitive conclusions about specific neurocognitive disorders within this population, this study sheds light on some of the specific deficits that geriatric homeless people may experience, which may inform clinical interactions and interventions with the population.

More specifically, frontal lobe deficits are likely to result in reduced executive functioning, including reduced ability to plan, organize, switch focus between different tasks, and inhibit socially inappropriate or otherwise inadvisable behaviors. This can affect not only the type of care that older homeless adults may need tailored to them, but also their interactions with the staff who are caring for them. The complex nature of caring for an older homeless adult with probable cognitive deficits, the barriers to fully assessing neurocognitive deficits, and the difficult interactions this can create for staff are illustrated in the following case example.

CASE EXAMPLE

The patient was a Caucasian homeless male in his mid-60s who presented to the hospital with complications and infection related to poorly managed HIV. He was in an inpatient medical unit for treatment; he ambulated with a wheelchair. He was well known to the hospital staff, as he had frequent stays for various HIV-related complications. While he was receiving medical care during his hospital stay, he was often openly hostile toward staff, for instance, by declining to offer crucial information to providers, expressing significant frustration at being asked questions, and leaving his hospital room to smoke cigarettes against medical advice. The hospital staff frequently entered his room to perform medical procedures, only to find him unexpectedly absent. When he was asked about these absences, he became visibly agitated and was less compliant with medical procedures following these discussions. Psychiatry was consulted to help facilitate better interactions between staff and patient and to assist in establishing appropriate aftercare so that he would be in an environment where he could successfully take his medications. His HIV infection had advanced to the stage where he required more intensive care and attentive medication adherence.

CASE DISCUSSION

Of immediate concern to the psychiatry staff was the patient's aftercare. When asked how he planned to care for himself and adhere to medical advice for HIV treatment, he stated plans to move to a different state to live with his sister, whom he stated would care for him. There were several obstacles to this plan; the client did not have any financial savings or means to pay for his travel out of state, nor did he have a way to contact his sister to notify her of his plans ahead of time. When the psychiatry staff attempted to discuss the details of this plan with the patient, he was unable to state any viable options and became increasingly agitated the longer the discussion continued.

The patient was not fully compliant with cognitive screeners, but the questions he was willing to answer indicated cognitive deficits. There were also behavioral indicators of cognitive deficits, including his demonstrated difficulty planning ahead and organizing a trip to live with his sister, which suggested possible frontal lobe deficits. Another indicator of frontal lobe deficits was his apparent inability to inhibit his frustration during interactions with medical staff, to such a degree that it was interfering with his ability to receive care. In addition, he had difficulty regularly taking his medications, stating that he frequently forgot to take them, and as a result was highly inconsistent in his medication regimen. This behavior was consistent with specific frontal lobe deficits, gross cognitive deficits, and the associated impairments in completing activities of daily living.

Because of the patient's difficult disposition and frequent unwillingness to work with hospital staff, the psychiatry staff's intervention was to facilitate discussion with the patient and medical staff present so that they could have productive discussions about future plans without the patient becoming so agitated he discontinued the conversation. Other interventions included having the patient describe his own medication schedule, the implications of not taking his medications, and his other aftercare plans. This allowed the hospital staff to ensure that the patient cognitively understood the severity of his illness and how to maintain his health, and to ensure his aftercare plans were reasonable, given his situation. By consulting with the psychiatry staff, the medical staff was better able to serve the patient, was able to tailor medical care to his cognitive abilities, and was able to incorporate his unique living situation into aftercare planning.

RELATED RESEARCH

The preceding case example is a helpful way to consider a real-world depiction of the existing research on neurocognitive disorders in the geriatric homeless population. However, due to the relative paucity of research on geriatric homeless individuals, it can be beneficial to also consider the research on neurocognitive disorders in the general adult homeless population in order to better understand characteristics and prevalence.

The state of neurocognitive disorders and deficits within the geriatric homeless population is especially pertinent when you consider the fact that the homeless population is steadily aging. Recent research suggests that the homeless population is aging as a whole, with older adults being overrepresented in homeless shelters (Culhane, Metraux, & Bainbridge, 2010). Furthermore, research suggests that there is a cohort effect among the homeless population, with the late half of the baby boomer generation being consistently disproportionately represented at homeless shelters (Culhane, Metraux, Byrne, Stino, & Bainbridge, 2013). As a result, the average age at homeless shelters is increasing. This means that those who are currently experiencing cognitive deficits and neurocognitive disorders as young and middle-aged adults are likely to continue experiencing similar or worsened deficits into older age, and that the already-high prevalence of neurocognitive disorders in the general adult population will likely result in even higher prevalence in the geriatric homeless population in the coming years. For these reasons, it is beneficial to review the literatureregarding the general homeless adult population, in order to understand the extent of the issue to inform care.

The relationship between global cognitive impairments and homelessness is more established among the general adult population. For instance, in a 2004 review, Spence, Stevens, and Parks (2004) found evidence of prevalent generalized cognitive impairments, typically measured with the MMSE. Many of the studies that examined more specific, focal cognitive impairments also found evidence that these cognitive impairments are highly prevalent (Spence et al., 2004). This review of literature established that cognitive deficits were common in homeless adults of all ages over a decade ago.

In a more recent paper, Ennis, Roy, and Topolovec-Vranic (2015) conducted a meta-analysis that examined memory impairments in homeless adults of all ages. This study defined memory problems as those measured by a validated neuropsychological test, rather than through other less rigorous measures such as the MMSE. The benefits of this approach include the ability to speak more specifically about types of cognitive deficits that are more common. Furthermore, the fact that the study was a meta-analysis allowed for broader exploration of various types of neuropsychological tests and neurocognitive domains, as well as populations in several cities.

Of note, Ennis et al. (2015) stated that studies that use validated neuropsychological tests are somewhat rare, further highlighting the difficulty of measuring and defining neurocognitive disorders within this population. However, they were able to examine 11 studies that occurred in both the United States and Canada, which fit their criteria, and they found that across the studies, cognitive deficits were common among homeless adults. More specifically, the researchers found consistent deficits in word-list cognitive tasks. Verbal memory deficits were present, but less consistent (Ennis et al., 2015). These types of cognitive deficits are likely to present as difficulty finding the word one wants to use in conversation, lack of diversity in words used in conversation, and difficulty remembering what has been said in previous conversations.

In addition to specific affected cognitive tasks, the researchers of this meta-analysis also examined factors potentially related to those cognitive deficits. They found that memory improved after participants received housing accommodations, and that it declined after becoming homeless. However, memory did not decline proportional to the length of homelessness, so the researchers were not able to more definitively link homelessness as a cause for the memory deficits (Ennis et al., 2015). This research is helpful, in that it highlights the benefits of using validated neuropsychological tests when examining memory and other cognitive deficits in this population. Doing so allows for more specific and nuanced examination and understanding of cognitive deficits among homeless adults. For instance, understanding that verbal memory deficits and word-list deficits are more common can provide information about the type of symptoms to be mindful of. This research also underscores the potential causal link between homelessness and neurocognitive impairments, suggesting that attempts to find housing for affected homeless patients may help improve neurocognitive deficits.

In another review of the research on neurocognitive impairments in homeless adults, Burra, Stergiopoulos, and Rourke (2009) looked at 22 homeless samples across North America, South America, Australia, and Europe. The researchers found evidence of widespread and prevalent cognitive deficits, but also noted that a wide range of neuropsychological tests was used. As a result, they were unable to make more specific conclusions, but their research still demonstrates that neurocognitive disorders are common in this population (Burra et al., 2009). This review demonstrates both that neurocognitive impairments are prevalent across cities in several countries on multiple continents, and that the inconsistency in measurements in the research again makes it difficult to make any conclusions about specific neurocognitive disorders among the general homeless adult population. Despite these limitations, it provides further evidence for the prevalence, and thus the likely increase in future prevalence among geriatric homeless adults.

Stergiopoulos et al. (2015) looked at more specific neurocognitive impairments in the general adult homeless population and found that such impairments were prevalent in their sample. Nearly three-quarters of the participants demonstrated neurocognitive deficits in general. More specifically, 48% had deficits in processing speed, 71% in verbal learning, 67% in recall, and 38% in executive functioning (Stergiopoulos et al., 2015). These deficits are likely to present as difficulty processing information quickly and making decisions based on it, difficulty learning and remembering what one is told, and difficulty organizing, planning, and completing other executive functioning tasks. The mean age of the sample was 41.1 years of age, which is notably younger than age 50. However, for those who are chronically homeless, these deficits will likely still be present, and may have worsened, by the time they reach the geriatric age of 50.

CONCLUSION

Neurocognitive disorders are difficult to measure accurately in geriatric homeless adults, but evidence suggests that they are highly prevalent in the population. Furthermore, the fact that neurocognitive deficits are prevalent among younger adults suggests that, as this population continues to age, the issue will become more widespread among geriatric homeless adults. As a result, the provision of medical, social, and other services to this population will likely be improved when providers are mindful of this, aware of what symptoms to look for, and include this knowledge into their provision of care. Understanding how this issue appears in clinical practice can help illuminate the research, and can provide practical instruction on how to work with an increasingly aging homeless population.

REFERENCES

Baggett, T. P., Hwang, S. W., O'Connell, J. J., Porneala, B. C., Stringfellow, E. J., Orav, E. J., . . . Rigotti, N. A. (2013). Mortality among homeless adults in Boston: Shifts in causes of death over a 15-year period. *JAMA Internal Medicine, 173*, 189–195. doi:10.1001/jamainternmed.2013.1604

Brown, R. T., Hemati, K., Riley, E. D., Lee, C. T., Ponath, C., Tieu, L., . . . Kushel, M. B. (2017). Geriatric conditions in a population-based sample of older homeless adults. *The Gerontologist, 57*(4), 757–766. doi:10.1093/geront/gnw011

Brown, R. T., Kiely, D. K., Bharel, M., & Mitchell, S. L. (2012). Geriatric syndromes in older homeless adults. *Journal of General Internal Medicine, 27*, 16–22. doi:10.1007/s11606-011-1848-9

Buhrich, N., Hodder, T., & Teesson, M. (2000). Lifetime prevalence of trauma among homeless people in Sydney. *The Australian and New Zealand Journal of Psychiatry, 34*(6), 963–966.

Burra, T. A., Stergiopoulos, V., & Rourke, S. B. (2009). A systematic review of cognitive deficits in homeless adults: Implications for service delivery. *The Canadian Journal of Psychiatry, 54*(2), 123–133. doi:10.1177/070674370905400210

Cohen, C. I. (1999). Aging and homelessness. *The Gerontologist, 39*(1), 5–15. doi:10.1093/geront/39.1.5

Culhane, D. P., Metraux, S., Byrne, T., Stino, M., & Bainbridge, J. (2013). The age structure of contemporary homelessness: Evidence and implications for public policy. *Analyses of Social Issues and Public Policy, 13*, 228–244. doi:10.1111/asap.12004

Culhane, D. P., Metraux, S., & Bainbridge, J. (2010). The age structure of contemporary homelessness: Risk period or cohort effect? *Penn School of Social Policy and Practice Working Paper*, 1–28. Retrieved from https://repository.upenn.edu/spp_papers/140

Ennis, N., Roy, S., & Topolovec-Vranic, J. (2015). Memory impairment among people who are homeless: A systematic review. *Memory, 23*, 695–713. doi:10.1080/09658211.2014.921714

Hategan, A., Tisi, D., Abdurrahman, M., & Bourgeois, J. A. (2016). Geriatric homelessness: Association with emergency department utilization. *Canadian Geriatrics Journal, 19*, 189–194. doi:10.5770/cgj.19.253

Rogoz, A., & Burke, D. (2016). Older people experiencing homelessness showed marked impairment on tests of frontal lobe function. *International Journal of Geriatric Psychiatry, 31*, 240–246. doi:10.1002/gps.4316

Spence, S., Stevens, R., & Parks, R. (2004). Cognitive dysfunction in homeless adults: A systematic review. *Journal of the Royal Society of Medicine, 97*, 375–379. doi:10.1258/jrsm.97.8.375

Stergiopoulos, V., Cusi, A., Bekele, T., Skosireva, A., Latimer, E., Schütz, C., . . . Rourke, S. B. (2015). Neurocognitive impairment in a large sample of homeless adults with mental illness. *Acta Psychiatrica Scandinavica, 131*, 256–268. doi:10.1111/acps.12391

4

Depression and Grief in Homeless Older Adults

Jeanne Maglione, Kristoffer Kalisuch, and Alana Iglewicz

As the general population ages, the proportion of older adults is also increasing over time. Older adults without stable housing represent a particularly vulnerable group with higher rates of mental health and medical conditions. Depression is common in older adults and associated with poor medical and mental health outcomes, including increased risk for suicide. Meanwhile, homelessness increases the risk for depressive syndromes. Barriers to adequate detection and treatment of depression in older homeless adults are discussed, as well as assessment and treatment strategies. Identification and treatment of grief are covered. Promising directions for future strategies to decrease depression among older homeless adults are also reviewed.

CLINICAL CASE EXAMPLE

Mr. A is a 72-year-old man who comes in to a community free clinic for evaluation of a nonhealing foot ulcer. He has been without shelter chronically over most of the past eight years since his house was foreclosed, although there were short periods of time in which he lived in shelters and emergency housing. His wife of 40 years died of myocardial infarction (MI) two years ago. He has a history of type 2 diabetes, hypertension, and hypercholesterolemia. He has been prescribed oral hypoglycemic medications and insulin in the past, but has not taken any of these in over a year. He appears frail and looks like a man in his eighties. Although he has not been weighing himself, he believes he has lost a significant amount of weight over the past year as evidenced by the fact that his clothes are now much more loose fitting. He reports daytime fatigue, poor sleep, and early morning awakening. Mr. A often lays awake at night wishing that he would not wake up the next morning, but he denies depressed mood. He has no active suicidal plan or intent. He used to enjoy walking on the beach, an activity he previously did on a daily basis with his wife. However, he can no longer find the motivation to go to the beach, let alone go for a walk on the beach. Although he used to be quite social, he says that he keeps to himself these days as he often feels irritated by people. Ruminating thoughts of guilt that he did not insist his wife was evaluated for her chest pain in the weeks that preceded her death preoccupy his mind. He also shares that it is not easy to maintain friendships on the streets. He has been concerned about his memory for more than a year. He does not like to come in to the clinic and has avoided it for many months.

DEPRESSION IN OLDER ADULTS

Depressive syndromes are common in older adults and represent a major public health concern. Major depressive disorder (MDD) is characterized by the presence of five depressive symptoms on most days over a period of at least two weeks, including low mood, anhedonia (decreased interest), or both, that result in functional impairment (5th ed.; *DSM-5*; American Psychiatric Association, 2013). Other depressive symptoms may include changes in appetite, poor psychomotor activity or slowing, trouble concentrating, changes in sleep, worthless feelings or inappropriate guilt, fatigue or loss of energy, or recurrent thoughts of death or suicide. MDD affects about 3% to 10% of older adults in primary care settings (Borson et al.,1986; Lyness, King, Cox, Yoediono, & Caine, 1999; Schulberg et al., 1998; Steffens et al., 2000). Subthreshold depressive syndromes (i.e., not meeting the full criteria for MDD) are much more common (9%–24%) in older adults (Judd & Akiskal, 2002; Judd et al., 1998a, 1998b; Lyness et al., 1999; Olfson et al., 1996). Depressive symptoms, even subthreshold symptoms, are associated with devastating consequences. In older adults, consequences include decreased quality of life (Meeks, Vahia, Lavretsky, Kulkarni, & Jeste, 2011), functional impairment (Bruce, 2001), increased burden of medical illness (Frasure-Smith, & Lesperance, 2003), risk for hospitalization (Prina, Deeg, Brayne, Beekman, & Huisman, 2012), disability (Alexopoulos, Vrontou, et al., 1996), and increased health services utilization (Unutzer et al., 1997; Vasiliadis et al., 2013). Further, increasing age is associated with higher rates of treatment refractoriness and less favorable outcomes (Mitchell & Subramaniam, 2005).

The diagnostic criteria for MDD are the same for older and younger adults. However, while younger adults more commonly present with affective symptoms, such as sad mood, worthlessness, and guilt, it is not uncommon for depressed older adults, like Mr. A, to present with weight loss, sleep complaints, trouble concentrating, fatigue, irritability, social withdrawal, and/or problems with self-care while denying depressed or sad mood (Table 4.1; Valiengo Lda, Stella, & Forlenza, 2016). A common presenting symptom in depressed older adults is cognitive impairment. In fact, up to 40% of older adults with major depression in the absence of a progressive neurocognitive disorder may exhibit cognitive deficits when tested (Alexopoulos, 2003; Alexopoulos, Gunning-Dixon, Latoussakis, Kanellopoulos, & Murphy, 2008; Lockwood, Alexopoulos, & van Gorp, 2002). Depressed older adults also exhibit deficiencies in verbal fluency, cognitive flexibility, and planning (Lim et al., 2013).

Multiple factors contribute to depression in late-life. Genetic factors play a role in depression occurring in later life, although not to the same extent as in younger life (Gatz, Pedersen, Plomin, Nesselroade, & McClearn, 1992). Psychosocial risk factors include stressful life events (Murphy, 1982), chronic stress, low socioeconomic status, poor perceived health, lack of social support, financial strain, and being single, widowed, or divorced (Doyi, Oppon, Glover, Gbeddy, & Kokroko, 2013). Protective factors include better socioeconomic status, a sense of mastery, social support, engagement with healthcare services, and perceived meaning in life (Fiske, Wetherell, & Gatz, 2009).

Late-life depression is heterogeneous and includes both chronic depressive disorders that develop earlier in life and depression presenting for the first time in later life. There is evidence to support the idea that depression developing late in life may be distinct in many ways from depression developing earlier in life. For example, some, but not all, studies have found associations between depression developing in later life and vascular risk factors such as hypertension and diabetes. Depression developing later in life has also been associated with vascular dementia, stroke, and white matter hyperintensities in multiple studies (Baldwin & O'Brien, 2002). It has been proposed that up to 50% of the cases of late-life depression may have

TABLE 4.1 *Common Presenting Symptoms in Depressed Older Adults Who Deny Depressed Mood*

Weight loss
Poor sleep
Memory/cognitive complaints
Fatigue
Irritability
Social withdrawal
Problems with self-care

Note: It is not uncommon for older adults to experience depression without depressed mood. The symptoms listed in this table can indicate the need for further assessment of mood.

a vascular component. This may explain, in part, late-life depression's high rates of recurrence and treatment refractoriness in comparison with those of depression beginning earlier in life (Souery, Papakostas, & Trivedi, 2006; Trivedi et al., 2006). A recent meta-analysis of 48 studies, including a total of 9,203 people with depression, found that depression was associated with higher levels of plasma endothelial biomarkers, white matter hyperintensities, cerebral microbleeds, and cerebral microinfarctions. Longitudinal data from eight of these studies showed that the white matter hyperintensities were associated with incident depression (van Agtmaal, Houben, Pouwer, Stehouwer, & Schram, 2017).

In summary, depressive symptoms are common in older adults, are difficult to treat, and are associated with poor outcomes. Subthreshold depressive syndromes (not meeting full criteria for a major depressive episode) are, by far, the most common form of depression in older adults and are also associated with poor outcomes. It may be more difficult to recognize depression in older adults particularly if symptoms are subthreshold or if sad or depressed mood is absent. Finally, some proportion of depression in older adults may have a vascular etiology, and this may have important implications for treatment and prognosis.

DEPRESSION AND HOMELESSNESS

The prevalence of MDD is likely elevated among homeless individuals, although this has not been adequately studied. Depending on the population studied and method of assessment used, estimates range from less than 2% to more than 40% (Fazel, Khosla, Doll, & Geddes, 2008). There have been even fewer studies of depression in elderly homeless populations. Barak and Cohen (2003) characterized a group of 98 homeless older adults (65 or more years of age) in Tel-Aviv, Israel, and found that 9.1% met criteria for MDD. Other studies have found depressive symptoms at moderate to severe levels in up to 30% of older individuals experiencing homelessness (Coohey & Easton, 2016). Based on studies of subthreshold depressive syndromes in nonhomeless older adults, it may follow that rates of subthreshold depressive symptoms are greater though well-designed studies are needed to confirm this.

Behavioral theories of depression propose that failure to engage in positive social interactions or enjoyable activities and/or engagement in negative or maladaptive activities results in decreased opportunities for positive outcomes. This, combined with self-critical cognitions, can then amplify avoidance of social interactions or enjoyable activities (Fiske, Wetherell, & Gatz, 2009). With his social isolation, decreased participation in previously enjoyable activities, and his self-critical thinking, we see both of these factors with the case of Mr. A. Both aging and homelessness increase the likelihood of decreased engagement in positive social interactions and enjoyable activities. Negative beliefs about aging and homelessness can lead to more self-critical thinking. Hence, the combination of aging and homelessness can be particularly detrimental in people with biological vulnerabilities.

At the same time, several studies support the idea that positive psychological traits can be protective against depression among homeless individuals. For example, one study of 168 homeless adults in Arkansas found that optimism and perceived support were both associated with decreased depression symptom levels (Fitzpatrick, 2017). Other forms of social capital may also be protective against depression occurring among homeless people (Fitzpatrick, 2017). Irwin and colleagues examined the relationship between social factors and depressive symptoms in a series of 155 homeless people with a mean age of 41 years. They found that, in addition to perceived social support, religious participation and trust were also reversely associated with depressive symptoms (Irwin, Lagory, Ritchey, & Fitzpatrick, 2008).

Though more study regarding depression in aging homeless populations is needed, taken together, the available data suggest that the combination of aging and homelessness could promote depression through decreased positive social interactions and engagement. Meanwhile, perceived social support and other forms of social capital may be protective.

SUICIDE

Suicide is the 10th leading cause of death in the United States and claims the lives of more than 800,000 people per year worldwide (World Health Organization, 2016). There are, on average, 121 completed suicides per day in the United States. Middle-aged adults are at the greatest overall risk for suicide, but suicide risk remains significant in older adults (Figure 4.1). Men are 3.5 times more likely to complete suicide. Figure 4.2 shows rates of suicides in adults over the age of 65 years by state. Studies suggest that older adults are more likely to use lethal means and suicidal behaviors are more likely to be lethal in older adults (Conwell & Thompson, 2008). At the same time, older adults are less likely to have reported suicidal thinking prior to a death by suicide (Blackmore et al., 2008) as compared to middle age and younger adults.

Homelessness is associated with a two- to five-fold increased risk for suicide (Arnautovska, Sveticic, & De Leo, 2014; Barak, Cohen, & Aizenberg, 2004; Sinyor, Kozloff, Reis, & Schaffer, 2017) and depressive symptoms are a major risk factor for suicidal thinking in homeless individuals (Noel et al., 2016). Morikawa and colleagues reported that 55.7% of homeless participants in Tokyo had suicidal thoughts and 31.6% had a history of suicide attempts

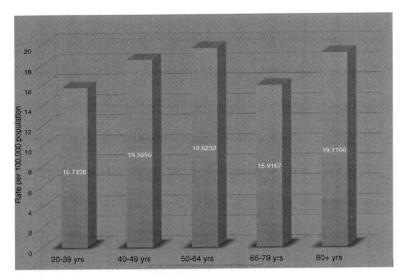

FIGURE 4.1   2015 U.S. suicide rates. Deaths by suicide per 100,000 people are shown by age group.

Source: Data from Centers for Disease Control, Fatal Injury Reports 1981–2015.

(Morikawa, Uehara, Okuda, Shimizu, & Nakamura, 2011). One study based on coroner reports of more than 3,300 people whose cause of death was reported to be a suicide found that homeless and precariously housed people

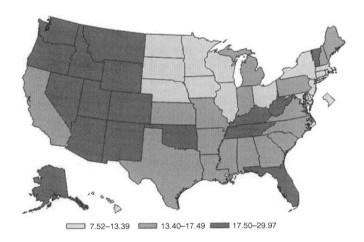

FIGURE 4.2   2008–2014 U.S. suicide rates. Deaths by suicide per 100,000 people aged 65 and older.

Source: Data from the Statistics, Programming, and Economics Branch of the National Center for Injury Prevention and Control; Centers for Disease Control and Prevention; National Center for Health Statistics, National Vital Statistics System; and the U.S. Census Bureau.

who died by suicide were more likely to be male and to die from a fall or jump and less likely to be married or to leave a suicide note (Sinyor et al., 2017). Another study of suicide among more than 1,100 homeless people in Israel found the most common cause of death to be hanging (Barak et al., 2004). In contrast, the most common method used for completed suicides among nonhomeless individuals is firearms.

Eviction and foreclosure are also suicide risk factors. A study comparing people served with an application for eviction from their home in Sweden between 2009 and 2012 with a random population sample found that eviction was associated with a four-fold increased risk for suicide (Rojas & Stenberg, 2016). Another study examined records from the National Violent Death Reporting System and found that increased eviction and foreclosure rates were both associated with increased rates of suicide (Fowler, Gladden, Vagi, Barnes, & Frazier, 2015). Like many homeless individuals, Mr. A has numerous suicide risk factors, including but not limited to his age, gender, death of his wife, passive suicidal ideation, homelessness secondary to home foreclosure, and social isolation.

Taken together, these studies suggest that aging, homelessness, and depression are all significant risk factors for suicide. Focus on interventions to reduce homelessness and to better treat depression among people without stable housing could decrease suicide rates in this vulnerable population.

DEPRESSION AND OTHER CHRONIC MEDICAL CONDITIONS

Biological age, also referred to as physiological or functional age, defines the health and functional status of an individual relative to peers who are the same chronological age. On the level of the individual, biological aging is associated with accumulation of chronic illnesses leading to functional decline. There are now multiple theories regarding the processes underlying biological aging. For example, the inflammatory theory of aging proposes a pro-inflammatory response contributes to multiple age-related diseases, including obesity, diabetes, and cardiovascular disease. The telomere attrition theory proposes that attrition of the protective end-complexes at the termini of eukaryotic chromosomes acts to promote the development of age-related diseases. The common thread to these theories is the idea that the same age-related biological processes may promote the development of multiple chronic medical illnesses.

Homelessness has been associated with accelerated aging. Age-adjusted mortality rates are nearly three times higher in homeless individuals than non-homeless people. While we are used to thinking of 65 years of age as a threshold between middle and older age, this may not be as applicable to homeless adults. Based on physical health characteristics, the biological (or physiological) age of homeless adults may be more similar to nonhomeless adults who are chronologically 10 years older (Grenier, Sussman, Barken, Bourgeois-Guerin, & Rothwell, 2016). Hence, with respect to physiological health, Mr. A's biological age may be more similar to the average nonhomeless man in his eighties. In a survey of 68 homeless people in the Toronto area, 50 years was the age at which participants generally started to consider themselves "old."

Depression and other chronic medical conditions often coexist and one complicates the other. Comorbid depression worsens outcomes of chronic medical disorders that are common in older adults, including stroke, cardiovascular disease, diabetes, and obesity. Poor access to healthcare and mental healthcare among homeless people complicates treatment of chronic illnesses, in turnleading to worse outcomes. This may be, in part, due to poor compliance, as both depression and homelessness are risk factors for medication noncompliance (Chong et al., 2014). Shared biological processes contributing to both depression and chronic medical conditions could also play a role.

Age, depression, and homelessness are all important risk factors for cardiovascular disease. Depression is an independent risk factor for incident coronary heart disease (CHD) in people with no CHD at baseline. Further, depression is a risk factor for all-cause and cardiac-related mortality in patients with an established history of CHD. A meta-analysis of 29 studies looking at the outcomes of depressed and nondepressed patients after an MI found depression was associated with a 2.7-fold increased risk for cardiac death and 2.3-fold increased risk of all-cause death during a two-year follow-up period (Meijer et al., 2011). More research is needed to completely elucidate the mechanisms underlying the association between depression and cardiovascular disease. However, multiple underlying mechanisms likely contribute (Carney & Freedland, 2017). Contributing biological factors could include cardiovascular autonomic dysregulation, inflammation, endothelial dysfunction, and platelet dysfunction. Behavioral factors contributing to the association may include medication noncompliance, poor diet, smoking behaviors, and exercise patterns. Homelessness is also a risk factor for cardiovascular disease. Cardiac risk factors such as noncontrolled hypertension, poorly treated high cholesterol, alcohol use, and smoking are more prevalent in homeless than in non-homeless populations (Asgary et al., 2016; Lee et al., 2005; Szerlip & Szerlip, 2002).

A complex relationship exists between tuberculosis (TB) and depression. Both homeless people and those with chronic mental health conditions are at greater risk for TB. Shelters and group housing arrangements increase the risk of transmission of TB, while both homelessness and depression tend to be obstacles to completing an adequate treatment course. Depression and homelessness are associated with risk factors for progression of TB, including smoking, poor nutrition, and other medical comorbidities, such as HIV infection and diabetes (Doherty et al., 2013). The reported incidence of depressive syndromes among persons with TB ranges from 52% to 75% (Doherty et al., 2013).

Studies regarding the prevalence of type 2 diabetes in homeless populations have reported inconsistent results. A recent meta-analysis did not find evidence to support the idea that the rates of diabetes among homeless populations are any different than among nonhomeless people. However, as in the case of Mr. A, individuals with depression and diabetes are less likely to achieve optimal glycemic control when diabetic (Arnaud, Fagot-Campagna, Reach, Basin, & Laporte, 2010), leading to increased likelihood of complications. Further, the interdisciplinary care required for adequate treatment of diabetes and its complications is rarely accessible to homeless individuals (Davis et al., 2017).

Depression is also commonly comorbid with other mental health conditions, especially substance-use disorders. People with substance-use disorders are at much higher risk of experiencing depression, and those with depression are at greater risk for substance-use disorders (Grant et al., 2016; Swendsen et al., 2010). This reciprocal relationship has been found broadly across different types of addictive substances, including alcohol, cannabis, opiates, and stimulants (Grant et al., 2016). When depression and substance-use disorders occur together, the clinical course tends to be more severe, outcomes tend to be worse, and risk for homelessness is increased (Briere, Rohde, Seeley, Klein, & Lewinsohn, 2014; Yoon, Petrakis, & Rosenheck, 2015). Comorbidity between depression and substance-use disorders is also associated with greater suicide risk (Farren, Snee, Daly, & McElroy, 2013; Hawton, Casanas, Haw, & Saunders, 2013). Although there is a gap in information about comorbid depression and substance-use disorders specifically in older adults, there are studies suggesting that older adults use drugs and alcohol at higher rates than previous generations (Blow & Barry, 2012). Therefore, assessment for substance-use disorders continues to be a critical element of depression assessment across the life span.

In summary, homeless adults are more likely to have a greater burden of chronic medical and mental health conditions, resulting in a biological age approximately 10 years older than nonhomeless people of the same chronologic age. Depression is frequently comorbid with chronic medical diseases, and when comorbidities occur, there tends to be worse outcomes both with respect to depression and other chronic medical diseases. This may be, in part, because biological processes related to aging contribute to both depression and chronic medical illnesses, and in partbecause people with depression tend to be less compliant with medical care and have more obstacles to obtaining adequate treatment. Comorbidity between depression and substance-use disorders is also particularly troublesome, leading to worse outcomes and increased rates of suicide. The significance of, comorbid medical and mental health conditions to the overall course and outcomes of depressive disorders underscores the need for a complete medical and mental health assessment when evaluating the older depressed and homeless individual.

DEPRESSION AND GRIEF

Another topic that warrants consideration in the diagnosis and treatment of depression in homeless older adults is grief. Grief is a universal human experience that is especially pertinent to the older homeless population. Homeless older adults grieve the loss of many things—their home, their dignity, their place in society, their social ties, and often the death of their loved ones. Mr. A's case highlights these multifarious losses. Disentangling grief and depression can be challenging, even for seasoned clinicians. From a symptom checklist perspective, symptoms of grief and depression overlap considerably. Sleep disturbances, mood changes, guilt, anhedonia, and even suicidal ideation are common symptoms of both grief and MDD (Lamb, Pies, & Zisook, 2010; Pies, 2009; Zisook, Reynolds, et al., 2010; Zisook, Simon, et al., 2010). However, qualitatively, grief and depression are quite distinct. A qualitative understanding of their symptoms is thus key to distinguishing between grief—a normal, adaptive human reaction to loss—and major depression—a serious, functionally impairing medical condition (Iglewicz, Seay, Zetumer, & Zisook, 2013). See Table 4.2 for a summary of the phenomenological distinctions between grief and MDD.

Sadness is typically present in both grief and depression. Yet, the nature of the sadness and its course with time distinguish between grief and depression. Loss and emptiness comprise the sadness in grief, whereas inability to anticipate pleasure or happiness and depressed mood comprise the sadness in depression. The sadness of grief is usually intermixed with humor and positive recollections of the deceased loved one. Also, the sadness of grief regularly decreases in intensity over days to weeks and comes in waves. Thoughts or reminders of the deceased loved one trigger these waves, also referred to as the pangs of grief. In contrast, the sadness of depression is pervasive (Lamb et al., 2010). Similarly, the anhedonia seen in grief is linked with longing for the deceased, whereas anhedonia seen in depression is pervasive. Both grieving individuals and individuals experiencing MDD have

TABLE 4.2 *Qualitative Differences Between Grief and Major Depressive Disorder (MDD)*

Symptom	Grief	MDD
Principal affect	Loss and emptiness	Persistent depressed mood
Emotional pain	Accompanied by positive emotions and memories	Pervasive unhappiness
Temporal pattern of sadness	Decreases in intensity over days to weeks; occurs in waves	Persistent
Anhedonia	Connected to longing for the deceased loved one	Pervasive
Suicidal ideation	Focus on life not being worth living without the deceased; common desire to join the deceased	Focus on ending one's own life because of worthlessness and the inability to cope with the suffering from the depression
Guilt	Focused on having let down or failed the deceased loved one	Focused on feelings of self-loathing and worthlessness
Content of thought	Preoccupation with memories and thoughts of the deceased	Negativistic and often self-critical ruminations

Note: Key symptoms of grief and major depressive disorder (MDD) are compared in this table.

preoccupying thoughts. In grief, thoughts are often preoccupied with yearning for their loved one. In juxtaposition, individuals with MDD often experience pessimistic and self-critical ruminations.

The content of guilty thoughts also helps disentangle grief from depression. In grief, thoughts of guilt focus on the "should haves," "could haves," and "what ifs"—essentially on thoughts about letting their loved one down (Iglewicz et al., 2013). Mr. A exemplifies this with his ruminations about not having insisted that his wife present for an evaluation of her chest pain prior to her death from an MI. In the absence of a co-occurring MDD, suicidal ideation is not a key feature of most people's grief. In fact, when it occurs, clinicians should highly consider MDD on the differential. However, there are times when suicidal thoughts are present with normal grief. In these instances, the suicidal thinking centers on the deceased loved one—that life is unbearable without their loved one's presence and/or that they desire to die in order to "join" their loved one (Zisook & Shear, 2009). In evaluating Mr. A, one would need to more fully understand his passive thoughts of suicide and determine whether these thoughts are linked to his wife's death.

On the whole, grief is a normal reaction to loss, and thus should not be medicalized. However, a form of grief called complicated grief (CG) (sometimes called pathological grief, traumatic grief, prolonged grief disorder (Prigerson, Horowitz, et al., 2009), or persistent complex bereavement disorder [American Psychiatric Association, 2013]) is highly comorbid with MDD, and when left untreated is associated with serious medical and mental health sequelae (Lichtenthal, Cruess, & Prigerson, 2004; Stroebe et al., 2007). Notably, when properly managed, people with CG can have promising prognoses (Shear et al., 2016).

In the usual healing process after a loss, "acute grief" transforms into what is called "integrated grief." In integrated grief, the grief takes up less emotional space with time, and the bereaved is able to integrate back into a meaningful life (Zisook & Shear, 2009). At times, factors interfere with this process and CG ensues. Common CG symptoms include yearning for the deceased; anger about the death; feelings of disbelief about the death; intrusive, self-blaming thoughts related to the death; intrusive images of the death; excessive avoidance of reminders of the loss; social isolation; loss of meaning in life; and suicidal ideation (Burg et al., 2005; Dell'Osso et al., 2011; Latham & Prigerson, 2004; Prigerson, Bridge, et al., 1999; Szanto, Prigerson, Houck, Ehrenpreis, & Reynolds, 1997; Szanto, Shear, et al., 2006). There are hints that Mr. A may be experiencing complicated grief—namely, his ruminating preoccupations of guilt that he did not bring his wife for treatment of her chest pain, ruminations that persist two years after her death. As part of his evaluation, it would be important to screen for other symptoms of CG. The detail that he has not been going for previously enjoyable walks on the beach may also be relevant. One possibility is that he has been avoiding the beach, as going there floods him with memories of his wife and painful reminders of her death. Although CG in the homeless population has not been adequately studied, CG is under-recognized, and thus undertreated, in the general population. This pattern is likely even more pronounced with the homeless older adult population.

While it is important to distinguish between the symptoms of grief or CG and MDD, it is also important to be aware of the co-occurrence of these conditions. Bereavement is a psychosocial stressor that can place certain vulnerable individuals at higher risk for developing MDD (Umberson, Wortman, & Kessler, 1992). In fact, a systematic review of risk factors for MDD in older adults found that recent bereavement was the strongest predictor of the development of a major depressive episode. Bereavement was an even stronger predictor than having had prior episodes of depression, disability, and sleep disturbance (Cole & Dendukuri, 2003). There is no need to have to choose between whether an individual has MDD **or** grief. Rather, it is more fruitful to think in terms of whether **both** can be present. When both grief and MDD occur together, one should approach the treatment as thoroughly, thoughtfully, and compassionately as one would the treatment of MDD alone.

BARRIERS TO CARE

Depression is underdiagnosed and often undertreated in older adults, even those with adequate housing. Many older adults do not receive any treatment for depression at all (Unutzer & Park, 2012; Wang et al., 2005). Compared with middle-aged adults, older adults who receive inadequate treatment may be more likely to relapse and have a worse prognosis (Kok & Reynolds, 2017; Mitchell & Subramaniam, 2005). Both aging and homelessness can make it more difficult to detect symptoms of depression in older adults. For example, decreased social engagement or participation in activities can be masked by retirement, loss of a spouse, or the presence of disabling comorbid medical conditions, all of which may be assumed to reasonably explain withdrawal behaviors. Similarly, people living without secure housing may be expected to have less opportunity to engage socially or participate in activities.

Co-occurring cognitive symptoms and medical comorbidities may prevent some older adults from adhering to the recommended treatment regimen (reviewed in Kok & Reynolds, 2017). Homeless older adults are often faced with additional obstacles, such as poor access to care and limited family and social supports.

Because of the relationship between depression and many other comorbid medical conditions, importance of psychosocial contributors, and increased risk of polypharmacy in older adults, it is ideal to treat depression in older adults utilizing a multidisciplinary team approach. This approach includes primary care providers, social workers, psychiatrists, psychologists, and other specialists as needed (e.g., pain management clinicians, pharmacists, neuropsychologists) (Kok & Reynolds, 2017). Unfortunately, homeless older adults often do not have access to this type of care. The most common location for delivery of care to homeless persons, regardless of the concern, is the emergency room (Ku, Scott, Kertesz, & Pitts, 2010). Emergency room care is fragmented, focused on crisis management, and inadequate to treat most conditions, especially depression (Wise & Phillips, 2013).

In summary, there are multiple layers of barriers preventing adequate detection and treatment of depression in older, homeless adults. Addressing these barriers will be critical to improving care, quality of life, and outcomes.

ASSESSMENT OF DEPRESSION

Standardized rating scales can be helpful for screening and following response to treatment. Screening protocols have not been specifically validated in homeless older adults. The Geriatric Depression Scale (GDS) has been validated in older adults. In addition to the original 30-item version of the GDS, there is evidence to support use of abbreviated 15-item and five-item versions, which are less cumbersome. The screening questionnaire with the greatest reported sensitivity in older adults is the PHQ-2 with a sensitivity of 100% and specificity of 77% (Li, Friedman, Conwell, & Fiscella, 2007). The U.S. Preventative Services Task Force, therefore, has recommended a two-level screen starting with the Patient Health Questionnaire (PHQ)-2 followed by additional screening if the PHQ-2 is positive using the GDS-15 or PHQ-9 (Maurer, 2012), which have better specificity (Maurer, 2012).

One of the most important components of the assessment of depressive symptoms is the clinical interview. It is important for clinicians to allow adequate time for discussion of depressive symptoms. One of the first steps is to distinguish between depressive symptoms and a major depressive episode. Many aspects of being homeless are "depressing." Not having a roof over one's head, experiencing social stigma, and struggling to meet one's basic needs are all near universal aspects of being homeless and are by nature "depressing." But, that does not mean that all homeless individuals are by proxy "depressed," aka experiencing an MDD. Sorrow, grief, and sadness are ubiquitous human experiences that should not be confused with the clinical disorder, MDD (Zisook, Pies, & Iglewicz, 2013). One way of distinguishing depressive symptoms from MDD is by using the three "Ps": persistent, pervasive, and pathological. MDD is more **persistent**, occurring most of the day for at least two weeks; more **pervasive**, affecting not only emotions, but also the way people think, behave, and interact with both others and themselves; and more **pathological**, triggering ongoing distress, suffering, and functional impairment (Iglewicz et al., 2013). Many aspects of Mr. A's life could be depressing: the death of his wife, the foreclosure of his house, his multiple medical conditions, and his social isolation. Yet, none of these depressing factors equate to an MDD. Rather, his many symptoms of depression, their duration, and his respective functional impairment do.

It is also important for clinicians to specifically inquire about suicidal thinking, including frequency and intensity of suicidal thinking and specifics about the content of those thoughts, intent, and plan. It is helpful to understand the time course of the symptoms and how it may relate to stressors, including housing status and availability of social support systems. As delineated earlier, it is also important to consider the role of grief in the depression. A mental health history, including history of prior treatments (successful or not), also provides critical information that may be used in treatment planning. Assessment for comorbid medical, mental health, and substance-use conditions is also important, as all are possible contributors to depressive symptoms. Because of the strong association between depressive symptoms and cognitive decline, assessing cognitive functioning is recommended. A review of medications should be done. Opiates, benzodiazepines, beta-blockers, and calcium channel blockers may contribute to depression in some individuals (Glover & Srinivasan, 2013).

PHARMACOTHERAPY

Available treatment options for depressive symptoms in older adults were recently reviewed (Kok & Reynolds, 2017; Pruckner & Holthoff-Detto, 2017). Available studies support the idea that response rates to selective serotonin reuptake inhibitors (SSRIs) (48%, 95% CI 46.1%-49.9%) are similar for younger and older adults (Kok, Nolen, & Heeren, 2012). Increasing evidence suggests that the effects of antidepressants on depression in older adults may be more modest than younger adults (Calati et al., 2013). Possible explanations include greater burden of comorbid medical conditions, neurodegenerative disorders, and treatment-level factors, such as decreased access to care and prescribing of suboptimal doses of antidepressants. The relationship between vascular pathology and late-life depression may also contribute. More research is needed in this area.

SSRIs and other second-generation antidepressants (serotonin–norepinephrine reuptake inhibitors (SNRIs), mirtazapine, and bupropion) are generally considered first-line treatments for depression in older adults. Side-effect profiles are similar in younger and older adults. Additional considerations in older adults include the association of SSRIs with increased risk of falls in older adults. The platelet inhibitory activity of SSRIs may be more of a concern for older adults who are at greater risk for bleeding and who may be more likely to be taking other blood-thinning medications. Any antidepressant has the potential to cause adverse effects related to polypharmacy.

Tricyclic antidepressants (TCAs) are no longer considered first-line treatments for depression in older adults due to increased associated risk for cardiac conduction abnormalities, sedative properties, and anticholinergic properties. Anticholinergic medications can contribute to constipation, urinary retention, and cognitive impairment, making them particularly problematic in older adults (Pruckner & Holthoff-Detto, 2017).

In general, strategies employed by clinicians to address treatment-resistant symptoms or a partial response include titration of the antidepressant to the maximum FDA recommended dose, switching to another antidepressant, combining two antidepressants, and augmentation (e.g., with lithium or aripiprazole). Referral to a psychiatrist or psychiatric nurse practitioner is recommended for patients who do not adequately respond to maximum doses of a single antidepressant. Very little published data is available to support one approach over another. Augmentation by lithium has been reported to improve symptoms in older adults with treatment-resistant depressive symptoms in multiple nonrandomized trials. A large placebo-controlled randomized trial examining the benefits of lithium augmentation in older adults has not yet been published. Treatment with lithium requires careful monitoring of side effects, medication interactions, and renal and thyroid functioning—all of which may be difficult in homeless patients whose care tends to be more fragmented. A randomized controlled trial (RCT) examining the benefits of augmentation of venlafaxine treatment with aripiprazole compared with placebo in 181 elderly patients over a 24-week period of time was done (Lenze et al., 2015). The authors reported a 44% remission rate among older adults with treatment refractory symptoms. The use of antipsychotic medications in older adults requires careful weighing of the possible benefits and risks, the latter of which include development of metabolic syndrome, extrapyramidal symptoms, tardive dyskinesia, and orthostatic hypotension (Jin, Meyer, & Jeste, 2004). Further, the FDA has issued warnings regarding increased risk for cerebrovascular adverse events (strokes and transient ischemic attacks) and mortality in older patients with progressive neurocognitive disorders treated with atypical antipsychotics. A psychiatrist or psychiatric nurse practitioner can help guide patients through evaluation of the risks and benefits of these augmentation strategies and assist with monitoring for adverse effects. Care management strategies could potentially help to provide the additional monitoring required to adequately treat more treatment-resistant forms of depression in homeless patients, but unfortunately they are not generally available currently.

NONPHARMACOLOGIC TREATMENT

Several specific therapies targeting depressive symptoms have been shown to be effective in older adults. These include cognitive behavioral therapy (CBT), problem-solving therapy (PST), and interpersonal therapy (IPT). The overall effect size of evidence-based nonpharmacological therapies in older adults is comparable to antidepressants, while medication side effects and increased risk for polypharmacy are only concerns with the latter (Pinquart, Duberstein, & Lyness, 2006). However, these therapies are often of little practical use for homeless individuals, as access to psychotherapy services is likely to be limited and other competing priorities, such as obtaining adequate food and shelter, can be barriers to attending regular therapy sessions.

Electroconvulsive therapy (ECT) has been shown to be effective in older adults, including those above the age of 80 years (Cattan et al., 1990; Tew et al., 1999). The response rate of ECT in patients who have not responded to pharmacotherapy for depression may be up to 80% (Avery & Lubrano, 1979). An initial course of ECT treatments is typically followed by maintenance ECT treatments and/or pharmacological therapy in order to reduce the chance of relapse. ECT may sometimes be done on an outpatient basis. However, in older homeless adults, we recommend ECT be done in the inpatient setting to allow for recovery in a safe location with the necessary support available.

There is growing evidence to support the idea that exercise benefits mood (Bridle, Spanjers, Patel, Atherton, & Lamb, 2012) in adults of all ages. A recent meta-analysis concluded that exercise interventions had a significant beneficial effect on mood. The evidence supported group-based mixed aerobic and anaerobic interventions at moderate intensity (Schuch et al., 2015, 2016). There have been no trials of exercise to treat depression in homeless older people, and investigation of implementable exercise strategies in this population would be of benefit.

Bright white light (BWL) therapy is a nonpharmacological treatment for depression with few side effects and a relatively rapid onset (days vs. weeks for pharmacotherapy or psychotherapy; Golden et al., 2005). Light therapy boxes are inexpensive and readily available for purchase from a number of marketers. They are also available through some healthcare systems. The efficacy of BWL was first established for seasonal affective disorder (SAS). A meta-analysis (Golden et al., 2005) and Cochrane review (Tuunainen, Kripke, & Endo, 2004) both concluded that BWL is also an effective treatment for non-seasonal depression with effect sizes similar to those in most antidepressant pharmacotherapy trials. Several studies have also shown that BWL is an effective treatment for depression in older adults (Lieverse et al., 2011; Sumaya, Rienzi, Deegan, & Moss, 2001; Wu, Sung, Lee, & Smith, 2015). Unfortunately, there are also barriers to the use of BWL for homeless older adults, namely, cost and daily access to electricity. Further investigation of implementable strategies to bring light therapy to homeless older people would be of benefit. For those who do not have access to a light therapy box, we recommend spending 30 minutes outdoors each day in the morning without sunglasses on.

TOWARD BETTER TREATMENT

Surveys of homeless people suggest that challenges with access and stigma associated with homelessness are important barriers preventing individuals from seeking healthcare. These may be particularly relevant to mental health needs where the establishment of trust with both the treating team and the healthcare system is critical. Several different groups have found that healthcare settings that were specifically tailored to meet the needs of homeless people decrease concerns related to stigma and result in increased satisfaction and utilization of care (Han & Wells, 2003; Kertesz et al., 2013). Peer navigators—individuals with a shared life experience—also address the barrier of stigma while helping homeless people navigate healthcare systems (Corrigan, Kraus, et al., 2017; Corrigan, Pickett, et al., 2017).

In the case of homeless older adults, improved care may require a program that is tailored to meet the needs of both homeless individuals and older adults. This could include access to a multidisciplinary team of primary care providers, social workers, psychiatrists, psychologists, and other specialists (e.g., neurologists, neuropsychologists, pain management specialists, pharmacists). Care management strategies to improve compliance for older homeless adults would be helpful to compensate for the effects of cognitive symptoms and high levels of disability. More research is needed in this area.

Additionally, providing stable housing may enable better outcomes. One prospective cohort study followed 250 homeless older adults in the Boston, Massachusetts, area over a 12-month period and found that the group that obtained housing had significantly fewer depressive symptoms than those who remained homeless (Brown et al., 2015). Several programs have attempted to address housing and mental health issues simultaneously with promising results. For example, the Housing First (HF) program, implemented in five Canadian cities, provides homeless adults with mental illness housing of their choosing along with mental health services and other supportive services without requiring residents to accept or engage in psychiatric care. HF has been shown to improve housing stability among homeless adults with a broad range of psychiatric diagnoses (Aubry et al., 2016; Collins, Malone, & Clifasefi, 2013), including adults over the age of 50 (Chung et al., 2017). Interestingly, improvements from baseline in mental health parameters and quality of life measures were greater among older homeless adults than their younger homeless counterparts, raising the possibility that improving housing stability may be especially critical for the older group (Chung et al., 2017).

In summary, in addition to more resources directed at providing adequate housing for older adults, programs specifically designed to meet the needs of older homeless people may encourage better engagement in care. More research is needed to determine what types of programs specifically meet the needs of older homeless adults.

CONCLUSION

Homeless older adults are at increased risk for developing depression. Untreated depression in homeless older adults leads to far-reaching consequences. These include poor medical and mental health outcomes, social isolation, impaired functioning, and, at times, suicide. The clinical presentation of depression in older adults and younger adults often differs. Having an appreciation for these differences allows clinicians to better diagnose and treat this vulnerable population. Additionally, nuanced intersections between grief and depression in the homeless older adult population are common. Unfortunately, clear barriers to the assessment and treatment of depression exist for homeless older adults.

Exploring the clinical case of Mr. A highlights common themes of the presentation, diagnosis, and treatment of depression in the homeless older adult population. While much is known about late-life depression and its treatment, much less is known about depression, specifically in homeless older adults. Assessment and treatment of depression in older adults, including homeless older adults, is a public health imperative. Research and advocacy are warranted to ensure that older homeless individuals with an MDD receive optimal assessment and treatment of their depression.

REFERENCES

Alexopoulos, G. S. (2003). Role of executive function in late-life depression. *The Journal of Clinical Psychiatry, 64*(Suppl. 14), 18–23.

Alexopoulos, G. S., Gunning-Dixon, F. M., Latoussakis, V., Kanellopoulos, D., & Murphy, C. F. (2008). Anterior cingulate dysfunction in geriatric depression. *International Journal of Geriatric Psychiatry, 23*(4), 347–355. doi:10.1002/gps.1939

Alexopoulos, G. S., Vrontou, C., Kakuma, T., Meyers, B. S., Young, R. C., Klausner, E., & Clarkin, J. (1996). Disability in geriatric depression. *American Journal of Psychiatry, 153*(7), 877–885. doi:10.1176/ajp.153.7.877

American Psychiatric Association. (2013). *Diagnostic and statistical manual of mental disorders* (5th ed). Arlington, VA: American Psychiatric Publishing. doi:10.1176/appi.books.9780890425596

Arnaud, A., Fagot-Campagna, A., Reach, G., Basin, C., & Laporte, A. (2010). Prevalence and characteristics of diabetes among homeless people attending shelters in Paris, France, 2006. *European Journal of Public Health, 20*(5), 601–603. doi:10.1093/eurpub/ckp197

Arnautovska, U., Sveticic, J., & De Leo, D. (2014). What differentiates homeless persons who died by suicide from other suicides in Australia? A comparative analysis using a unique mortality register. *Social Psychiatry and Psychiatric Epidemiology, 49*(4), 583–589. doi:10.1007/s00127-013-0774-z

Asgary, R., Sckell, B., Alcabes, A., Naderi, R., Schoenthaler, A., & Ogedegbe, G. (2016). Rates and predictors of uncontrolled hypertension among hypertensive homeless adults using New York City shelter-based clinics. *Annals of Family Medicine, 14*(1), 41–46. doi:10.1370/afm.1882

Aubry, T., Goering, P., Veldhuizen, S., Adair, C. E., Bourque, J., Distasio, J., . . . Tsemberis, S. (2016). A multiple-city RCT of housing first with assertive community treatment for homeless Canadians with serious mental illness. *Psychiatric Services, 67*(3), 275–281. doi:10.1176/appi.ps.201400587

Avery, D., & Lubrano, A. (1979). Depression treated with imipramine and ECT: The DeCarolis study reconsidered. *The American Journal of Psychiatry, 136*(4B), 559–562.

Baldwin, R. C., & O'Brien, J. (2002). Vascular basis of late-onset depressive disorder. *The British Journal of Psychiatry: The Journal of Mental Science, 180,* 157–160. doi:10.1192/bjp.180.2.157

Barak, Y., & Cohen, A. (2003). Characterizing the elderly homeless: A 10-year study in Israel. *Archives of Gerontology and Geriatrics, 37*(2), 147–155. doi:10.1016/S0167-4943(03)00043-8

Barak, Y., Cohen, A., & Aizenberg, D. (2004). Suicide among the homeless: A 9-year case-series analysis. *Crisis, 25*(2), 51–53. doi:10.1027/0227-5910.25.2.51

Blackmore, E. R., Munce, S., Weller, I., Zagorski, B., Stansfeld, S. A., Stewart, D. E, . . . Conwell, Y. (2008). Psychosocial and clinical correlates of suicidal acts: Results from a national population survey. *The British Journal of Psychiatry: The Journal of Mental Science, 192*(4), 279–284. doi:10.1192/bjp.bp.107.037382

Blow, F. C., & Barry, K. L. (2012). Alcohol and substance misuse in older adults. *Current Psychiatry Reports, 14*(4), 310–319. doi:10.1007/s11920-012-0292-9

Borson, S., Barnes, R. A., Kukull, W. A., Okimoto, J. T., Veith, R. C., Inui, T. S., . . . Raskind, M. A. (1986). Symptomatic depression in elderly medical outpatients. I. Prevalence, demography, and health service utilization. *Journal of the American Geriatrics Society, 34*(5), 341–347. doi:10.1111/j.1532-5415.1986.tb04316.x

Bridle, C., Spanjers, K., Patel, S., Atherton, N. M., & Lamb, S. E. (2012). Effect of exercise on depression severity in older people: Systematic review and meta-analysis of randomised controlled trials. *The British Journal of Psychiatry: The Journal of Mental Science. 201*(3), 180–185. doi:10.1192/bjp.bp.111.095174

Briere, F. N., Rohde, P., Seeley, J. R., Klein, D., & Lewinsohn, P. M. (2014). Comorbidity between major depression and alcohol use disorder from adolescence to adulthood. *Comprehensive Psychiatry, 55*(3), 526–533. doi:10.1016/j.comppsych.2013.10.007

Brown, R. T., Miao, Y., Mitchell, S. L., Bharel, M., Patel, M., Ard, K. L., . . . Steinman, M. A. (2015). Health outcomes of obtaining housing among older homeless adults. *American Journal of Public Health, 105*(7), 1482–1488. doi:10.2105/AJPH.2014.302539

Bruce, M. L. (2001). Depression and disability in late life: Directions for future research. *American Journal of Geriatric Psychiatry, 9*(2), 102–112. doi:10.1097/00019442-200105000-00003

Burg, M. M., Barefoot, J., Berkman, L., Catellier, D. J., Czajkowski, S., Saab, P., . . . ENRICHD Investigators. (2005). Low perceived social support and post-myocardial infarction prognosis in the enhancing recovery in coronary heart disease clinical trial: The effects of treatment. *Psychosomatic Medicine, 67*(6), 879–888. doi:10.1097/01.psy.0000188480.61949.8c

Calati, R., Salvina Signorelli, M., Balestri, M., Marsano, A., De Ronchi, D., Aguglia, E., & Serretti, A. (2013). Antidepressants in elderly: Metaregression of double-blind, randomized clinical trials. *Journal of Affective Disorders, 147*(1–3), 1–8. doi:10.1016/j.jad.2012.11.053

Carney, R. M., & Freedland, K. E. (2017). Depression and coronary heart disease. *Nature Reviews Cardiology, 14*(3), 145–155. doi:10.1038/nrcardio.2016.181

Cattan, R. A., Barry, P. P., Mead, G., Reefe, W. E., Gay, A., & Silverman, M. (1990). Electroconvulsive therapy in octogenarians. *Journal of the American Geriatrics Society, 38*(7), 753–758. doi:10.1111/j.1532-5415.1990.tb01465.x

Chong, M. T., Yamaki, J., Harwood, M., d'Assalenaux, R., Rosenberg, E., Aruoma, O., & Bishayee, A. (2014). Assessing health conditions and medication use among the homeless community in Long Beach, California. *Journal of Research in Pharmacy Practice*, *3*(2), 56–61. doi:10.4103/2279-042X.137073

Chung, T. E., Gozdzik, A., Palma Lazgare, L. I., To, M. J., Aubry, T., Frankish, J., . . . Stergiopoulos, V. (2017). Housing First for older homeless adults with mental illness: A subgroup analysis of the At Home/Chez Soi randomized controlled trial. *International Journal of Geriatric Psychiatry*. Advance online publication. doi:10.1002/gps.4682

Cole, M. G., & Dendukuri, N. (2003). Risk factors for depression among elderly community subjects: A systematic review and meta-analysis. *The American Journal of Psychiatry*, *160*(6), 1147–1156. doi:10.1176/appi.ajp.160.6.1147

Collins, S. E., Malone, D. K., & Clifasefi, S. L. (2013). Housing retention in single-site housing first for chronically homeless individuals with severe alcohol problems. *American Journal of Public Health*, *103*(Suppl. 2), S269–S274. doi:10.2105/AJPH.2013.301312

Conwell, Y., & Thompson, C. (2008). Suicidal behavior in elders. *The Psychiatric Clinics of North America*, *31*(2), 333–356. doi:10.1016/j.psc.2008.01.004

Coohey, C., & Easton, S. D. (2016). Distal stressors and depression among homeless men. *Health & Social Work*, *41*(2), 111–119. doi:10.1093/hsw/hlw008

Corrigan, P. W., Kraus, D. J., Pickett, S. A., Schmidt, A., Stellon, E., Hantke, E, . . . Lara, J. L. (2017). Using peer navigators to address the integrated health care needs of homeless African Americans with serious mental illness. *Psychiatric Services*, *68*(3), 264–270. doi:10.1176/appi.ps.201600134

Corrigan, P. W., Pickett, S., Schmidt, A., Stellon, E., Hantke, E., Kraus, D, . . . Community Based Participatory Research Team. (2017). Peer navigators to promote engagement of homeless African Americans with serious mental illness in primary care. *Psychiatry Research*, *255*, 101–103. doi:10.1016/j.psychres.2017.05.020

Davis, J. A., Tsui, I., Gelberg, L., Gabrielian, S., Lee, M. L., & Chang, E. T. (2017). Risk factors for diabetic retinopathy among homeless veterans. *Psychological Services*, *14*(2), 221–228. doi:10.1037/ser0000148

Dell'Osso, L., Carmassi, C., Rucci, P., Ciapparelli, A., Conversano, C., & Marazziti, D. (2011). Complicated grief and suicidality: The impact of subthreshold mood symptoms. *CNS Spectrums*, *16*(1), 1–6. doi:10.1017/S1092852912000090

Doherty, A. M., Kelly, J., McDonald, C., O'Dywer, A. M., Keane, J., & Cooney, J. (2013). A review of the interplay between tuberculosis and mental health. *General Hospital Psychiatry*, *35*(4), 398–406. doi:10.1016/j.genhosppsych.2013.03.018

Doyi, I., Oppon, O. C., Glover, E. T., Gbeddy, G., & Kokroko, W. (2013). Assessment of occupational radiation exposure in underground artisanal gold mines in Tongo, Upper East Region of Ghana. *Journal of Environmental Radioactivity*, *126*, 77–82. doi:10.1016/j.jenvrad.2013.07.007

Farren, C. K., Snee, L., Daly, P., & McElroy, S. (2013). Prognostic factors of 2-year outcomes of patients with comorbid bipolar disorder or depression with alcohol dependence: Importance of early abstinence. *Alcohol and Alcoholism*, *48*(1), 93–98. doi:10.1093/alcalc/ags112

Fazel, S., Khosla, V., Doll, H., & Geddes, J. (2008). The prevalence of mental disorders among the homeless in western countries: Systematic review and meta-regression analysis. *PLOS Medicine*, *5*(12), e225. doi:10.1371/journal.pmed.0050225

Fiske, A., Wetherell, J. L., & Gatz, M. (2009). Depression in older adults. *Annual Review of Clinical Psychology*, *5*, 363–389. doi:10.1146/annurev.clinpsy.032408.153621

Fitzpatrick, K. M. (2017). How positive is their future? Assessing the role of optimism and social support in understanding mental health symptomatology among homeless adults. *Stress and Health: Journal of the International Society for the Investigation of Stress*, *33*(2), 92–101. doi:10.1002/smi.2676

Fowler, K. A., Gladden, R. M., Vagi, K. J., Barnes, J., & Frazier, L. (2015). Increase in suicides associated with home eviction and foreclosure during the US housing crisis: Findings from 16 National Violent Death Reporting System States, 2005–2010. *American Journal of Public Health, 105*(2), 311–316. doi:10.2105/AJPH.2014.301945

Frasure-Smith, N., & Lesperance, F. (2003). Depression: A cardiac risk factor in search of a treatment. *Journal of the American Medical Association, 289*(23), 3171–3173. doi:10.1001/jama.289.23.3171

Gatz, M., Pedersen, N. L., Plomin, R., Nesselroade, J. R., & McClearn, G. E. (1992). Importance of shared genes and shared environments for symptoms of depression in older adults. *Journal of Abnormal Psychology, 101*(4), 701–708. doi:10.1037/0021-843X.101.4.701

Glover, J., & Srinivasan, S. (2013). Assessment of the person with late-life depression. *The Psychiatric Clinics of North America, 36*(4), 545–560. doi:10.1016/j.psc.2013.08.004

Golden, R. N., Gaynes, B. N., Ekstrom, R. D., Hamer, R. M., Jacobsen, F. M., Suppes, T., . . . Nemeroff, C. B. (2005). The efficacy of light therapy in the treatment of mood disorders: A review and meta-analysis of the evidence. *The American Journal of Psychiatry. 162*(4), 656–662. doi:10.1176/appi.ajp.162.4.656

Grant, B. F., Saha, T. D., Ruan, W. J., Goldstein, R. B., Chou, S. P., Jung, J., . . . Hasin, D. S. (2016). Epidemiology of *DSM-5* drug use disorder: Results from the National Epidemiologic Survey on Alcohol and Related Conditions-III. *JAMA Psychiatry, 73*(1), 39–47. doi:10.1001/jamapsychiatry.2015.2132

Grenier, A., Sussman, T., Barken, R., Bourgeois-Guerin, V., & Rothwell, D. (2016). 'Growing old' in shelters and 'On the street': Experiences of older homeless people. *Journal of Gerontological Social Work, 59*(6), 458–477. doi:10.1080/01634372.2016.1235067

Han, B., & Wells, B. L. (2003). Inappropriate emergency department visits and use of the Health Care for the Homeless Program services by homeless adults in the northeastern United States. *Journal of Public Health Management and Practice, 9*(6), 530–537. doi:10.1097/00124784-200311000-00014

Hawton, K., Casanas, I. C. C., Haw, C., & Saunders, K. (2013). Risk factors for suicide in individuals with depression: A systematic review. *Journal of Affective Disorders, 147*(1–3), 17–28. doi:10.1016/j.jad.2013.01.004

Iglewicz, A., Seay, K., Zetumer, S. D., & Zisook, S. (2013). The removal of the bereavement exclusion in the DSM-5: Exploring the evidence. *Current Psychiatry Reports, 15*(11), 413. doi:10.1007/s11920-013-0413-0

Irwin, J., Lagory, M., Ritchey, F., & Fitzpatrick, K. (2008). Social assets and mental distress among the homeless: Exploring the roles of social support and other forms of social capital on depression. *Social Science & Medicine, 67*(12), 1935–1943. doi:10.1016/j.socscimed.2008.09.008

Jin, H., Meyer, J. M., & Jeste, D. V. (2004). Atypical antipsychotics and glucose dysregulation: A systematic review. *Schizophrenia Research, 71*(2–3), 195–212. doi:10.1016/j.schres.2004.03.024

Judd, L. L., & Akiskal, H. S. (2002). The clinical and public health relevance of current research on subthreshold depressive symptoms to elderly patients. *The American Journal of Geriatric Psychiatry, 10*(3), 233–238. doi:10.1097/00019442-200205000-00002

Judd, L. L., Akiskal, H. S., Maser, J. D., Zeller, P. J., Endicott, J., Coryell, W., . . . Keller, M. B. (1998a). A prospective 12-year study of subsyndromal and syndromal depressive symptoms in unipolar major depressive disorders. *Archives of General Psychiatry, 55*(8), 694–700. doi:10.1001/archpsyc.55.8.694

Judd, L. L., Akiskal, H. S., Maser, J. D., Zeller, P. J., Endicott, J., Coryell, W., . . . Keller, M. B. (1998b). Major depressive disorder: A prospective study of residual subthreshold depressive symptoms as predictor of rapid relapse. *Journal of Affective Disorders, 50*(2–3), 97–108. doi:10.1016/S0165-0327(98)00138-4

Kertesz, S. G., Holt, C. L., Steward, J. L., Jones, R. N., Roth, D. L., Stringfellow, E, . . . Pollio, D. E. (2013). Comparing homeless persons' care experiences in tailored versus nontailored primary care programs. *American Journal of Public Health, 103*(Suppl. 2), S331–S339. doi:10.2105/AJPH.2013.301481

Kok, R. M., Nolen, W. A., & Heeren, T. J. (2012). Efficacy of treatment in older depressed patients: A systematic review and meta-analysis of double-blind randomized controlled trials with antidepressants. *Journal of Affective Disorders, 141*(2–3), 103–115. doi:10.1016/j.jad.2012.02.036

Kok, R. M., & Reynolds, C. F., 3rd. (2017). Management of depression in older adults: A review. *Journal of the American Medical Association, 317*(20), 2114–2122. doi:10.1001/jama.2017.5706

Ku, B. S., Scott, K. C., Kertesz, S. G., & Pitts, S. R. (2010). Factors associated with use of urban emergency departments by the U.S. homeless population. *Public Health Reports, 125*(3), 398–405. doi:10.1177/003335491012500308

Lamb, K., Pies, R., & Zisook, S. (2010). The bereavement exclusion for the diagnosis of major depression: To be, or not to be. *Psychiatry, 7*(7), 19–25.

Latham, A. E., & Prigerson, H. G. (2004). Suicidality and bereavement: Complicated grief as psychiatric disorder presenting greatest risk for suicidality. *Suicide & Life-Threatening Behavior, 34*(4), 350–362. doi:10.1521/suli.34.4.350.53737

Lee, T. C., Hanlon, J. G., Ben-David, J., Booth, G. L., Cantor, W. J., Connelly, P. W., & Hwang, S. W. (2005). Risk factors for cardiovascular disease in homeless adults. *Circulation, 111*(20), 2629–2635. doi:10.1161/CIRCULATIONAHA.104.510826

Lenze, E. J., Mulsant, B. H., Blumberger, D. M., Karp, J. F., Newcomer, J. W., Anderson, S. J., . . . Reynolds, C. F., 3rd. (2015). Efficacy, safety, and tolerability of augmentation pharmacotherapy with aripiprazole for treatment-resistant depression in late life: A randomised, double-blind, placebo-controlled trial. *Lancet, 386*(10011), 2404–2412. doi:10.1016/S0140-6736(15)00308-6

Li, C., Friedman, B., Conwell, Y., & Fiscella, K. (2007). Validity of the Patient Health Questionnaire 2 (PHQ-2) in identifying major depression in older people. *Journal of the American Geriatrics Society, 55*(4), 596–602. doi:10.1111/j.1532-5415.2007.01103.x

Lichtenthal, W. G., Cruess, D. G., & Prigerson, H. G. (2004). A case for establishing complicated grief as a distinct mental disorder in *DSM-V. Clinical Psychology Review, 24*(6), 637–662. doi:10.1016/j.cpr.2004.07.002

Lieverse, R., Van Someren, E. J., Nielen, M. M., Uitdehaag, B. M., Smit, J. H., & Hoogendijk, W. J. (2011). Bright light treatment in elderly patients with nonseasonal major depressive disorder: A randomized placebo-controlled trial. *Archives of General Psychiatry, 68*(1), 61–70. doi:10.1001/archgenpsychiatry.2010.183

Lim, J., Oh, I. K., Han, C., Huh, Y. J., Jung, I. K., Patkar, A. A., . . . Jang, B. H. (2013). Sensitivity of cognitive tests in four cognitive domains in discriminating MDD patients from healthy controls: A meta-analysis. *International Psychogeriatrics, 25*(9), 1543–1557. doi:10.1017/S1041610213000689

Lockwood, K. A., Alexopoulos, G. S., & van Gorp, W. G. (2002). Executive dysfunction in geriatric depression. *The American Journal of Psychiatry, 159*(7), 1119–1126. doi:10.1176/appi.ajp.159.7.1119

Lyness, J. M., King, D. A., Cox, C., Yoediono, Z., & Caine, E. D. (1999). The importance of subsyndromal depression in older primary care patients: Prevalence and associated functional disability. *Journal of the American Geriatrics Society, 47*(6), 647–652. doi:10.1111/j.1532-5415.1999.tb01584.x

Maurer, D. M. (2012). Screening for depression. *American Family Physician, 85*(2), 139–144.

Meeks, T. W., Vahia, I. V., Lavretsky, H., Kulkarni, G., & Jeste, D. V. (2011). A tune in "a minor" can "b major": A review of epidemiology, illness course, and public health implications of subthreshold depression in older adults. *Journal of Affective Disorders. 129*(1–3), 126–142. doi:10.1016/j.jad.2010.09.015

Meijer, A., Conradi, H. J., Bos, E. H., Thombs, B. D., van Melle, J. P., & de Jonge, P. (2011). Prognostic association of depression following myocardial infarction with mortality and cardiovascular events: A meta-analysis of 25 years of research. *General Hospital Psychiatry, 33*(3), 203–216. doi:10.1016/j.genhosppsych.2011.02.007

Mitchell, A. J., & Subramaniam, H. (2005). Prognosis of depression in old age compared to middle age: A systematic review of comparative studies. *The American Jjournal of Psychiatry, 162*(9), 1588–1601. doi:10.1176/appi.ajp.162.9.1588

Morikawa, S., Uehara, R., Okuda, K., Shimizu, H., & Nakamura, Y. (2011). [Prevalence of psychiatric disorders among homeless people in one area of Tokyo]. [Nihon koshu eisei zasshi] *Japanese Journal of Public Health, 58*(5), 331–339.

Murphy, E. (1982). Social origins of depression in old age. *The British Journal of Psychiatry: The Journal of Mental Science, 141*, 135–142. doi:10.1192/bjp.141.2.135

Noel, F., Moniruzzaman, A., Somers, J., Frankish, J., Strehlau, V., Schutz, C., & Krausz, M. (2016). A longitudinal study of suicidal ideation among homeless, mentally ill individuals. *Social Psychiatry and Psychiatric Epidemiology, 51*(1), 107–114. doi:10.1007/s00127-015-1142-y

Olfson, M., Broadhead, W. E., Weissman, M. M., Leon, A. C., Farber, L., Hoven, C., . . . Kathol, R. (1996). Subthreshold psychiatric symptoms in a primary care group practice. *Archives of General Psychiatry, 53*(10), 880–886. doi:10.1001/archpsyc.1996.01830100026004

Pies, R. (2009). Depression or "proper sorrows"—have physicians medicalized sadness? *Primary Care Companion to the Journal of Clinical Psychiatry, 11*(1), 38–39. doi:10.4088/PCC.08l00618

Pinquart, M., Duberstein, P. R., & Lyness, J. M. (2006). Treatments for later-life depressive conditions: A meta-analytic comparison of pharmacotherapy and psychotherapy. *The American Journal of Psychiatry, 163*(9), 1493–1501. doi:10.1176/ajp.2006.163.9.1493

Prigerson, H. G., Bridge, J., Maciejewski, P. K., Beery, L. C., Rosenheck, R. A., Jacobs, S. C., . . . Brent, D. A. (1999). Influence of traumatic grief on suicidal ideation among young adults. *The American Journal of Psychiatry, 156*(12), 1994–1995.

Prigerson, H. G., Horowitz, M. J., Jacobs, S. C., Parkes, C. M., Aslan, M., Goodkin, K, . . . Maciejewski, P. K. (2009). Prolonged grief disorder: Psychometric validation of criteria proposed for *DSM-V* and *ICD-11. PLOS Medicine, 6*(8), e1000121. doi:10.1371/journal.pmed.1000121

Prina, A. M., Deeg, D., Brayne, C., Beekman, A., & Huisman, M. (2012). The association between depressive symptoms and non-psychiatric hospitalisation in older adults. *PLOS ONE, 7*(4), e34821. doi:10.1371/journal.pone.0034821

Pruckner, N., & Holthoff-Detto, V. (2017). Antidepressant pharmacotherapy in old-age depression—a review and clinical approach. *European Journal of Clinical Pharmacology, 73*(6), 661–667. doi:10.1007/s00228-017-2219-1

Rojas, Y., & Stenberg, S. A. (2016). Evictions and suicide: A follow-up study of almost 22,000 Swedish households in the wake of the global financial crisis. *Journal of Epidemiology and Community Health, 70*(4), 409–413. doi:10.1136/jech-2015-206419

Schuch, F. B., Vancampfort, D., Richards, J., Rosenbaum, S., Ward, P. B., & Stubbs, B. (2016). Exercise as a treatment for depression: A meta-analysis adjusting for publication bias. *Journal of Psychiatric Research, 77*, 42–51. doi:10.1016/j.jpsychires.2016.02.023

Schuch, F. B., Vasconcelos-Moreno, M. P., Borowsky, C., Zimmermann, A. B., Rocha, N. S., & Fleck, M. P. (2015). Exercise and severe major depression: Effect on symptom severity and quality of life at discharge in an inpatient cohort. *Journal of Psychiatric Research, 61,* 25–32.

Schulberg, H. C., Mulsant, B., Schulz, R., Rollman, B. L., Houck, P. R., & Reynolds, C. F., 3rd. (1998). Characteristics and course of major depression in older primary care patients. *International Journal of Psychiatry in Medicine, 28*(4), 421–436. doi:10.2190/G23R-NGGN-K1P1-MQ8N

Shear, M. K., Reynolds, C. F., 3rd, Simon, N. M., Zisook, S., Wang, Y., Mauro, C., . . . Skritskaya, N. (2016). Optimizing treatment of complicated grief: A randomized clinical trial. *JAMA Psychiatry, 73*(7), 685–694. doi:10.1001/jamapsychiatry.2016.0892

Sinyor, M., Kozloff, N., Reis, C., & Schaffer, A. (2017). An observational study of suicide death in homeless and precariously housed people in Toronto. *Canadian Journal of Psychiatry Revue Canadienne de Psychiatrie, 62*(7), 501–505. doi:10.1177/0706743717705354

Souery, D., Papakostas, G. I., & Trivedi, M. H. (2006). Treatment-resistant depression. *The Journal of Clinical Psychiatry, 67*(Suppl. 6), 16–22.

Steffens, D. C., Skoog, I., Norton, M. C., Hart, A. D., Tschanz, J. T., Plassman, B. L., . . . Breitner, J. C. (2000). Prevalence of depression and its treatment in an elderly population: The Cache County study. *Archives of General Psychiatry, 57*(6), 601–607. doi:10.1001/archpsyc.57.6.601

Stroebe, M., Boelen, P. A., van den Hout, M., Stroebe, W., Salemink, E., & van den Bout, J. (2007). Ruminative coping as avoidance: A reinterpretation of its function in adjustment to bereavement. *European Archives of Psychiatry and Clinical Neuroscience, 257*(8), 462–472. doi:10.1007/s00406-007-0746-y

Sumaya, I. C., Rienzi, B. M., Deegan, J. F., 2nd, & Moss, D. E. (2001). Bright light treatment decreases depression in institutionalized older adults: A placebo-controlled crossover study. *The Journals of Gerontology Series A, Biological Sciences and Medical Sciences, 56*(6), M356–M360. doi:10.1093/gerona/56.6.M356

Swendsen, J., Conway, K. P., Degenhardt, L., Glantz, M., Jin, R., Merikangas, K. R., . . . Kessler, R. C. (2010). Mental disorders as risk factors for substance use, abuse and dependence: Results from the 10-year follow-up of the National Comorbidity Survey. *Addiction, 105*(6), 1117–1128. doi:10.1111/j.1360-0443.2010.02902.x

Szanto, K., Prigerson, H., Houck, P., Ehrenpreis, L., & Reynolds, C. F., 3rd. (1997). Suicidal ideation in elderly bereaved: The role of complicated grief. *Suicide & Life-Threatening Behavior, 27*(2), 194–207.

Szanto, K., Shear, M. K., Houck, P. R., Reynolds, C. F., 3rd, Frank, E., Caroff, K., . . . Silowash, R. (2006). Indirect self-destructive behavior and overt suicidality in patients with complicated grief. *The Journal of Clinical Psychiatry, 67*(2), 233–239. doi:10.4088/JCP.v67n0209

Szerlip, M. I., & Szerlip, H. M. (2002). Identification of cardiovascular risk factors in homeless adults. *The American Journal of the Medical Sciences, 324*(5), 243–246. doi:10.1097/00000441-200211000-00002

Tew, J. D., Jr., Mulsant, B. H., Haskett, R. F., Prudic, J., Thase, M. E., Crowe, R. R., . . . Sackeim, H. A. (1999). Acute efficacy of ECT in the treatment of major depression in the old-old. *The American Journal of Psychiatry, 156*(12), 1865–1870.

Trivedi, M. H., Rush, A. J., Wisniewski, S. R., Nierenberg, A. A., Warden, D., Ritz, L., . . . STAR*D Study Team. (2006). Evaluation of outcomes with citalopram for depression using measurement-based care in STAR*D: Implications for clinical practice. *The American Journal of Psychiatry, 163*(1), 28–40. doi:10.1176/appi.ajp.163.1.28

Tuunainen, A., Kripke, D. F., & Endo, T. (2004). Light therapy for non-seasonal depression. *The Cochrane Database of Systematic Reviews,. 2004*(2), CD004050.

Umberson, D., Wortman, C. B., & Kessler, R. C. (1992). Widowhood and depression: Explaining long-term gender differences in vulnerability. *Journal of Health and Social Behavior, 33*(1), 10–24. doi:10.2307/2136854

Unutzer, J., & Park, M. (2012). Older adults with severe, treatment-resistant depression. *Journal of the American Medical Association, 308*(9), 909–918. doi:10.1001/2012.jama.10690

Unutzer, J., Patrick, D. L., Simon, G., Grembowski, D., Walker, E., Rutter, C., & Katon, W. (1997). Depressive symptoms and the cost of health services in HMO patients aged 65 years and older. A 4-year prospective study. *The Journal of the American Medical Association, 277*(20), 1618–1623. doi:10.1001/jama.1997.03540440052032 doi:10.1001/jama.277.20.1618

Valiengo Lda, C., Stella, F., & Forlenza, O. V. (2016). Mood disorders in the elderly: Prevalence, functional impact, and management challenges. *Neuropsychiatric Disease and Treatment, 12*, 2105–2114. doi:10.2147/NDT.S94643

van Agtmaal, M. J. M., Houben, A., Pouwer, F., Stehouwer, C. D. A., & Schram, M. T. (2017). Association of microvascular dysfunction with late-life depression: A systematic review and meta-analysis. *JAMA Psychiatry, 74*(7), 729–739. doi:10.1001/jamapsychiatry.2017.0984

Vasiliadis, H. M., Dionne, P. A., Preville, M., Gentil, L., Berbiche, D., & Latimer, E. (2013). The excess healthcare costs associated with depression and anxiety in elderly living in the community. *The American Journal of Geriatric Psychiatry, 21*(6), 536–548. doi:10.1016/j.jagp.2012.12.016

Wang, P. S., Schneeweiss, S., Brookhart, M. A., Glynn, R. J., Mogun, H., Patrick, A. R., & Avorn, J. (2005). Suboptimal antidepressant use in the elderly. *Journal of Clinical Psychopharmacology, 25*(2), 118–126. doi:10.1097/01.jcp.0000155819.67209.e5

Wise, C., & Phillips, K. (2013). Hearing the silent voices: Narratives of health care and homelessness. *Issues in Mental Health Nursing, 34*(5), 359–367. doi:10.3109/01612840.2012.757402

World Health Organization. (2016). Suicide fact sheet. Retrieved from http://www.who.int/mediacentre/factsheets/fs398/en

Wu, M. C., Sung, H. C., Lee, W. L., & Smith, G. D. (2015). The effects of light therapy on depression and sleep disruption in older adults in a long-term care facility. *International Journal of Nursing Practice, 21*(5), 653–659. doi:10.1111/ijn.12307

Yoon, G., Petrakis, I. L., & Rosenheck, R. A. (2015). Correlates of major depressive disorder with and without comorbid alcohol use disorder nationally in the veterans health administration. *The American Journal on Addictions, 24*(5), 419–426. doi:10.1111/ajad.12219

Zisook, S., & Shear, K. (2009). Grief and bereavement: What psychiatrists need to know. *World Psychiatry, 8*(2), 67–74. doi:10.1002/j.2051-5545.2009.tb00217.x

Zisook, S., Pies, R., & Iglewicz, A. (2013). Grief, depression, and the *DSM-5*. *Journal of Psychiatric Practice, 19*(5), 386–396. doi:10.1097/01.pra.0000435037.91049.2f

Zisook, S., Reynolds, C. F., 3rd, Pies, R., Simon, N., Lebowitz, B., Madowitz, J., . . . Shear, M. K. (2010). Bereavement, complicated grief, and *DSM*, part 1: Depression. *The Journal of Clinical Psychiatry, 71*(7), 955–956. doi:10.4088/JCP.10ac06303blu

Zisook, S., Simon, N. M., Reynolds, C. F., 3rd, Pies, R., Lebowitz, B., Young, I. T., . . . Shear, M. K. (2010). Bereavement, complicated grief, and *DSM*, part 2: complicated grief. *The Journal of Clinical Psychiatry, 71*(8), 1097–1098. doi:10.4088/JCP.10ac06391blu

5

Ethical and Legal Issues in the Geriatric Homeless

Yash Joshi and Kristin Beizai

Changing demographics worldwide show that the number of adults aged 65 years and older will increase from 600 million presently to nearly 1.6 billion by 2050, accounting for 12% of the total population (He, Goodkind, & Kowal, 2016). In the United States, similar trends are projected, with the number of Americans 65 years and older doubling from 46 to 96 million from present day to 2060, which will represent one out of four individuals at that time. Epidemiological data suggests these trends are also occurring in the homeless population. From the early 1990s to mid-2000s, the median age of homeless individuals increased by about 10 years, from 37 to 46, with those who were aged 50 years and over nearly tripling from 11% to 32% (Hahn, Kushel, Bangsberg, Riley, & Moss, 2006), and today, it is estimated that half of single homeless adults are aged 50 years and older (Culhane, Metraux, Byrne, Stino, & Bainbridge, 2013).

Homelessness by itself increases the overall mortality risk three- to four-fold, with the presence of serious health issues, substance-use and dependence, unemployed status, and age over 60 years portending early death (Schinka et al., 2016). The average life expectancy is estimated to be reduced as well by about 12 years on average, from the national U.S. average of 78.8 years to 66.5 years for homeless people (Metraux, Eng, Bainbridge, & Culhane, 2011). Homeless adults also experience an accelerated burden of aging-associated illness—for example, in a recent sample of older homeless adults, the prevalence and impact of limitations in homeless adults in their late fifties were more severe than in the housed population in their eighties (Brown, Kiely, Bharel, & Mitchell, 2012; Brown, Hemati, et al., 2017). Those homeless adults were more impaired in completing activities of daily living, including bathing, dressing, and managing their finances, and had cognitive impairment, visual impairment, and urinary incontinence at a much greater rate than their housed counterparts.

This increased risk of geriatric syndromes in the homeless occurs in the context of higher rates of comorbid serious mental illness and psychosocial stressors. A review of the prevalence of serious mental disorders in the homeless revealed the most common disorder to be alcohol and substance-use disorders, with the prevalence of psychosis at least as high as depression (up to 42%), and substantially higher than the community estimates (Fazel, Khosla, Doll, & Geddes, 2006). Homelessness is associated with a low quality of life, increased risk of assault, early death, and lack of insurance and resources (Folsom et al., 2005). Homelessness with onset before the age of 50 years is associated with more adverse life experiences, including lower educational attainment, increased risk incarceration, increased risk childhood abuse or neglect, mental health and substance-use problems, and lower attainment of life milestones (marriage and full-time employment; Brown, Hemati, et al., 2017).

The ethical and legal issues that arise in the care of the geriatric homeless population, therefore, are complex not only because they involve nuances unique to either population, but because the combination of being undomiciled and aged leads to significant unique vulnerability. This confluence of medical illness, mental illness, and psychosocial distress leads to greater bioethical conundrums, with high stakes for patients, more stakeholders involved in their care, and greater system resource utilization to lead to optimal outcomes.

The usual dilemmas in geriatrics of creating an acceptable process for informed consent, judging adequate decision-making capacity for treatment acceptance and refusal, determining appropriate substitute decision makers, preserving privacy and confidentiality, promoting advance care planning, and allocating healthcare resources are made more challenging in the homeless. Attention to applicable laws in the jurisdiction of practice is required, which may differ greatly in scope even across narrow geographic areas. Complicating factors often include ongoing psychiatric comorbidities and serious medical illnesses, which change a patient's mentation and cognitive capacities.

Therefore, appropriate assessment and treatment in these complex cases no doubt requires input from an interprofessional team, including geriatricians, psychiatrists, ethicist consultants, risk management, legal counsel, specialists, social workers, nurses, and other allied staff. Here we present a case with changing psychiatric, ethical, and legal issues to illustrate how such complex tensions arise and may be resolved in a homeless geriatric patient.

CASE: PART I

Mr. R, a 57-year-old male, homeless for many years, with no prior psychiatric history and a past medical history of left middle cerebral artery stroke with residual aphasia and right-sided hemiparesis, hypertension, and diabetes mellitus type 2, was admitted with altered mental status and hypertensive emergency. After his blood pressure was stabilized, he continued with fluctuating lethargy and stupor and was intermittently agitated, with assaultive behavior. MRI revealed acute infarcts of right internal capsule, right globus pallidus, and left superior cerebellum.

Psychiatry was consulted regarding Mr. R's agitation and repeated attempts to elope and sign out against medical advice. He was diagnosed with delirium, determined to lack medical decision-making capacity, and was placed on a 72-hour psychiatric hold for grave disability. As he was exhibiting diffuse paranoia and agitation, treatment with olanzapine and valproic acid (for mood stabilization and psychosis) was initiated.

An immediate and perhaps the most proximal concern at the start of this case is the ability of Mr. R to make autonomous choices and participate in informed consent. The process of informed consent requires the provision of available relevant information (the nature of the illness, proposed intervention, and related risks and benefits), decision-making capacity on the part of the patient, and voluntary agreement (or refusal), without coercion. Decision-making capacity requires the expression of a consistent choice, comprehension of relevant information, appreciation of the situation and its consequences, and the ability to manipulate the information rationally or use reasoning.

It is critical to understand that determining *capacity* to make healthcare choices is completely distinct from determining *competency* to do so (Ganzini, Volicer, Nelson, Fox, & Derse, 2004). Capacity may be assessed by clinicians and includes understanding whether a patient has the ability to comprehend the nature of his or her healthcare decisions and to formulate and communicate decisions about his or her care. Any physician may determine whether or not a patient has the capacity to make decisions over specific healthcare issues. In more complex cases, especially involving patients who have psychiatric illness (i.e., schizophrenia, bipolar disorder, depression, etc.) or cognitive disorders (dementias, delirium, other states of altered mentation), psychiatrists are frequently asked to provide second opinions. In cases when patients decline medically indicated life-saving or life-altering care, or when patients accept radical care with serious potential consequences (i.e., treatment plans with limited clinical trials, heroic or unusual care for orphan/rare diseases, novel or unproven medical devices or technology), multidisciplinary teams are usually required. Competency, on the other hand, is legally determined by courts, queries whether an individual is capable of making valid decisions, and may be assessed when patients are thought to have a *profound* and *permanent* impairment in their decision making. As a legal process, the determination of incompetency may be costly in terms of time and finances, and similar in terms of resource requirements to the guardianship process.

However, the mere presence of any cognitive impairment or any degree of psychiatric comorbidity does not mean that patients, therefore, have compromised decision-making ability. While appropriate cognitive functioning or absence of psychiatric decompensation is inherently linked to the ability to make autonomous decisions, there is a wide range in terms of scope and magnitude of healthcare decisions that patients may make, and equally broad is the impact of cognitive impairment and mental illness. While no single instrument is acceptable for all contexts, well-published tools for assessing cognitive impairment and thought or mood disorders exist and can be a useful aid in documenting severity of illness.

In a similar vein, patients who are not *adequately* informed, or who have not been given consistent information by clinicians about healthcare decisions, are *de facto* not able to act autonomously. The burden is on those who provide healthcare to be able to communicate effectively with patients, keeping in mind their educational background and health literacy, and the reality that patients see multiple different providers of health information, and that treatment recommendations may be shifting faster than patients can account for. Assessing decision-making capacity appropriately means acknowledging not only that patients may freely act against best-practice medical advice (and refuse care or treatment), but patients who superficially appear to acquiesce to medical advice may lack a critical understanding of what they are agreeing to. Agreement does not equate to capacity.

Assessment of decision-making capacity is commonly performed in the aged, in contexts outside of healthcare. As shown in Table 5.1, formal scales and procedures have been developed for assessing everyday decision making, finances, driving, sexual relations, voting, and providing testimony.

In geriatric populations, specialized instruments have been developed to assess healthcare decision-making capacity, including the MacArthur Competence Assessment Tool for Treatment (MacCAT-T), the Hopemont Capacity Assessment Interview (HCAI), and the Competency to Consent to Treatment Interview (CCTI). The literature has not yet matured enough to

TABLE 5.1 *Methods of Assessing Capacity in Domains Not Associated With Healthcare-Related Decision Making in Older Individuals*

Capacity	How to Assess
Everyday decision making and ability to live independently	Structured assessment of functional abilities (e.g., The Kohlman Evaluation of Living Skills) and executive function (e.g., Executive Interview) may help detect elders needing higher level of care. The Assessment of Capacity for Everyday Decision-Making assesses specific capacities. Screen for self-neglect.
Finances	Both self- and informant reports of financial abilities may be inaccurate. The Financial Capacity Instrument allows structured assessment of financial knowledge, skills, and judgment.
Driving	Patients who have mild cognitive impairments and early dementia should be monitored carefully, and formal driving skills evaluation should be considered. Patients who have moderate or more severe dementia should not drive.
Sexual relations	Evaluate the patient's awareness of the relationship, capacity to avoid exploitation, and awareness of potential risks.
Voting	Patients who have severe dementia are unlikely to have capacity. The Competence Assessment Tool for Voting can be used to assess capacity in mild to moderate stages. Ensure that older adults who have capacity actually can cast a ballot.
Testamentary capacity	The Hopkins Competency Assessment is designed specifically to evaluate capacity to execute an advance directive.

Source: Adapted from Walaszek, A. (2009). Clinical ethics issues in geriatric psychiatry. *Psychiatric Clinics of North America, 32*(2), 343–359. doi:10.1016/j.psc.2009.02.004

use them as more than aids in assessing capacity, rather than a formal litmus test. Others have pushed for more qualitative, process-oriented approaches to assess decision making in older adults who have cognitive impairment, including asking questions to assess adequacy on domains of understanding medical information and appreciating how the facts pertain to their beliefs, how patients reason in comparing options, and how they communicate a choice, as shown in Table 5.2 (Appelbaum, 2007; Karlawish, 2008).

On the other hand, "sliding-scale" assessments of capacity, where there is a higher bar for patients to consent to high-risk interventions, or to refuse intervention where lack of interventions would lead to serious consequences to the patient, are widely accepted. In the medically ill, decision-making capacity may fluctuate related to delirium, and efforts to identify and treat contributors to delirium are rewarded when patients regain decision-making capacity.

When cognitive impairment is suspected, there exist a variety of relatively short standardized bedside assessments that can be performed by any

TABLE 5.2 *Clinical Assessment of Medical Decision-Making Capacity in Older Adults*

Decisional Ability	How to Assess
Understanding	After disclosing clinical information (e.g., risks and benefits of a specific treatment), the clinician asks the patient to repeat, in his/her own words, the information.
Appreciation	The clinician ascertains how well the patient accepts that the facts presented actually apply to the patient by probing the patient's beliefs about his/her diagnoses and about the possible benefits from treatment.
Reasoning	The clinician assesses the patient's ability to compare options, patient's ability to infer how a particular choice will affect the patient, and the logical consistency of these answers.
Expressing choice	The clinician determines whether the patient can communicate a consistent decision about treatment.

Source: Adapted from Walaszek, A. (2009). Clinical ethics issues in geriatric psychiatry. *Psychiatric Clinics of North America, 32*(2), 343–359. doi:10.1016/j.psc.2009.02.004, using data from Moye, J., Karel, M. J., Azar, A. R., & Gurrera, R. J. (2004). Hopes and cautions for instrument-based evaluation of consent capacity: Results of a construct validity study of three instruments. In M. B. Kapp (Ed.), *Ethics, Law, and Aging Review* (Vol.10, pp. 39–61). New York, NY: Springer Publishing, and approach from Karlawish, J. (2008). Measuring decision-making capacity in cognitively impaired individuals. *Neurosignals, 16*, 91–98. doi:10.1159/000109763

clinician or allied staff that requires only brief training. Three popular assessments are the St. Louis University Mental Status assessment, the Montreal Cognitive Assessment, and the Mini-Mental State Examination. Any impairment found on these assessments should be followed-up by a deeper investigation by specialists such as psychiatrists, neurologists, or psychologists.

In the preceding case, on initial contact, Mr. R was in a medical crisis (hypertensive emergency), which could end in death if untreated, with a developing stroke syndrome, leading to delirium, a medical condition that alters cognition and mentation to a profound degree. During a medical emergency, consent is presumed, and the informed consent process is waived. However, as his altered mentation persisted over days, and his medical status was judged to be non-emergent, an assessment for his ability to participate in the informed consent process was required. His repeated request to leave in the context of significant medical risk required a very high level of decision-making capacity. Mr. R was not able to show understanding of his condition and understanding of the consequences of his refusal of care, nor was he able to show clear reasoning in reaching his decision. He was determined to lack decision-making capacity, to leave against medical advice, and to refuse recommended medical interventions.

Additionally, because he exhibited symptoms of psychiatric illness (intense paranoia and agitation) without any known past psychiatric history, it was not clear to the treatment team whether a psychiatric diagnosis had been missed in the past or whether this paranoia was associated with delirium, a not uncommon occurrence. Nevertheless, given there was some suspicion of unappreciated mental illness, which satisfied probable cause, he was also placed on an involuntary psychiatric hold for grave disability. Using both the previously mentioned rationales, he was initiated on psychotropic medication targeting his delirium, paranoia, and agitation. Giving the appropriate medications provides treatment to reduce the severity and time course of the delirium, the paranoia, and the agitation. A second gain would be the improvement of his decision-making capacity, so he could begin to participate in shared decision making.

CASE: PART II

Social work consultation was requested to identify a surrogate decision maker for medical decisions, as there was no identified family or advance care directive. Mr. R failed a swallowing test as he had significant dysphagia and dysarthria. He was placed on oral food and water restriction, a nasogastric tube was placed, and tube feeds were initiated. He persistently demanded food and had significant anger and behavioral issues associated with being denied this request.

As his mentation improved, he provided a contact number for a Mr. A. Mr. A was the son of a bar owner the patient used to work for. Over the years, the patient had continued to do odd jobs for Mr. A and to use his house to store his tent, clothes, and bank card, and receive his mail. The ethics team was consulted to address the question "Is it ethically justifiable to place a feeding tube against the patient's wishes?"

The hospital policy supported the use of a friend as a surrogate (in a hierarchy) and though the patient was not considered capacitated to make complex medical decisions, he was consistent in his wish that Mr. A be his surrogate, frequently pointing to a piece of paper with Mr. A's name and phone number. Mr. A agreed to serve this role. He made his decisions based upon Mr. R's long and strongly held values of independence and minimal medical intervention. One example of the patient's need for independence was his persistent refusal of housing. Though there was no clear documented psychiatric history, the patient had a history of some alcohol usage, being a loner over the years, and with paranoia about people interfering in his affairs.

The decision was made with the surrogate decision maker to remove the nasogastric tube and allow oral intake despite the risk of aspiration. Mr. R was placed on a 14-day psychiatric hold, as he was assessed as continuing to meet the standard for grave disability.

Part II of the case describes a scenario not uncommonly encountered in healthcare settings. A medical illness takes away the ability of a patient to make healthcare decisions and a surrogate decision maker is not available, not known, or not able to be emergently reached.

Once a patient has been determined to lack decision-making capacity, the next dilemma: Who should be making decisions on the patient's behalf?

Consistent with the hospital protocol, the attending physician and the chief of service took the role of substitute decision maker while a surrogate decision maker was sought. Input from the ethics team, which any treatment team member can call, was also requested. In our case, appropriate psychotropic medication consent was not possible in a patient with delirium, and therefore the treatment team, by virtue of wanting to act in the best interests of this patient, offered him these medications, which he accepted.

Determining who may be an appropriate substitute decision maker *after* the patient is stabilized and there is no medical emergency, *and* the process by which that determination occurs, however, can be less straightforward. Ideally, family members who understand the patient's values and wishes are ready to offer guidance with *the patient's values*—not their own—in mind (Dunn & Alici, 2013). These decisions can be made clearer with advance directives detailing who may serve as a healthcare proxy or who is designated to have power of attorney (DPOA), where the patient, prior to losing decision-making capacity, can clearly describe his or her preferences both in general and about specific healthcare choices to those individuals (such as the level of medical intervention at the end of life). However, the scope of healthcare decisions is ever expanding, and not everything that could possibly be relevant to future events can be clearly expressed ahead of crises. Not uncommonly, conflict may arise if there is a perceived discrepancy among family members and close relations about who knows the patient's values most clearly, and who is able to act with that in mind, even if advance directives are known and healthcare proxies or DPOAs have been designated. Little is illuminated in terms of legal guidelines in the United States (local, state, and federal laws) to address such difficulties, and therefore institutions and healthcare systems generally develop internal policies and procedures when such issues arise (Brendel & Schouten, 2007).

Limited data on the homeless regarding views on death suggest fear of anonymous death, fear of not receiving treatment due to stigma of homelessness, and fear of a lonely, prolonged, or painful death are principle concerns. Barriers to advance care planning among the homeless include personal factors (prioritization to day-to-day survival, negative experiences with healthcare), systemic factors (lack of housing, lack of continuity of care), provider behavior (lack of knowledge, communication skills, stereotyping of homeless), and financial limitations (insufficient funds for end-of-life care or burial plan). As opposed to nonhomeless persons, surveys have shown homeless adults have different preferences for surrogate decision makers, generally selecting alienated family members, friends, or homeless service providers (National HCH Council, 2016). A 2014 study by Ko and Nelson-Becker (2014) also found that homeless patients have a preference for physicians to be their surrogate decision maker due to expertise.

In our case Mr. R, who was determined to lack decision-making capacity to oppose oral food and water restriction, as well as the placement of a nasogastric tube, insisted that a nonrelated acquaintance, Mr. A, be used as a substitute decision maker. Indeed, patients who lack decision-making capacity for specific healthcare decisions may still retain the capacity to appoint others as substitute decision makers (Moye, Sabatino, & Brendel, 2013). Mr. R demonstrated this by being consistent in his efforts, which was confirmed when the treatment team spoke with Mr. A. And Mr. A completed shared decision making with the team to remove the nasogastric tube and allow oral intake, with full understanding of the associated risks (aspiration pneumonia) and based on his understanding of Mr. R's values.

CASE: PART III

Mr. R progressed to a pureed diet, but began demanding discharge and declined a post-stroke rehabilitation admission. Cognitive improvement and delirium resolution continued slowly. He began to repeatedly write "go home!" and "don't want!"

He declined all referrals (stroke rehabilitation, mental health, speech therapy, physical therapy, and homeless resources) and expressed the consistent desire to be discharged and remain homeless. He was able to express how he would get food and where he would sleep. His surrogate, Mr. A, was in support of his making the decision and felt that it was consistent with Mr. R's long-held values and behaviors. Mr. R was determined to have medical decision-making capacity.

He was not felt to meet criteria for a psychiatric conservatorship or legal guardianship. The psychiatric hold was lifted, and he was discharged against medical advice, per his request.

The explicit goal of healthcare providers is to deliver the best care possible to their patients. It comes as no surprise, then, that when patients do not want interventions that are medically indicated and known to reduce morbidity and mortality, clinicians feel the imperative to change minds. Nevertheless, when a patient is determined to have decision-making capacity; has been educated about the risks, benefits, and alternatives to treatment; and expresses a consistent choice, in line with his or her long-standing beliefs, these choices must be honored. While Mr. R in the case presented was exhibiting poor judgment and declining interventions that improve post-stroke functioning, which would ultimately improve his ability to maintain his preferred independent lifestyle, this was not grounds to continue a psychiatric hold, nor a reason to not support his restored ability to make autonomous choices. To argue the opposite point—to force compulsory medical and psychiatric treatment—would mean that a psychiatric conservatorship or guardianship would need to be enacted—a lengthy process that, in this case, is inappropriate. Further, the legal process for a psychiatric conservatorship requires a psychiatric diagnosis, exempting major neurocognitive disorder and delirium, and in our jurisdiction, guardianship can only be applied for in cases where the patients have assets to support the cost. This essentially makes guardianship not a viable option for our significantly cognitively impaired geriatric homeless adults.

Of course, this respect for autonomous choice is made more challenging in situations where there is a perception (and perhaps the reality too) that homeless aged patients are "difficult." Indeed, separate lines of evidence show that clinicians have negative attitudes toward both homeless persons (Fine, Zhang, & Hwang, 2013) and the aged (Samra et al., 2015). On the other hand, homeless individuals are more likely to have maladaptive coping skills, as well as disinhibition, apathy, and executive dysfunction, which can lead to a challenging therapeutic encounter, particularly in crisis or extremis (Pluck et al., 2011; Samuel, Connolly, & Ball, 2012). This tension is reflected aptly in the seminal piece by Groves, who described the "hateful" patient, a patient who clinicians dread to care for, who are dependent "clingers," entitled demanders, manipulative help-rejecters, and self-destructive deniers (Groves, 1978). Groves describes that for clinicians who want to treat their patients fairly, realizing when these interactions are occurring is crucial to being psychologically minded enough to not let it affect clinical decision making. In disenfranchised populations, especially the geriatric homeless, this awareness may help obviate ethical pitfalls, especially as it relates to when individuals accept or refuse care. In fact, allowing a patient the right to refuse treatment when he or she is capacitated, despite the clinician's misgiving, is the most appropriate way to support respect for the autonomy of the patient. Providing compassionate care and increasing positive interactions between the healthcare system and homeless individuals may promote engagement and more successful outcomes.

CASE CONCLUSION

Mr. R returned several times with aspiration pneumonia for brief admissions (related to his swallowing difficulties), each time shortly thereafter demanding to leave and declining ongoing outpatient care. The third time, he presented with a sandwich in hand, having vomited on his shirt, and requested an admission to help him with his swallowing. He was admitted for stroke rehabilitation.

This case highlights the psychiatric, ethical, and legal issues in a case where diagnosis, treatment, and decision-making agency fluctuate in a homeless aged person. While the initial contact with this patient was frustrating to healthcare providers due to lack of optimizing a good aftercare plan, we respected the patient's wishes and allowed him to discharge to his own recognizance. In the end, this patient was accepting of the original treatment plan and presented to the hospital seeking this after he found that living with his disability was more burdensome and disruptive to his life than accepting stroke rehabilitation.

No ethical framework or algorithm can appropriately capture the ethical and legal challenges faced in complex cases such as these. However, we have found that using the "four topics" approach, as popularized by Jonsen and colleagues (Jonsen, Siegler, & Winslade, 2010), can be a comprehensive start (see Table 5.3). The four topics approach was developed in order to provide clinicians with a framework for evaluating and focusing on specific aspects of clinical ethics cases, linking clinical context to ethical principles. While it is relatively simplistic, it is straightforward and is relevant to the vast majority of ethical conflicts that arise in clinical care. In our case, the consensus agreement to focus on the patient's preferences and his interpretation of the best quality of life for him ultimately led to an increased trust in his healthcare providers and an improved clinical outcome.

TABLE 5.3   The Four Topics Approach to Clinical Ethics and Ethical Decision Making

Medical Indications

What are the facts of medical history/condition?
Medical condition diagnosis and prognosis?
Treatment
  Past and present
  Risks/Benefits
  Pain and adverse effects
Symptoms
Curative or reversible component of illness
Past experiences with the healthcare system
Functional level

(continued)

TABLE 5.3   The Four Topics Approach to Clinical Ethics and Ethical Decision Making (*continued*)

Patient Preferences

Is the patient competent? Does he or she comprehend the situation? Does the patient have capacity?
If YES
   Goals regarding treatment? Goals for the rest of life?
   How can the team help achieve goals?
   What is the patient's understanding of palliative care/procedures?
   How does the patient make decisions?
   Is there a health proxy? A living will? Who can be the best advocate?
   Is consent freely acquired? Is there coercion? Is there bias?
If NO
   Who has the legal authority to decide on the patient's behalf?
   How does this authority change as the patient's health status changes?
   What are the ethical and legal limits of such an authority?

Quality of Life

What does quality of life mean to the patient?
How can this be interpreted in the context of a terminal or life-altering illness?
What brings meaning to the patient's life?
What physical, social, psychological, and spiritual factors are at play?
Are there circumstances under which the patient would consider stopping all medications or treatments? If so, when?
How do persons other than the patient perceive the patient's quality of life and of what ethical relevance are their perceptions?
What can be achievable (given the patient's preferences)?

Contextual Features

What family issues are present that could influence treatment decisions? Whose other interests are affected?
What resources are available to the patient (economic, financial, insurance, physical, emotional, societal, etc.)?
Is the illness/condition terminal or catastrophic? If so, are there avenues for palliation or options for home/hospice/hospital-based care?
What are the relevant laws that are applicable? How do these laws impact treatment decisions?
How does the healthcare team feel about the treatment plan? Is there a consensus? Are all members comfortable with the treatment plan?
Are there any institutional or personal conflicts of interest at play?

Source: Jonsen, A. R., Siegler, M., & Winslade, W. J. (2010). *Clinical ethics: A practical approach to ethical decisions in clinical medicine* (7th ed., p. 238). New York, NY: McGraw-Hill.

REFERENCES

Appelbaum, P. S. (2007). Clinical practice. Assessment of patient's competence to consent to treatment. *New England Journal of Medicine, 357*(18), 1834–1840. doi:10.1056/NEJMcp074045

Brendel, R. W., & Schouten, R. (2007). Legal concerns in psychosomatic medicine. *Psychiatric Clinics of North America, 30*, 663–676. doi:10.1016/j.psc.2007.07.010

Brown, R. T., Hemati, K., Riley, E. D., Lee, C. T., Ponath, C., Tieu, L., Guzman, D., & Kushel, M. B. (2017). Geriatric conditions in a population-based sample of older homeless adults. *Gerontologist, 57*(4), 757–766. doi:10.1093/geront/gnw011

Brown, R. T., Kiely, D. K., Bharel, M., & Mitchell, S. L. (2012). Geriatric syndromes in older homeless adults. *Journal of General Internal Medicine, 27*(1), 16–22. doi:10.1007/s11606-011-1848-9

Culhane, D. P., Metraux, S., Byrne, T., Stino, M., & Bainbridge, J. (2013). The age structure of contemporary homelessness: Evidence and implications for public policy. *Analyses of Social Issues and Public Policy, 13*, 228–244. doi:10.1111/asap.12004

Dunn, L. B., & Alici, Y. (2013). Ethical waves of the silver tsunami: Consent, capacity and surrogate decision-making. *The American Journal of Geriatric Psychiatry, 21*(4), 309–313. doi:10.1016/j.jagp.2013.01.023

Fazel, S., Khosla, V., Doll, H., & Geddes, J. (2006). The prevalence of mental disorders among the homeless in western countries: Systematic review and meta-regression analysis. *PLOS Medicine, 5*(12), e255. doi:10.1371/journal.pmed.0050225

Fine, A. G., Zhang, T., & Hwang, S. W. (2013). Attitude towards homeless people among emergency department teachers and learners: A cross-sectional study of medical students and emergency physicians. *BMC Medicine Education, 13*, 112. doi:10.1186/1472-6920-13-112

Folsom, D., Hawthorne, W., Lindamer, L, Gilmer, T., Bailey, A., Golshan, S., ... Jeste, D. V.. (2005). Prevalence and risk factors for homelessness and utilization of mental health services among 10,340 patients with serious mental illness in a large public mental health system. *American Journal of Psychiatry, 162*(2), 370–376. doi:10.1176/appi.ajp.162.2.370

Ganzini, L., Volicer, L., Nelson, W. A., Fox, E., & Derse, A. R. (2004). Ten myths about decision making capacity. *Journal of the American Medical Directors Association, 5*(4), 263–267. doi:10.1016/j.jamda.2005.03.021

Groves, J. E. (1978). Taking care of the hateful patient. *New England Journal of Medicine, 298*, 883–887. doi:10.1056/NEJM197804202981605

Hahn, J. A., Kushel, M. B., Bangsberg, D. R., Riley, E., & Moss, A. R. (2006). Brief report: The aging of the homeless population: Fourteen-year trends in San Francisco. *Journal of General Internal Medicine, 21*(7), 775–778. doi:10.1111/j.1525-1497.2006.00493.x

He, W., Goodkind, D., & Kowal, P. (2016). *An aging world: 2015* (International Population Reports, P95/16-1). Washington, DC: U.S. Government Publishing Office. Retrieved from https://www.census.gov/content/dam/Census/library/publications/2016/demo/p95-16-1.pdf

Jonsen, A. R., Siegler, M., & Winslade, W. J. (2010). *Clinical ethics: A practical approach to ethical decisions in clinical medicine* (7th ed., p. 238). New York, NY: McGraw-Hill.

Karlawish, J. (2008). Measuring decision-making capacity in cognitively impaired individuals. *Neurosignals, 16*, 91–98. doi:10.1159/000109763

Ko, E., & Nelson-Becker, H. (2014). Does end-of-life decision making matter? Perspectives of older homeless adults. *American Journal of Hospice and Palliative Medicine, 31*(2), 183–188. doi:10.1177/1049909113482176

Metraux, S., Eng, N., Bainbridge, J., & Culhane, D. P. (2011). The impact of shelter use and housing placement on mortality hazard for unaccompanied adults and adults in family households entering New York shelters: 1990–2002. *Journal of Urban Health, 88*(6), 1091–1104. doi:10.1007%2Fs11524-011-9602-5

Moye, J., Sabatino, C. P., & Brendel, R. (2013). Evaluation of capacity to appoint a health-care proxy. *The American Journal of Geriatric Psychiatry, 21*(4), 326–336. doi:10.1016/j.jagp.2012.09.001

Moye, K., Karel, M. J., Azar, A. R., & Gurrera, R. J. (2004). Hopes and cautions for instrument-based evaluation of consent capacity: Results of a construct validity study of three instruments. In M. B. Kapp (Ed.), *Ethics, Law, and Aging Review* (Vol. 10, pp. 39–61). New York, NY: Springer Publishing. doi:10.1093/geronb/62.1.P3

National Health Care for the Homeless Council. (2016). Advance Care Planning for Individuals Experiencing Homelessness. *inFocus, 4*(2). Retrieved from https://www.nhchc.org/wp-content/uploads/2016/06/in-focus-advance-care-planning-final-for-posting.pdf

Pluck, G., Lee, K. H., David, R., Macleod, D. C., Spence, S. A., & Parks, R. W. (2011). Neurobehavioural and cognitive function is linked to childhood trauma in homeless adults. *British Journal of Clinical Psychology, 50*, 33–45. doi:10.1348/014466510X490253

Samra, R., Griffiths, A., Cox, T., Conroy, S., Gordon, A., & Gladman, J. R. F. (2015). Medical students' and doctors' attitude towards older patients and their care in hospital settings: A conceptualization. *Age and Ageing, 44*, 776–783. doi:10.1093/ageing/afv082

Samuel, D. B., Connolly, A. J., & Ball, S. A. (2012). The convergent and concurrent validity of trait-based prototype assessment of personality disorder categories in homeless persons. *Assessment, 19*, 287–298. doi:10.1177/1073191112444461

Schinka, J. A., Curtiss, G., Leventhal, K., Bossarte, R. M., Lapcevic, W., & Casey, R. (2016). Predictors of mortality in older homeless veterans. *The Journals of Gerontology, 72*(6), 1103–1109. doi:10.1093/geronb/gbw042

Walaszek, A. (2009). Clinical ethics issues in geriatric psychiatry. *Psychiatric Clinics of North America, 32*(2), 343–359. doi:10.1016/j.psc.2009.02.004

Housing and Social Issues in Homeless Care

Helena Harvie and Robert Rumore

When analyzing the housing and social issues that are being faced by the homeless population, it is best to know what resources are currently available and how they are being utilized. Although a variety of housing options and community programs are available, these resources often do not fit well for the elderly homeless population. In this chapter, we will briefly revisit the issues, discussed in other chapters, constituting the main causes of homelessness among the geriatric population, with special attention to people who became homeless due to economic factors, substance abuse, mental illness, or all of these reasons. We will begin with a description of a general distinction within the geriatric homeless population followed by an overview of housing, shelter, and community programs that are available in most major cities. Not every region or city will have all cited resources available, and some might be called a different name. The chapter will end with a series of case studies. Each one will demonstrate a different social issue facing a geriatric homeless person and how it impacts an older adult in locating housing and/or social services. During our discussion, examples of services and cases from several cities will be cited.

TYPOLOGY OF THE GERIATRIC HOMELESS POPULATION

It is helpful to distinguish between two general types of geriatric homeless persons, related to time of onset, which could present distinct barriers to their receiving services. Some geriatric homeless individuals have "aged into" their geriatric status while they were homeless; others have become homeless after they aged.

Individuals in the first group were once young homeless people. Persistent mental health, substance abuse, and health issues have contributed to their instability and caused them to become long-term chronic homeless individuals. While they are far more impaired than they were in their youth, they have become accustomed to their lifestyle, and regardless of how difficult their lives are, change of any kind can be a struggle. They may have what they consider to be social supports in place, while being homeless, and may find it more difficult to leave those supports behind.

The second group is those who become homeless after the age of 50, often due to their geriatric condition. While it is difficult for anyone at any age to become homeless and adjust to that lifestyle or accomplish what it takes to reverse that situation, it is far more difficult for someone whose physical and/or mental condition has deteriorated to a point of chronicity or irreversibility.

FINANCIAL ISSUES

Many homeless individuals were leading normal productive lives before they became homeless. There were no apparent mental health or substance-abuse issues that led to their homelessness; however, there may have been a precipitating social factor. For instance, they may have simply lost their job and had difficulty finding a new one. Perhaps they lacked the social support necessary to stay with family or friends through this difficult period. Perhaps this is where latent psychiatric or substance-abuse issues—which had not presented a serious issue in the past—came to the surface, such as a "functioning" alcoholic losing a constructive activity or a relationship that helped keep his alcoholism "in check" or the person whose situation in life causes him/her to fall into a state of depression. After all, housing can be expensive and the loss of a job and the end of a relationship, besides causing financial strain, are traumatic events that can be the cause of homelessness.

Regardless, the reasoning goes, if a person's reason for homelessness was strictly financial, then the route out of homelessness would be financial as well; the person needs simply to obtain and maintain a new job and take time to save money to rent an apartment or buy a home.

HOMELESS RESOURCES

There are two different categories of resources that are currently used to assist homeless individuals: social services and housing options. Among the latter, there are community programs such as emergency shelters and transitional housing. These programs are often funded by national grants through the Department of Housing and Urban Development (HUD) and through local donations. Federal funding for these programs is provided through the Homeless Emergency Assistance and Rapid Transition to Housing (HEARTH) Act of 2009, which was signed into law on May 20, 2009. The HEARTH Act is a reauthorization of HUD's McKinney-Vento Homeless Assistance program, which was last authorized in the Housing and Community Development Act of 1992 (National Alliance to End Homelessness, 2008).

SHELTERS

Emergency shelters can be found in most large towns and cities. In some areas of the country, there are no qualifiers for shelter other than showing up at the door, nor are there restrictions on shelter users and the amount of times that shelter can be accessed; this is referred to as a "right to shelter." Shelter is available for all those who need it without any question.

In many locations, however, some homeless shelters will have user requirements such as barring anyone who has a lease or housing agreement. Others will have an income limit or residency requirements. Some will exclude individuals based on sex-offender status. Some shelters exercise zero tolerance for substance abuse, while others might accept substance abusers, but mandate treatment. Other rules include having curfews and not allowing people to stay in a shelter during the day. Some shelters have mandates on the duration of stay or the frequency with which someone can use the shelter, while others do not have limits, but encourage people to move on to other housing.

Many shelters are also only nighttime shelters, which means an individual has to leave every morning and then return at night to wait in line to see about bed availability. Such policy and practice can lead to the stress of a person's uncertainty of having a stable place to live and also forces individuals to spend the daylight hours in the same area in order not to miss the line at night.

All of the these requirements can be different across shelters and can be unique to different cities, however, all shelters must follow the rules set out in the Emergency Solution Grants Program, which outlines program and facility requirements to make sure the shelters are safe (U.S. Department of Housing and Urban Development, 2015).

In some places, and in some times, homelessness has been viewed simply as an economic problem (albeit often one of individual failing). Therefore, the prevailing opinion and practice in how to address homelessness—the cure—was simply to have someplace for homeless people to stay. This is often heard to be described negatively as "warehousing" homeless people. If all that is needed is for someplace to stay, then shelters certainly do fulfill that purpose.

Some people will just need to get their lives together and move on; a shelter, at its most basic level, was considered a starting point for doing that.

However, that is not always enough. Therefore, a more enlightened view became that to erradicate homelessness you have to start by providing *decent shelter*. That is a term and concept that can be very subjective, and not all shelters can be considered to be decent living environments. At best, this situation could be the result of practical and impartial forces such as lack of funding and staffing. More cynically, there is and has been, in some places and at some times, a public attitude and opinion that shelters should not be comfortable places to stay. It is an opinion that "you get what you pay for," and if a shelter is too comfortable, then people will not want to leave. It has even been considered that there are people who will enter a shelter just for a free place to stay or to receive the housing available to those who are homeless. It is highly unlikely, though, that a geriatric person would want to become homeless just for the housing he or she may receive. Regardless of the reason, shelters have not always been considered to be the most hospitable places.

In contrast, many locations have taken steps over the years to progressively create a more hospitable shelter environment. Again, this evolved along with other attitudes and opinions related to homelessness, largely the recognition that homelessness is not an isolated condition of lack of a home/shelter, but rather a function of other social, economic, and individual factors. Therefore, if you address the underlying cause(s) of the homelessness, not just the need for shelter, then the person will be able to overcome the resulting homeless condition.

It serves to follow that the most cost-effective and efficient way to address homelessness would be to merge the service and shelter together. One step toward this was to contract the shelters to private social services agencies whose specialty was to address the issue in question. Another step was to create specialty shelters, a practice which results in the compartmentaliza-tion of populations and specialization of services within shelters. For exam-ple, in New York City, there are several categories of the shelters, including mental health, substance abuse, employment, veteran, disabled, and medi-cally frail and elderly shelters. The idea is that a person will do much better if surrounded by other like-minded individuals with similar circumstances and needs. Compartmentalizing homeless populations can make address-ing the homeless issue more manageable and success more measurable. Theoretically, for every person who is affected by an issue that caused his or her homelessness, there is a corresponding route out of homelessness, and it is up to the service provider to provide that route. The specialized shelter can start people out on that path.

As an example, for many years the New York City shelter system has operated on a three-step system. Everyone goes through a central intake location and is subsequently sent to an assessment shelter. During an average two-week stay, these individuals are assessed by a team of social workers, case managers, and medical and psychiatric staff who designate to which program shelter they will be sent for their own specialized needs. An otherwise stable homeless person who is experiencing a stretch of bad luck would be sent to an employment shelter.

If a person with a work history, and no apparent substance abuse or mental health issues, is placed into a shelter environment where his or her cohort is acting responsibly, abstaining from substance use, and not experiencing some of the crises associated with people with mental health issues, that person will do much better. In employment shelters, residents will more likely keep their areas clean, and everyone will have a single-minded focus on vocational training and job-seeking activities. The staff will focus on vocational training and support groups. Once residents obtain employment, the staff can focus on money management and savings goals. The clients can establish social connections within the shelters, and perhaps even meet roommate material, someone they can share an apartment with.

These individuals will reverse their homelessness by obtaining financial stability and return to the open market of housing. Affordable housing will certainly be an issue for someone taking this route. However, there are programs in many communities that set aside affordable housing, and again, there would be the possibility of connecting with a roommate. Therefore, the route to housing for such individuals would, theoretically, be through intensive vocational programs and community housing resources based solely on income such as HPD, HUD, and state or local public housing, if these options are available in their area. If a program was to be creative, perhaps an ancillary service that could assist would be some sort of roommate-matching service.

A shelter like that, for an individual whose main reason for homelessness is financial, sounds good in theory, and it works for some people. However, it is a lot less likely to work for someone who is geriatric. In this scenario, the sole reason for homelessness is that the person could have retired or lost his or her job at an age close to retirement and can no longer afford to own a home. These individuals would gladly work, but are no longer marketable due to their age. Geriatric populations also have a greater chance of lacking social support. Many of the friends or relatives who can be relied upon by a younger person might not be available to a geriatric whose families may have moved away to live separate lives and whose age cohort is deceased. While an employment shelter might be a more ideal location for an elderly person, it would not likely produce a route out of homelessness.

TRANSITIONAL HOUSING

Most transitional housing programs will have set criteria for a specific population they are trying to assist; however, the services provided and the specific rules can be different between each program (National Alliance to End Homelessness, 2008). For example, there are transitional housing options that are intended for substance abusers (sober living facilities) or for veterans who suffer from mental health and substance abuse (dual diagnosis). There are others that are intended for domestic violence victims or individuals being released from prison. Transitional housing can be in many different forms from a large program serving over 100 people at one site to a small house for four or six residents. Each program also has a different time limit. Some can be up to two years, while others can be limited to 90 days. There are some programs that will assist individuals with locating more permanent housing and will often employ social workers or case managers to assist them (U.S. Department of Housing and Urban Development, 2015). Others provide only a short-term housing option for an individual and will not provide any employees to assist with resources. Another common requirement for transitional housing is that an individual has to be independent with his or her activities of daily living (ADLs), which are toileting, showering, and eating. The ADL requirement may be a particularly challenging one for the geriatric homeless population. There are often no resources available in a transitional housing program to get that level of assistance (McInnis-Dittrich, 2013).

The concept behind the continuum of transitional to permanent housing is based on the idea that homeless persons coming out of the shelter system may need a trial period to see whether they can make it on their own, especially in regard to a person who is mentally ill. The thought is that such individuals did not "fall" into their position overnight; their homelessness is the culmination of years of issues that arose around their mental health status. Therefore, they cannot necessarily re-enter housing without first re-building independent living skills. Indeed, many persons in the shelter system have never maintained their own apartment. Therefore, before moving into more independent housing, they will spend two years in transitional housing learning the skills necessary to live on their own, and additionally, assuring that they are following up with their mental health treatment. Once the client has been monitored, observed, and assisted, over a two-year (or less) period, the person can be referred to more independent housing.

Whereas transitional housing is staffed 24 hours per day, once in "permanent" supported housing, the individual lives independently and only receives periodic case management visits. Housing within this system can sometimes be for people with substance-abuse issues, but is overwhelming for people with mental health issues.

Most of the time, and under ideal circumstances, the continuum of housing would include both of these steps and the client would move through the shelter, into transitional housing, and on to more independence. However, for a variety of reasons (sometimes not optimal), there are individuals who skip over the transitional step. Sometimes, the person really is able to go straight from the shelter to a more independent environment. Other times, however, a shelter resident may refuse a staffed residence and a less-structured environment is available. Under pressure to move people due to time constraints, the need to free up space in a shelter for others, and in keeping with a client's right to choose his or her destiny, the client may skip over more appropriate housing. This might also happen at a transitional residence under which there are time limits to move people into permanent housing. Housing exists through a patchwork of various funding sources, each with their own requirements for qualifying. This means that people are not always being placed in the location that is the best fit for them.

For the geriatric population, some clients are qualified on paper, but in reality are not ready for living independently. While some people can be successfully situated, other people "fall through the cracks" such as those who are qualified for independent living based on a grant that provided "Housing First" for the substance-abusing population. One could argue that no one should be denied housing, regardless of substance abuse. However, placing elderly, substance-abusing clients into an apartment unattended with no onsite staff or support can become counterproductive; such apartments generally come to resemble the street. In order to supplement the services for this type of client, some places have the option to turn to a network of service providers to include home attendants, but that might not always be available to them.

While transitional housing would seem to be an optimal environment for the geriatric population due to its 24-hour staffing and hands-on approach, this also has its flaws in both the ability to obtain this type of housing and the need for the resident to move on once he or she is there; after all, it is "transitional" housing.

One problem encountered, from the perspective of a referring shelter working with the geriatrics population, is that this housing is specifically for mentally ill individuals. As it turns out, not all geriatric/elderly people have mental health issues that qualify them for this type of housing. Clients whose diagnosis features dementia and who could benefit from the type of housing available to people who are mentally ill are selected out. Conversely, there is housing for elderly people (which will be outlined in a later section) for which many geriatric homeless could qualify; these locations do not accept individuals with mental health diagnoses and certainly not people who are currently abusing substances and/or drinking alcohol.

The geriatric population seems to do quite well in the transitional setting; they have their own apartment and also have access to staff 24 hours/per day. They have someone who can monitor their taking of medication, psychiatric as well as medical. Still, these locations are not designed or meant to provide hands-on care; the elderly people placed in these locations still require extra services. In order to supplement their service needs, some programs can also call upon outside providers such as home health aides. Some providers have added medical/nursing staff and specialized social workers such as geriatric social workers to their facilities. Because any one facility may not be capable of accommodating a full salary for these professionals, another option is to have a shared professional staff among several facilities.

Having geriatric social workers with specific expertise and connections in the field can be very effective in placing clients into geriatric facilities. Limitations include the fact that many of these facilities are resistant to accepting persons with a psychiatric diagnosis such as cognitive dysfunction. Also, many clients do not wish to go to a place that is referred to as a skilled nursing facility (SNF) or nursing home.

In the end, in transitional housing, there is always the expectation that the person will transition out. Clients are put into independent living in order to meet the requirements of the funders and a mandate by the government to end homelessness. Although in principle everyone deserves a home, it does not mean that everyone can maintain a home. A home can mean something different to different people. Such is the case with many in the geriatric population. Fortunately, these mandates are flexible, and there are often geriatric clients who are allowed to age into their "transitional" homes. Still, the regulation remains even though it seems like the transitional model for permanent housing might be a more viable alternative for the geriatric population.

RECUPERATIVE CARE/MEDICAL RESPITE

Another program that is found in some cities is called "Recuperative Care" (sometimes referred to as medical respite), which provides medical care to homeless persons recovering from an acute illness or injury, no longer in need of acute care, but unable to sustain recovery if living on the street or other unsuitable place (Bruno, 2012). This program was piloted in Los Angeles in late 2007, when news reports of several hospitals purportedly "dumping" patients in the skid row area. This led to the Los Angeles City Attorney proposing, and the city council adopting, an ordinance that makes it illegal for a hospital to discharge a patient to downtown Los Angeles (Bruno, 2012). This type of program would fall into transitional housing as it is not permanent. It is intended to assist homeless individuals who are getting out of the hospital and cannot return to the streets for a medical reason but do not need SNF level of care. Individuals in these programs can often receive home healthcare, but are still required to be able to complete all of their ADLs (Wacker & Roberto, 2013).

Programs such as these do not exist throughout the country and would be of great assistance if they were more widespread because a large portion of the geriatric population becomes homeless, or returns to homelessness, following discharge from hospitals.

OUTREACH

Before discussing some other developments in options available to the homeless, notice should be given to a key element of homeless services not previously mentioned, namely, outreach. Although there are a variety of transitional as well as permanent housing options, as demonstrated earlier and next, not all homeless people accept them. Some persons, though aware of the options, choose not to accept them. Others may be new to homelessness, and in need of someone to guide them.

The concept of homeless outreach is simple. Stripped of all of its nuances, it is simply going out, picking up homeless people, and bringing them into the shelters that are available for them. With outreach, more people get into shelters and off of the streets. Outreach has evolved over time in an attempt to become more effective. There are various types and levels of services available to homeless individuals, so rather than just bringing people to shelter, the outreach team, in a larger city with more services, can be equipped with the information needed to set the client in the proper direction. The outreach teams also get to know the clients out in the street and can be instrumental in matching the right client with the right service location. They can also follow up with the client after they are placed to provide some continuity and a familiar face in a new environment.

SAFE HAVENS

Safe havens were created as an alternative to a traditional shelter. The idea is not new, but safe havens have been growing in acceptance and practice. The concept for safe havens grew out of the philosophy that no one should be denied shelter with the acknowledgment that not everyone will accept shelter for various, often legitimate, reasons.

When asked what keeps some of the "chronic" homeless people out on the streets, most outreach workers will provide the same answers. Largely, people want freedom to come and go as they please. They do not want a curfew, and they want to stay in as they please. They do not want to be sent off to wander the street during the day. Finally, they do not want to be pressured or forced to engage in services. Finally, homeless shelters already have bad reputations. However much homeless shelters may have improved, people still remember their bad reputation; the older someone is, the further back he or she can recall and the more ingrained the perception.

In a city like New York, to enter a safe haven, a client does not have to go through the normal bureaucracy that he or she would typically have to go through to get into a shelter. Rather, a chronically homeless person will be brought to a safe haven directly by the outreach team that encounters the individual on the street and with whom he or she is familiar. From an outreach perspective, even asking a person if he or she wants to go to a safe haven instead of a shelter makes a big difference, simply by having it called something else. Safe havens are generally smaller than shelters, and many of them actually have separate rooms for the clients. They have as many or more ancillary services attached to them as a shelter, but no one is pressuring the person to accept these services. Engagement is subtle, and by the client's choice, and follows the philosophy of working with the client at their level of readiness and at their own pace in his or her familiar environment. By not forcing the services and treatment on the individual and by still allowing him or her to stay, you create a "captive audience" with whom to engage and work. When an individual chooses to engage in services, it makes the services a lot more effective.

Not all of society looks upon the safe haven or Housing First concepts and philosophy favorably. There is sometimes a prevailing attitude that the client is getting too much for nothing. Even the staff may find it difficult to adjust to their way of thinking, feeling that the client is "getting away with too much" or that a disservice is being done to him or her by not imposing rules or the staff's will upon the client.

However, this approach works, and it works for the geriatric population as well as anyone else. Individuals who had been intoxicated in the morning, noon, and night—lying on the sidewalk, urinating, and defecating on themselves for years—who would rarely enter the shelter system entered safe havens and have been transformed. They may not have stopped drinking, but they were no longer waking up on the sidewalk—feeling extremely hung-over and facing the shame of being in public—and wanting to drink to forget it. Those same clients could now wake up inside, in a comfortable bed with a clean bathroom nearby. They are not asked to leave during the day, but to have a meal and a shower right there where they awakened. They can sit and watch TV, socialize with friends, and, most importantly, see a case manager, psychiatrist, doctor, or nurse; without being forced to, most of them will go. Importantly, these clients experience a huge improvement in self-esteem.

Finally, a safe haven can be more cost-effective to society in general. Prior to entering the safe haven, these clients might not have used shelter, but they did use the emergency department for their multiple medical issues, and they did enter detox just to get off the street, though they had no intention of recovery. Sometimes, a sympathetic public will intervene and call an ambulance to pick people up because they feel sorry for someone; this is common among the geriatric population. This was also very expensive. If the client is safely inside a safe haven, it can greatly reduce the use of emergency services, a fact that can be used to influence public opinion in their favor.

The safe haven model is not specific to the geriatric population and is most often targeted for chronically homeless individuals. The geriatric population is well represented among the chronically homeless population for obvious reasons; many chronically homeless individuals are geriatric because chronic homelessness is something that you need to age into and because the extra dimension of geriatric conditions risks the geriatric persons becoming part of the chronically homeless population. However, not all geriatric clients are chronically homeless. Having a similar program focused on the geriatric population, chronic or not, that does not screen out individuals for active substance abuse and lack of treatment compliance would be an effective addition to geriatric homeless services.

SECTION 8

Low-income housing that is subsidized by the federal government is often called Section 8. There are two types: project-based assistance and the housing choice voucher program. In project-based assistance, rental subsidies are given to property owners who agree to rent to low-income individuals and families. Properties are usually dedicated to this type of housing. Residents have to pay 30% of their adjusted income, and the rent has to be fair market. About one-half of the project-based Section 8 housing is dedicated to elderly households (Wacker & Roberto, 2013). In the housing choice voucher program, individuals and families find their own housing, including single-family homes, town houses, and apartments. As long as the property meets program requirements, an individual is allowed to rent there and pay 30% of his or her income. However, if rent is above the fair market value, the individual is responsible for the difference (Wacker & Roberto, 2013).

GERIATRIC HOUSING OPTIONS

There are many housing resources that are available to homeless individuals and for seniors. Some of these resources involve independent living facilities (ILF), assisted living facilities (ALFs), board and care, and SNFs. Each of these resources requires an individual to be at a certain level of care. The level of care a person qualifies for can be determined by a doctor, physical therapist, or psychiatrist and is often based on how an individual completes his or her ADLs. "Assessing an older adult's competence in the ADLs determines his or her ability to complete the basic tasks of self-care, such as eating, toileting, ambulating, and transferring, bathing, dressing and grooming" (McInnis-Dittrich, 2013, p. 93). Levels of care are determined based on how well an individual can do his or her ADLs. Another category of ADLs is instrumental ADLs (IADLs), which are more complicated than basic ADLs. However, these tasks are considered necessary to managing a household, such as using a telephone or preparing meals (McInnis-Dittrich, 2013). IADLs may also include cleaning the house, arranging transportation, administration of medications, and managing money.

The first level of care is an ILF. An individual must be able to do all ADLs on his or her own. ILFs are often private homes, where the owner rents out a room; however, it can be in a senior community or a more institutionalized setting that has easy access when it is required. An ILF can serve as a residential community. ILFs can offer a safe living environment, but with minimal assistance, as there is usually no assistance with medications or any ADLs unless in an emergency. Rent will depend on whether it is a single room or shared room, whether food is provided, and the location.

The next level is an ALF. "Assisted living is defined as a residential, long term arrangement designed to promote maximum independent functioning among frail older adults while providing in home support services" (McInnis-Dittrich, 2013, p. 10). These can be more institutionalized and may be part of a senior community. Average assisted living facilities can have about 54 units, with some much larger and some much smaller. These facilities will often provide medication assistance and can provide some minor assistance in emergencies. These are often intended for people who still want their own space, but need some assistance with IADLs. Rent can increase depending on how much care is offered. The average cost of an ALF across the country is $3,628 (Genworth Financial, 2016). There are many ways that an assisted living facility can be paid for. These include savings, some long-term care insurance policies, financial benefits from the Department of Veterans Affairs, and other personal funds a person might have. Medicare coverage for an ALF can be very limited, as well as Medicaid, whose coverage can vary from state to state (Botek, 2013).

The two highest levels of care are board and care and SNFs. Board and care facilities are privately funded and are intended for individuals who need help with ADLs. They do not provide 24-hour nursing care, but do provide 24-hour assistance as needed (McInnis-Dittrich, 2013). These board and care facilities can often cost over $2,000. In some instances, Medicaid may cover the cost of a board and care, but that varies from state to state (Wacker & Roberto, 2013). Board and care facilities can range in size and can span from very small, family style in single-family homes to much larger, more institutional settings.

SNFs, on the other hand, are institutional in nature. They provide 24 hours of nursing care and can assist with wound care and physical therapy. They often will provide long-term care for individuals who cannot do their ADLs and require nursing assistance. The median cost of SNFs across the country for a semi-private room is $6,844, and $7,698 for a private room (Genworth Financial, 2016). "There are four sources of payment of nursing home costs: Medicare, Medicaid, out of pocket, and long-term care insurance" (Wacker & Roberto, 2013, p. 396). Most SNFs receive reimbursements from the Centers for Medicare and Medicaid Services (CMS). To qualify for reimbursements, the individual must be qualified for Medicare and Medicaid, and the facility must be certified by CMS (Wacker & Roberto, 2013). Homeless individuals are often unable to afford out-of-pocket costs on their own and are forced to utilize Medicaid or other long-term care insurance to assist with payment. Costs of an SNF are dependent on location and services provided.

Another housing resource that many seniors use is single-room occupancy hotels (SROs). "Typically, SRO provides residents with a private room and a shared kitchenette and a bathroom with a shower" (Wacker & Roberto, 2013, p. 319). These are often motels that provide month-to-month leases. Rooms are considered studios and can range from 80 sq. ft. to 150 sq. ft. Some have their own bathroom, while others may have communal bathrooms with a mini kitchen in each room. SROs were built to be cheaper housing options that were located in local business centers. Most also do not do background checks, which can make them desirable for individuals that have bad credit or evictions on their record. Services provided to tenants can range from nothing to highly managed care. Sometimes, SROs will offer limited security, light housekeeping, or an errand service (Wacker & Roberto, 2013).

While most elderly individuals are able to utilize the aforementioned resources, there are many reasons why an individual may not. Some choose not to utilize the aforementioned resources due to cost and not having enough income to support it. Some do not qualify for these services, and others do not have the services available to them in their location. The following case studies will show a variety of housing and social issues that elderly homeless individuals face and why they may not qualify or utilize the previously mentioned resources. Rather than being based on any one person, each case study is a composite of different clients from the field.

VEHICLE/HIGHER LEVEL OF CARE

Mr. Hoss is a 68-year-old African American who has been living in a van for the past 20 years. Mr. Hoss has a past medical history of congestive heart failure, morbid obesity, and two past strokes within the past five years. While Mr. Hoss has been living out of a van, he did not consider himself homeless. He was able to have a bed in the back with connections for electricity and water. Mr. Hoss was able to connect to TV in the back of his van and was able to drive to different locations.

After Mr. Hoss's first stroke, he was forced to use a wheelchair. Mr. Hoss was able to buy a wheelchair that was small and easily foldable to fit in the back of his van. However, Mr. Hoss had to rely on strangers to get him in and out of his wheelchair and back to his van. Mr. Hoss would pay an individual $25 to assist him with transferring. Due to the small size of his van, Mr. Hoss was able to move around inside very easily.

Due to worsening medical conditions, Mr. Hoss needed more assistance with his daily needs than he could do on his own. Unfortunately, no home health agency would come to a vehicle to provide care. Mr. Hoss was forced to give up his van and was forced into an SNF. He could not afford any other housing options based on his income of $1,075 a month from Social Security retirement. Mr. Hoss chose to go into an SNF because he could receive daily physical therapy where he hoped he could improve enough to go back to his van. After multiple readmissions to the hospital, Mr. Hoss eventually passed away and was never able to return to his van.

Many homeless individuals reside in vehicles, trailers, and recreational vehicles (RVs); however, these vehicles are not meant for human habitation. Other places individuals stay that are not meant for human habitation include parks, sidewalks, abandoned buildings, tent encampments, or directly on the street (Regional Task Force on the Homeless, 2016). Some individuals choose to live in vehicles because they want to live a lifestyle like Mr. Hoss, and some because they are forced to. The 2015 Point-In-Time Count (PITC) showed "Two-thirds of chronically homeless individuals (or 54,815 people) were staying in unsheltered locations such as under bridges, in cars, or in abandoned buildings. This is more than twice the national rate for all homeless people (31%)" (Henry, Shivji, de Sousa, & Cohen, 2016, p. 60).

Anyone who resides in a vehicle that is not meant for habitation, even if modified, is considered to be homeless. These individuals are often very hesitant to leave their vehicle, as they fear the vehicle being towed or broken into. Individuals who have also been living in their vehicles for a significant period of time may find it more difficult to locate a place to live. If an individual has to rent an apartment or room, most landlords would want a rental history. If Mr. Hoss had wanted to find a place to rent, he would have been unable to produce a rental history. This is one factor that is often overlooked for individuals who choose to locate to more stable housing after living in their vehicles.

Care of these individuals can be complicated as stated earlier; no home health agency can come to a vehicle. Trailers and RVs have to be parked in a stable location with connections before an in-home agency can come and assist. In-home care is often provided to individuals to assist with getting stronger through physical therapy, and home health aides can assist with ADLs. Mr. Hoss could have benefited from these services due to his growing need for assistance with ADLs. Mr. Hoss was happy living in his vehicle, but his care became too much for him to handle. It was not sustainable for Mr. Hoss to keep locating strangers to get him in and out of his vehicle. In cases like these, individuals are often left in their vehicles or wheelchair for hours longer than they should due to not being able to locate anyone. This can be very dangerous for individuals with serious medical conditions.

Due to these medical conditions, Mr. Hoss could not go to any place that did not provide some assistance with ADLs. This led to an SNF placement. If Mr. Hoss had already had his own apartment or had already been in an ALF, he could have received assistance in the home. It is incredibly hard to find an apartment when someone has to help you with your ADLs. Oftentimes, these individuals end up in SNFs and often stay there longer than they would like or end up living there for the rest of their lives.

Mr. Hoss was never able to regain his strength enough to do his own ADLs and remained at an SNF for the rest of his life. If Mr. Hoss had been able to get stronger and do his ADLs on his own, he may have qualified for an ALF or a board and care. However, due to his income, he did not earn enough to afford it. If Mr. Hoss no longer qualified for SNF care, the SNF would have been forced to either find placement for him, such as an ILF, or would return Mr. Hoss to his van. More often than not, individuals are returned to their prior residence, whether that was a vehicle or the street, from an SNF.

When determining the level of care, it can be difficult for medical personnel because a person may be appropriate for more than one but unable to afford the one most appropriate. A physician can determine that an individual would benefit from living in an ALF, but if a person cannot afford it, then he or she will often either go to an SNF or back to the community. The following case study will continue to focus on how income will determine placement.

LIVING ON A FIXED INCOME

Mr. May is an 81-year-old Caucasian male who has been residing in a two-bed-room apartment for the past 10 years in San Diego, California. Prior to that, he resided with his spouse in their own home. When his spouse died, Mr. May was forced to leave his home and move into an apartment as he could no longer afford the mortgage payments. Mr. May only receives $1,100 from Social Security once a month.

He received a two-month notice of eviction, as the landlord had elected to sell the residence and no longer rent it out. Mr. May could not locate another apartment to rent on his fixed income in those two months. He had thought about going to an ILF, but the cheapest he could find was for a shared room at $750. Mr. May knew he could not share a room with anyone due to past mental health issues, which included anxiety and post-traumatic stress disorder (PTSD). Due to stress, Mr. May became sicker and eventually went to the hospital the day before his eviction.

After physical therapy evaluated him, he was deemed to need SNF level of care and was forced to go to an SNF. After he became stronger, the only options presented to him were an ILF or the streets. Mr. May chose to go to the streets as he knew living with others would be more detrimental to him than living on the streets.

"Over 25 million Americans aged 60+ are economically insecure—living at or below 250% of the federal poverty level (FPL) ($29,425 per year for a single person)" (National Council on Aging, 2016, p. 1). The vast majority of these individuals live on a fixed income of either Social Security retirement, supplemental Social Security, or Social Security disability. That means they received a set amount every month either from Social Security or a pension. Among the elderly beneficiaries who are receiving Social Security benefits, 21% of the married couples and about 43% of the unmarried persons rely on Social Security for 90% or more of their income (Social Security Administration, 2017). The average retired worker will receive on average $1,360 per month and a disabled person will receive $1,171 on average per month (Social Security Administration, 2017).

Not having enough income is one of the greatest issues facing elderly individuals who are homeless. If an individual requires a higher level of care, he or she will most likely not be able to afford it. If a person does not need a higher level of care and can technically afford a $750 ILF on a $1,171 per month income, it does not leave much room for food or any other bills. Other individuals may not be able to maintain the housing they are residing in due to a decrease in income. Due to this, some individuals choose to go to the streets, because they do not want to be in any debt and do not want to live above their means.

If older adults chose to locate work to supplement their income, they would find many barriers in place. The Age Discrimination in Employment Act, which was signed in 1967, prohibits the discrimination of any older adult over the age of 40; however, many older adults over 55 who have wanted to work remain unemployed far longer than their younger counterparts.

First, while some companies value older employees, many others view them as being unable to learn new things or unwilling to use computer technology. Older adults may have to utilize job training programs or take classes to keep up with newer technologies in their chosen field. Others may choose to pursue an encore career, which is a second career later in life. "Most older adults currently in encore careers are leading-edge baby boomers who came from professional and white collar jobs, have at least some college education, are women and live in cities or suburbs" (Wacker & Roberto, 2013, p. 154). Another issue is that, if an individual is residing in subsidized housing, his or her rent may go up with the added income. This can be a detriment for individuals to seek out employment in order to make their lives better.

Mr. May attempted to locate an apartment, but due to the high cost of living in San Diego, he could not locate an affordable one. If he chose to move to a place that he could afford, he may have not been able to afford to move or relocate. Due to this, many individuals are stuck where they reside. Adults may also not want to leave an area where they are comfortable and have family/friends.

Mr. May also could not utilize homeless resources until he was officially evicted or had the letter of eviction. Mr. May would not have been eligible to go to a local shelter until he had been on the streets and no longer had a rental agreement. There are other services in certain cities called rapid re-housing, which can provide short-term rental/case management assistance. However, Mr. May would eventually have to pick up where a program like this leaves off and would be unable to afford the payments on his own.

Individuals who reside on a fixed income are most appropriate for housing vouchers through the HUD's Section 8 program. This would allow Mr. May to obtain an apartment and pay only 30% of his income toward rent. Unfortunately, in some cities, the wait for a Section 8 voucher can be multiple years. In San Diego county, approximately 46,000 households are on a waiting list to obtain a federal housing choice voucher (Section 8). The average wait to obtain a housing voucher is 8 to 10 years (San Diego Housing Commission, 2017). In other locations, a Section 8 voucher can be obtained much more easily.

SUBSTANCE ABUSE

Mr. Thompson is a 68-year-old Caucasian male, who has been homeless for most of his life. Mr. Thompson has been an alcoholic for over 40 years and claims his greatest joys in life are vodka, coffee, cigarettes, then food/water, in that order. Mr. Thompson has been unable to maintain any housing due to excessive alcohol use.

Mr. Thompson also has serious medical problems, which include chronic osteomyelitis and pressure ulcers. He has been wheelchair-bound for the past 10 years. He has a chronic ostomy bag, which he cannot take care of when he is using any substances.

Due to medical issues, Mr. Thompson is in and out of hospitals. He does have Medicare and Medicaid. Social workers have placed Mr. Thompson multiple times into an SNF as he requires supervision due to wound care and medical issues.

Over the years, Mr. Thompson has left multiple SNFs against medical advice (AMA) due to wanting to drink alcohol when he wants to. He will often find himself back on the streets and, within a short period of time, back in a hospital.

While other chapters have discussed substance abuse, this case study shows how it can affect housing issues. Mr. Thompson would have qualified for any number of housing programs that focus on substance abuse; however, Mr. Thompson did not want to stop using, and that is an important distinction. Resources are available for individuals who want to stop using substances in facilities from treatment centers to transitional housing. However, not all resources are available for individuals who require the medical assistance that they require.

Mr. Thompson required some assistance with ADLs, which eliminated shelters, transitional housing, and ILFs. This only left environments where an individual had to live with others either in a small house or in an institution. There are no housing options for an individual who wants to drink to the point of belligerence and still remain housed in a community setting. This is due to the safety of the individual and other residents in the community.

Individuals like these will often come back to emergency departments and will be admitted for placement into an SNF. This cycle will repeat until either Mr. Thompson finds an SNF that he likes or ends up dying on the streets or in a hospital. No facility can force someone into care unless he or she is under guardianship/conservatorship. "A conservatorship is a court case where a judge appoints a responsible person or organization (called the "conservator") to care of another adult (called the "conservatize") who cannot care for himself or herself or manage his or her own finances" (Judicial Council of California, n.d., para. 1). A case could be made to place such a restriction on Mr. Thompson; however, the Lanterman–Petris–Short (LPS) conservatorships are intended for individuals with a serious mental illness. It is not intended for individuals whose main mental illness is substance abuse (Judicial Council of California, n.d.). Individuals will often need assistance if they are under the influence and unable to take care of themselves; however, once someone becomes free of whatever substance he or she is using, the individual is usually able to take care of himself or herself. Putting someone under guardianship/conservator-ship is equivalent to taking that person's rights away. This process can take a long time to get through, as it involves the court system.

Individuals like Mr. Thompson will often end up back on the streets due to their own choices. Someone with an addiction will often choose the streets rather than not being able to use substances or being forced to an environment where he or she is monitored every day. Even if there were programs that assisted individuals with substance abuse and with complex medical care, a person would still have to want to participate in those programs. For the safety of other residents and employees, it would probably involve some rules and regulations. For an individual like Mr. Thompson, a program like that would probably not be enough to keep him there.

HOUSING PEOPLE WITH SUBSTANCE-ABUSE ISSUES

Substance abuse is a major reason why people become homeless, and, as mentioned earlier, it can be a symptom of homelessness after the fact. Even someone who becomes homeless for other reasons could succumb to substance abuse due to fewer controlling factors. Therefore, it would make sense that the best way to re-house someone and to assure that a person maintains his or her stability and housing would be to remove the reason, that is, the person's substance abuse.

Once again, this sounds great in theory. Depending on which substance a person is using, the process of becoming sober would begin with the person's entry into a detoxification regimen or program. Sometimes, detox is looked at as an end in and of itself. Rather than being looked at as an initial step in the person's road to recovery, a way of getting him or her through the physically dangerous period when the individual first stops using the substance, detox is sometimes perceived and presented as an end in itself.

However, detox is technically only the time needed for an individual to be medically cleared of the abused substance(s). After that, it is within the client's means to extend the length of his or her sobriety by entering rehabilitation. Entering rehabilitation will not solve the problem of homelessness, because 28 days will not be enough to assure that the person gets housed. In fact, homelessness itself can serve as a barrier to entering rehabilitation. Many rehabilitation programs will not want to accept a homeless person due to the potential for being "stuck with" that client once the rehab is completed. This creates a dilemma whereby something that could extend the client's stability and assure his or her greater potential for successfully maintaining housing can be denied to that person due to his or her homelessness.

However, the further alternative, the most efficient way to get a homeless substance abuser housed, is to enter residential substance abuse treatment. Not only does this extend the person's sobriety, so that he or she will be better prepared to develop the skills for continued stability after completing the program, but it is, by definition, housing. Often the client can extend this (depending on payment constraints due to how they are funded), but at the very least, they will be there long enough for the onsite staff to seek housing for them (as opposed to the time-limited, 28-day rehabilitation).

The problem with this route for an elderly client is that he or she might tend to have extra health issues that will complicate his or her treatment. More importantly, a client needs to agree to enter one of these programs. Psychologically, many people in general, let alone the homeless, appreciate their freedom and would not necessarily want to give up a year of their life. It might work for someone who has just hit "rock bottom" and wants to get back on his or her feet and for whom little "damage" has been done...it is easier to claw back after not falling so far. However, for a client who has been homeless for years, this may seem too insurmountable a task. This is further compounded for the geriatric population. You might know intuitively that you will have a greater chance of stability and success if you dedicate yourself to entering a program. However, if you are already elderly, you would probably not want to spend any part of your remaining days in a program that might feel like incarceration.

While good intentioned, ultimately this approach can be counterproductive. Telling someone that he or she can be housed by going this route can be overwhelming. Faced with this daunting task of undergoing detoxification, completing rehabilitation, and going through a residential substance abuse program, many people simply give up.

HOUSING PEOPLE WITH MENTAL ILLNESS

Just as no one wants to be homeless, no one wants to be mentally ill. Still, mental illness is considered to be a major cause of homelessness, and consequently, there is a great deal of focus on housing the mentally ill. There are many housing options available to individuals with mental health issues on the local as well as the federal level. However, before reaching that step, many individuals with mental illness end up in the shelter system.

In a system such as New York City's, where there are employment shelters, so too are there mental health shelters. In a mental health shelter, the process for housing consists of completing a housing application that will include a psychiatric evaluation from a psychiatrist and a psychosocial evaluation that can be completed by a social worker or case manager. Having a doctor perform a physical examination is also recommended, as medical diagnoses or conditions could influence the type of housing appropriate to that individual. The diagnoses that are most appropriate and will result in housing through HRA (human resource administration) are schizophrenia, schizoaffective disorder, bipolar disorder, and major depression. HRA evaluates clients' applications on criteria such as diagnosis, homeless history, and reported ability to perform routine tasks, including the access to and engagement in mental health services and the ability to take medication independently. Clients whose application indicates a need for assistance with the latter will be approved for 24-hour-staffed transitional programs.

Clients who are deemed already to be capable of more independent living may be referred to a variety of programs considered to be "permanent" supported housing with only intermittent staff visits. These types of housing programs are described in more detail next.

REGISTERED SEX OFFENDERS

Mr. Hawthorne is a 78-year-old Asian male who is a registered sex offender. He receives $1,800 from Social Security retirement. Mr. Hawthorne became a sex offender when he was 60 years old. Mr. Hawthorne served 11 years in prison for his crimes and was released when he was 71. Due to his registration status, Mr. Hawthorne was unable to go to any shelters and was placed in a transitional housing program following his prison stay. Not willing to have roommates, Mr. Hawthorne initially chose to live on the streets and eventually rented a room in an SRO. The rent was $750 for a 100 sq. ft. room.

After a school was built down the street, Mr. Hawthorne was forced to leave the SRO and search for a new one. Due to limited income, Mr. Hawthorne could not locate another SRO to live in and ended up on the streets. Due to his status, there were no programs that were available to him in the area in which he resided, including local shelters. He also could not locate any ILFs that would take registered sex offenders nor could he qualify for Section 8 housing.

After a year of living on the street, Mr. Hawthorne became gravely ill. He was taken to the local hospital where he passed away.

Before 1994, there were only a few states that required sex offenders to register addresses with local law enforcement. The Jacob Wetterling Crimes Against Children and Sexually Violent Offender Regulation Act in 1994 changed that. It required states to implement a sex-offender registration program, and in 1996 Wetterling was amended by Megan's Law. This required all states to conduct community notification and required the creation of Internet sites containing state sex-offender information. However, Megan's Law did not set any requirements for how states needed to conduct those notifications or the methods and forms (Office of Justice Programs, 2017). The Adam Walsh Child Protection and Child Safety Act of 2006 established uniform and comprehensive sex-offender registration and notification requirements across all 50 states and territories and the District of Columbia (Office of Justice Programs, 2017). Due to online registries and restrictive ordinances at the state and/or local level that range from 500 to 2,500 ft. from schools, childcare facilities, playgrounds, and parks, homelessness is one of the largest issues facing registered sex offenders (Barnes, Dukes, Tewksbury, & De Troye, 2009).

Mr. Hawthorne was unable to escape his sex-offender status and was unable to locate appropriate housing that he could afford. The city that Mr. Hawthorne was residing in did not provide any emergency shelters or services to registered sex offenders. Often this is done because large shelters will have a family section on the premises or be within distance of a school.

If Mr. Hawthorne had been well enough to go to an SNF, he would have faced difficulty in locating one that would take him. Most SNFs are also close to schools and often have children present who visit with their families, which would break the restrictive residency requirements set out by several states. Facilities also must be careful on who they take, as a U.S. Government Accountability Office report in 2006 showed the facilities contacted do not have separate requirements, areas, or supervision for residents solely based on a past conviction, which could put other residents in danger. Facilities will often only put these requirements on residents based on the behaviors of residents. Also, facilities often are not aware of a person's registration status upon admission and cannot take precautions (U.S. Government Accountability Office, 2006).

Due to these concerns, registered sex offenders are usually forced to remain in the hospital until they become strong enough to live on their own.

Mr. Hawthorne had to leave his residence when a school was built in his area. "Most states ban sex offenders from living within 1,000 feet of areas populated by children, such as schools, parks, bus stops, and day care centers. Some states, such as New Jersey, have expanded the distance to 2,500 feet, making it even more difficult to find permanent housing. In a study by Robbers, 35% of registered sex offenders reported having to leave their residences because their landlords or communities discovered their offender status" (Schultz, 2014, p. 69). These restrictive ordinances limit the areas an individual can live and forces them out of populated areas. This can hinder them from receiving proper services.

Federal guidelines also prohibit sex offenders from utilizing some services. In 1998, Section 8 housing became banned for all registered sex offenders who are required to register for life (42 U.S.C. §13663). They cannot be in other federally funded programs either such as transitional housing that is paid for through HUD grants. Oftentimes, this is because the community program is receiving federal funds or the program's location conflicts with a restrictive ordinance. Most of these individuals will reside either on the street, in motels, or in SROs.

THE GAP

Ms. Johnson is a 75-year-old female who has been living on the streets for the past eight years. Prior to that, she was living with her boyfriend in a one-bedroom apartment. She was forced to leave after he passed away, and she could no longer afford the rent on her own. She currently receives $800 per month from SSI. She does not qualify for Social Security retirement or disability, because she never worked enough hours to contribute. For the past year, she has been able to sleep in a friend's garage on an old cot. This garage is not insulated and does not have running water.

Ms. Johnson recently went to the local urgent care center due to a growing lump in her breast. She was then taken to a local hospital where she was diagnosed with breast cancer. During treatment, Ms. Johnson was deemed not to need SNF level of care and would be more appropriate for home health. She was referred to a recuperative care placement and went. However, after receiving radiation, she became sicker and was deemed to need more care than they could provide. She was sent back to the hospital.

Upon admission, physicians evaluated her and determined that she did not need an inpatient hospital stay; however, she could not be discharged to the street as she could not take care of herself. An inpatient social worker assisted her with applying for Medicaid, and she was referred to local SNFs. Ms. Johnson decided she did not need an SNF and chose to return to the garage. Due to the living situation, she could not receive any home health or in-home assistance. She stated, "I've been doing this a long time. I can take care of myself."

After six months, Ms. Johnson was brought back to the local hospital where it was discovered that her cancer had returned. She was transferred to a palliative care unit where she passed away.

Women and families are the fastest-growing segment of the homeless population, with one-third of the total homeless population composed of families spearheaded by women (The National Center on Family Homelessness, 2011). Ms. Johnson was fortunate enough to find a place to live that was not in the streets and where she would be able to be relatively safe. However, the garage did not allow her to receive any assistance in the home, and she was forced to either enter an SNF or do without that assistance.

Ms. Johnson initially utilized the recuperative care resource that is available in some cities. However, she was unable to stay there due to them recommending a higher level of care. Instances like these can be very common. Most community programs are not equipped to deal with older adults that need ADL assistance. Other times, a program may recommend a higher level of care, due to liability issues, if they feel a person is unsafe in their program.

Due to limited income, she was also unable to afford a board and care or an ALF, which would have been an appropriate level of care. There are some public payment options for ALFs such as supplemental payments to the facility for services for Supplemental Security Income (SSI) clients, reimbursement by Medicaid, Medicaid waiver, or state long-term care programs, or some combination of these sources (Wacker & Roberto, 2013). However, Ms. Johnson was unable to take advantage of these resources due to a lack of facilities in her area and a lack of facilities that would take these types of payments. There is unfortunately a large gap in services for low-income individuals who do not need an SNF, but also need some assistance with their ADLs. This is across the country and is demonstrated by a large number of people either living in SNFs or living on the streets at an older age.

Ms. Johnson did not need to be homeless or living in a garage for the end of her life, but she chose that over going to an SNF. Many individuals make a choice like this due to freedom and not wanting a restrictive environment. She also could not go to a community program like a shelter or transitional housing due to her needing assistance with ADLs. Often individuals may need assistance with their ADLs, but will figure out creative ways to do them without assistance.

VETERANS AND PRIDE

Mr. Smith is a 75-year-old African American, Marine Corps veteran. He served 20 years in the service in the infantry. After discharging from the service, he worked as an accountant. Upon his retirement at 65, he started to increase his drinking due to an increase in his PTSD symptoms, which he received from his service in Vietnam. From pension and retirements, he earns $3,000 per month.

Mr. Smith became homeless after his excessive drinking led him to miss rent payments on his apartment. He was served with an eviction notice, which has hindered him from locating any other place to live. To get help, he went to the local Veterans Affair (VA) hospital where he was evaluated by a social worker for homeless resources and substance-abuse resources. Mr. Smith said he was too old to start substance-abuse treatment now and refused to go to any program, including transitional housing, as they had rules and a curfew that he would have to follow. Mr. Smith would often say, "I served 20 years in the service. Why would I go someplace that will make me have a curfew like a child? I want my freedom."

Mr. Smith elected to go back to the streets. He was unable to go to any local shelters as he earned too much money. After repeated hospital admissions for alcohol detox, Mr. Smith realized that he needed assistance and chose to go to a program that provided housing assistance and substance-abuse resources. Once stable, the community agency was able to assist Mr. Smith into locating his own apartment through HUD Veterans Affairs Supportive Housing (VASH).

"Veterans in general are overrepresented in the U.S. homeless population and women veterans are 3 to 4 times more likely to become homeless than their civilian counterparts" (Gamache, Rosenheck, & Tessler, 2003; Rubin, Weiss, & Coll, 2013). In January 2014, communities across America identified 49,933 homeless veterans during Point-In-Time Counts (PITCs), which represents 8.6% of the total homeless population; as of 2015, there was an estimate of 18.9 million veterans (National Alliance to End Homelessness, 2015; National Center for Veterans Analysis and Statistics, 2017). Due to these statistics, it is important to discuss veterans' issues as they do make up such a large portion of older adults.

There are many programs that can assist veterans; however, there are many reasons why this subgroup has a higher rate of homelessness than other community groups. Veterans often have a higher rate of mental illness with PTSD and substance abuse (Rubin et al., 2013). Mr. Smith had evidence of both these diseases. Even though he was able to be successful, he continued to abuse alcohol and never treated his PTSD symptoms.

Veterans have many programs to help with homelessness; however, the vast majority of VA medical centers rely on community partners to assist with homelessness. For example, Housing and Urban Development VA Supportive Housing (HUD VASH) involves not only a Section 8 voucher, but also social work case management, mental health services, addiction therapists, and employment services, which accompany HUD VASH (Rubin et al., 2013). Veterans also utilize transitional housing through community programs. Some VA medical centers may have a domiciliary on their campus, but most will utilize a community partner to assist with providing that level of care (Rubin et al., 2013).

Mr. Smith had issues utilizing these services, however, due to his income. In some states, $3,000 per month will put an individual over the income limit on shelters and transitional housing. It may even put an individual over the income limit for HUD VASH. Due to a large cost of living disparity across the country, income requirements are based on percentages relative to the poverty level of the area. HUD has different requirements for every area of the country, but takes individuals who fall into very low-income, low-income standards, or extremely low-income limits. HUD calculates this by counting individuals in the household, income, poverty line, and cost of living in the area (Rubin et al., 2013).

Mr. Smith was fortunately in an area where he fell below that percentage line and was able to utilize HUD VASH. However, this was only after Mr. Smith was willing to go to services. Veterans and other elderly individuals are often resistant to go to programs where they will have to follow rules such as curfews and restrictions on substance abuse. This is often due to individuals feeling that they have lived their own life and deserve to do what they want. It can be incredibly humbling for any individual to have to not only ask for help, but then to go to a program. Mr. Smith was unable to initially go to a program like this until he failed many times on his own.

Mr. Smith was a perfect storm of PTSD, substance abuse, and elderly pride, which hindered him from being housed and receiving services sooner. Many of these individuals fall through the cracks and are often why there are so many homeless veterans still on the street. Homeless veterans are also not immune to any of the other issues that face civilians, which have been discussed in this chapter.

GERIATRIC HOMELESSNESS

One case that illustrates a spectrum of issues that affect the geriatric population, even in a more advanced service delivery system, is the case of Mr. W, an 81-year-old male of Chinese ancestry who neither spoke nor understood English. His residency status was unknown, and he had no known next of kin. He had arrived after being brought in by the police after they found him wandering around on the street.

Having a translator did not help because Mr. W had advanced dementia and was a very poor historian. Fortunately for Mr. W, he had ended up in a shelter with an empathic staff that included a small medical and psychiatric clinic. However, this original shelter was an assessment shelter, and therefore not intended for clients to stay for the long term.

The shelter staff made exceptions for Mr. W. The rule was that, unless clients were seeing a clinical staff member, they needed to be out during the day. Not only was he not made to leave, but the staff struggled to keep him from leaving the building. At the same time, the staff also wanted him to get his fresh air, so they took him for walks. This was a great strain of time and effort for the staff, which was not designed to exert so much one-on-one effort with clients. It was a very busy shelter where all front-line staff were always occupied maintaining security and operations. In fact, Mr. W was generally left to sit, in eyesight of the staff, while they went about doing other business. Often, this was in front of the medical office where the doctor and nurses kept an eye on him.

Throughout the day, he would stand up and begin walking toward the door where a staff person would chase him.

Despite staff efforts and their perception that their shelter was the best place for him, Mr. W did not belong in an assessment shelter, but rather in a specialized shelter that serviced the fragile and elderly. The assessment shelter did have medical and psychiatric staff, but their main purpose, as was the shelter's, was to assess and distribute residents out to specialty shelters. The medical and psychiatric teams evaluated clients and diagnosed them mainly for the purpose of placement in a mental health, medical, or other shelter. In the process, they would complete documentation required for clients to be housed. They could start the client on medication, but that would invariably be continued elsewhere after a client's transfer. The medical and psychiatric staff often provided the first care that some clients had received for long periods, but invariably they diagnosed individuals and began treatment but only to decide that they needed a medical shelter—or hospital, rehab, or palliative care—before moving them on.

Mr. W could not be accepted in one of the previously mentioned medical facilities due to his lack of documentation, including insurance. Therefore, after several weeks, Mr. W was sent to a shelter for frail and elderly clients intended to meet his needs on a more continual basis.

Approximately a week or so later, Mr. W returned to the assessment shelter with the police. It was the only address that he had when they found him again wandering the streets after leaving that shelter. The shelter that he had been sent to was not being neglectful; they were just not designed to monitor clients that closely. They were designed to isolate frail and elderly clients from the more active and potentially troublesome general population. They had medical staff on site too, and they specialized in finding housing for frail and elderly clients. However, they did not provide hands-on care and one-on-one monitoring. People come and go from the shelters all of the time.

Following that episode, Mr. W stayed at the assessment shelter for several months. During that time, he was continually sent to the hospital and many times needed to stay, sometimes more than a month. However, without insurance, he was invariably sent back, usually before he fully recovered. Hospitals could not *place him in a geriatric or medical facility despite his great need and could not keep him on their units forever. Eventually, Mr. W's health condition deteriorated to a point where he could no longer function, and there was no question that he could not return. He was designated a "charity case" by the city hospital system and eventually was placed in a nursing home to live out his days. However, the case demonstrates how—with even the most advanced system of care—a client can fall through the cracks. For most of his time in the shelter, Mr. W did not need to be locked away somewhere for his own protection, but neither should he have been in a shelter. What Mr. W needed was to be in a place where he had some right to privacy and (supervised) independence, but a caring 24-hour staff, regardless of his documentation or insurance coverage.*

CONCLUSION

While there are many resources available for elderly homeless individuals, there are also many reasons why an individual may not be able to utilize them. Some of the aforementioned resources that were discussed were shelters, transitional housing, and recuperative care programs. For housing resources, there are ILFs, ALFs, board and care facilities, and SNFs. There are also programs that assist with locating permanent housing such as Section 8 through the Department of Housing and Urban Development, and there are programs such as rapid rehousing that can assist an individual with short-term assistance with locating housing available.

Unfortunately, many people are not able to take advantage of these resources either because they do not have an income to support the housing options that provide the level of care they need, they are sex offenders, or they have a mental health or substance-abuse problem that hinders them from either accepting assistance with locating those resources or maintaining that housing once they are able to locate housing that might be available to them.

Looking at best-case scenarios and programs that have worked, there are philosophies and practices that, though they may not be specific to the geriatric population, seem to work well for all populations, including the geriatric populations that are served by them.

Compartmentalizing homeless populations and services seems to work well. In the example of the homeless veteran, compartmentalizing the population and creating specialized services for them, including housing, have been very effective. A focus on that population has, according to the U.S. Department of Veterans Affairs, resulted in a 50% reduction in the homeless veteran population from 2010 to 2016 based on the annual PITC homeless count. This has, of course, been beneficial to the geriatric population due to their representation among veterans, as outlined earlier, but not all veterans are geriatric.

Having onsite services and ancillary services connected to shelters and to housing programs has also been very effective. However, too few of those housing options come with the services attached to the programs and rely on the creativity of those staff involved to obtain them.

Safe havens, which are low demand and high threshold, but with easily accessible services, have been very effective in engaging and servicing chronically homeless individuals. They accept everyone regardless of their issues and treatment compliance. However, not all geriatric people are chronically homeless.

Transitional housing, where people have their own apartment, but benefit from staff 24 hours/day, could be optimal places for the homeless geriatric population, but they are rarely based on the person's age and are not always hands-on and intensive. Their transitional nature does not always allow people to "age in place" where they are.

Nursing homes and ALF can have extensive hands-on assistance, care, and monitoring for the elderly. Such facilities have specialized staff and equipment to tend to their residents' medical needs. However, not all forms of elderly housing will accept homeless people.

Creating a system that combines the beneficial characteristics of all the previously mentioned programs would be the most effective way to treat the geriatric homeless population, provided it would allow the person to age in place. It makes sense for clients who are capable of moving on to a greater level of independence to do so with the right support systems in place. Many clients will achieve that level of stability and have a desire to move on. However, for many within the geriatric homeless population, that is not always a viable alternative. Many have medical, neurological, social, and psychological needs that might inhibit their ability to live independently. As demonstrated earlier, many lack the means, qualification, or desire to engage in treatment that is mandatory to obtain available housing and services.

No one wants homeless people to languish in shelters, but given this reality, the most obvious solution would be for geriatric shelter facilities to be equipped with all that this population might need right from the start.

Geriatric homeless people should be in a safe, comfortable environment from the beginning, be allowed to remain there, and have appropriate services built up around them during their stay. If that place receives any clients, regardless of whether they are using substances, take psychiatric medication, have serious medical needs, or lack insurance, then no one should fall through the cracks. People will not need to move on because their initial placement has everything in place that will ever be needed.

Returning to the example of veterans, the reduction in homeless veterans occurred largely because veterans are a sympathetic population who the public sees as deserving of greater assistance. This allows for an increase in funding and a consequent increase in service provision and housing across the country. Focusing on that population and providing all the necessary support resulted in that reduction.

In that same way, the elderly are sympathetic figures as well. A public service campaign to focus on them as a subpopulation could go a long way toward ensuring their care as well.

While this chapter points out different areas where individuals may have issues getting out of homelessness, there is still a lot more that can be discussed on how to solve homelessness. Oftentimes, these solutions will require programs that are not available in certain areas and will require community resources and involvement. Unfortunately, homelessness is on the rise for elderly individuals. Many individuals were hit by the recession in 2008 and were unable to recover. There are fewer programs available, and when resources become scarce, it is often the most vulnerable individuals who suffer the most. Individuals who are elderly and homeless are some of the most vulnerable individuals in our society. As the nation, states, and localities address the overall issue of homelessness, programs need to be designed, and thus made available, keeping this most vulnerable group in mind.

REFERENCES

Barnes, J. C., Dukes, T., Tewksbury, R., & De Troye, T. M. (2009). Analyzing the impact of a statewide residence restriction law on South Carolina sex offenders. *Criminal Justice Policy Review, 20*(1), 21–43. doi:10.1177/0887403408320842

Botek, A.-M. (2013). 3 Key differences between independent living and assisted living. Retrieved from https://www.agingcare.com/articles/difference-between-independent -living-and-assisted-living-168142.htm

Bruno, K. (2012). *Recuperative care 2012 summary report.* Retrieved from https://www. nhfca.org/reports/Recup%20Report%20final%208%2012.pdf

Gamache, G., Rosenheck, R., & Tessler, R. (2003). Over-representation of women veterans among homeless women. *American Journal of Public Health, 93*(7), 1132–1136. doi:10.2105/AJPH.93.7.1132

Genworth Financial. (2016). Genworth 2016 Cost of Care Survey: Home care providers, adult day health care facilities, assisted living facilities, and nursing homes. Retrieved from https://www.genworth.com/dam/Americas/US/PDFs/Consumer /corporate/131168_050516.pdf

Henry, M., Shivji, A., de Sousa, T., & Cohen, R. (2016). *The 2015 Annual Homeless Assessment Report (AHAR) to Congress.* Retrieved from https://www.hudexchange.info/ resources/documents/2015-AHAR-Part-1.pdf

Jacob Wetterling Crimes Against Children and Sexually Violent Offender Registration Act, Public Law 103-322 (1994).

Judicial Council of California. (n.d.). Conservatorship. Retrieved from http://www.courts.ca.gov/selfhelp-conservatorship.htm

McInnis-Dittrich, K. (2013). *Social work with older adults* (4th ed.). New York, NY: Pearson.

National Alliance to End Homelessness. (2008). *Homeless assistance reauthorization.* Washington, DC: Author.

National Alliance to End Homelessness. (2015). *Fact sheet: Veteran* homelessness. Retrieved from http://www.endhomelessness.org/library/entry/fact-sheet-veteran-homelessness

National Center for Veterans Analysis and Statistics. (2017). *Profile of veterans: 2015.* Retrieved from https://www.va.gov/vetdata/docs/SpecialReports/Profile_of_Veterans_2015.pdf

The National Center on Family Homelessness. (2011, December). The characteristics and needs of families experiencing homelessness. Retrieved from http://mha.ohio.gov/Portals/0/assets/Initiatives/TIC/Homeless/The%20Characteristics%20and%20Needs%20of%20Families%20Experiencing%20Homelessness.pdf

National Council on Aging. (2016). Economic security for senior facts. Retrieved from https://www.ncoa.org/wp-content/uploads/NCOA-Economic-Security.pdf

Office of Justice Programs. (2017). Legislative history of federal sex offender registration and notification.) Retrieved from . https://ojp.gov/smart/legislation.htm

Regional Task Force on the Homeless. (2016). *We all count Point-In-Time Count 2016 San Diego County.* San Diego, CA: Regional Task Force on the Homeless.

Rubin, A., Weiss, E., & Coll, J. (Eds.). (2013). *Handbook of military social work.* Hoboken, NJ: Wiley.

San Diego Housing Commission. (2017). Waiting list applicants. Retrieved from http://www.sdhc.org/Rental-Assistance/Waiting-List-Applicants

Schultz, C. (2014). The stigmatization of individuals convicted of sex offenses: Labeling theory and the sex offense registry. *Themis: Research Journal of Justice Studies and Forensic Science, 2*(1), Article 4. Retrieved from http://scholarworks.sjsu.edu/themis/vol2/iss1/4

Social Security Administration. (2017, January 01). Fact sheet Social Security. Retrieved from https://www.ssa.gov/news/press/factsheets/basicfact-alt.pdf

U.S. Department of Housing and Urban Development. (2015). *Emergency Solutions Grants (ESG) program.* Washington DC: U.S. Department of Housing and Urban Development. Retrieved from https://www.hudexchange.info/programs/esg/esg-law-regulations-and-notices

U.S. Government Accountability Office. (2006). *Long-term care facilities: Information on residents who are registered sex offenders or are paroled for other crimes.* Washington DC: U.S. Government Accountability Office.

Wacker, R., & Roberto, K. (2013). *Community resources for older adults* (4th ed.). New York, NY: Sage.

7

Infectious Diseases in Homeless Geriatrics Population: Part I: Viral

Roxana Aminbakhsh, Roger A. Strong, Diane Chau,
Ashkan Vafadaran, and Elham Faroughi

EXPLORING INFECTIOUS DISEASE PROBLEMS AMONG HOMELESS ELDERLY

Roxana Aminbakhsh

Homelessness is a rising healthcare problem. Secondary to poor living situations and limited access to healthcare services, homeless people are at increased risk for exposure to various communicable diseases (Badiaga, Raoult, & Brouqui, 2008). As a result, the homeless population has a higher prevalence of many infectious diseases.

Per the Centers for Disease Control and Prevention (CDC), epidemiology studies of the homeless population showed 6.2% to 35% HIV infection, 17% to 30% for hepatitis B infection, 12% to 30% for hepatitis C infection, 1.2% to 6.8% for active tuberculosis, 3.8% to 56% for scabies, 7% to 22% for body lice infestation, and 2% to 30% for *Bartonella quintana* infection, which is the most louse-borne infection in urban homeless (Badiaga et al., 2008). Homelessness, on one hand, increases the prevalence of infectious diseases, and aging, on the other hand, makes the elderly more vulnerable to infections.

The result of a study published in the *Journal of General Internal Medicine*, which was conducted on 531 homeless persons (13.9% of them older than 50 years of age), showed that older homeless individuals tend to be in poorer health. They were 3.6 times more likely to report a chronic medical condition than the younger population, and they tended to use shelter-based clinics and street outreach teams more commonly as their source of usual care.

Older homeless adults have a greater disease burden than their younger counterparts (Garibaldi, Conde-Martel, & O'Toole, 2005).

The human body undergoes multiple changes through aging, which decreases the elderly's immunity and makes them vulnerable to infections. The elderly's compromised immunity is multifactorial, resulting from immune senescence, chronic diseases, medications, malnutrition, and functional declines. T-cell production and proliferation decrease with aging, which causes decreased cell-mediated immunity and decreased response to new antigens. Elderly also experience thinning of skin, diminished cough reflex, enlarged prostate, and other changes, which will make them more prone to infections. Also, chronic diseases like diabetes and dementia can predispose them to infections (Strausbaugh, 2001).

In a closer look, we can see a difference in prevalence of infectious diseases among the elder homeless population compared with the younger homeless group. For example, in many countries with low to moderate tuberculosis (TB) incidence, there is a shift of cases to the elderly. In a study conducted in Japan, 14.4 TB cases/100,000 population were reported in 2015. A small percentage of these cases was related to those who were foreign-born (6.4%) and patients with HIV (<0.1%), who thus are not considered significant in transmission of this disease. However, 71.8% of the reported cases were elderly (>60 years of age). Considering the high incidence of TB in Japan until the 1970s, reactivation of remotely acquired latent TB makes the elderly a vulnerable group to this infectious disease (Seto et al., 2017).

Not only is the prevalence of some infectious diseases higher among elderly homeless persons, but providing appropriate care for the elder population is also a challenge. For example, growing older with HIV/AIDS is creating new public health challenges. At present, the healthcare infrastructure is not well equipped to provide care that is needed for HIV-positive older adults. Training of elder service providers is needed for the appropriate care of HIV-positive older adults as the population ages (Cahill & Valadéz, 2013).

Barriers to healthcare access among groups of vulnerable, homeless persons were examined in a study. It showed that the main barriers included lack of insurance, lack of appropriate transportation, stigma, not respecting healthcare providers, confusion, not knowing where to go, or being too sick to look for help (Martens, 2009). There is a need for specific and targeted outreach to connect older homeless persons to appropriate services (Garibaldi et al., 2005).

Among numerous healthcare services that need to be provided for homeless persons, vaccination is one of the most important measures that can decrease the rate of communicable diseases in this vulnerable population. However, studies have shown that simply offering vaccination to the homeless population might not be very successful. Other strategies like providing education about vaccinations and discussing risks and benefits with homeless persons can increase the rate of acceptance of vaccination. In addition to educational incentives, monetary incentives have been used in some cases with success. Providing a combination of easy access, incentives, and coping strategies can increase the rate of vaccination in the homeless population (Wood, 2012).

Besides vaccination, there are many other aspects that should be considered to decrease infectious diseases in this population. Evidence has shown that appropriate public health interventions can decrease the spread of many infectious diseases. However, these interventions should be tailored to each individual group. These interventions include, but are not limited to, improvement of personal clothing and bedding hygiene, providing Ivermectin to treat pruritus secondary to scabies or body lice infestation, supervision on syringes and needles in patients with HIV, and treatment of hepatitis C. Success in implementation of appropriate procedures needs a national preventive public health program for the homeless (Badiaga et al., 2008). In order to make any improvements in a geriatric patient's homeless situation, further information through research is needed. However, there are insufficient studies in this field. In Chapters 7 and 8, we will discuss common infectious diseases in the geriatrics homeless population.

DISEASES FOUND IN THE HOMELESS POPULATION

Roger A. Strong

As with the United States population generally, the homeless population is aging. This is reflected in the changes in the U.S. homeless population ages, with about 11% of single homeless adults being above age 50 in 1990 to about 50% in 2013 (Brown et al., 2017). The median age shifted from about 35 years in 1990 to about 50 years in 2010 (Knopf-Amelung, 2013). This rate of range is expected to continue, and Sermons and Henry (2010) created the graph shown in Figure 7.1 to illustrate this, showing the increase in absolute numbers of the elderly homeless.

With increasing age, it is not surprising that the elderly homeless also have increasing experience with various geriatric conditions. However, and importantly, there is a higher prevalence of various geriatric conditions in those who are homeless and 50 years or older compared to those who are housed and 75 years or older (Brown et al., 2017; Inouye, Studenski, Tinetti, & Kuchel, 2007). Clearly, homelessness leads to a type of accelerated aging and the risks that come with it.

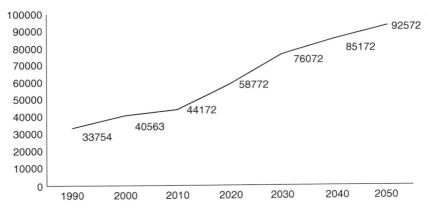

FIGURE 7.1 Project of elderly homelessness.

Source: Sermons, M.W., & Henry, M. (2010). *Demographics of Homelessness Series: The rising elderly population.* Washington, DC: Homelessness Research Institute. Retrieved from https://endhomelessness.org/resource/the-rising-elderly-population

With the comorbidities and metabolic changes that come with aging, aging itself renders individuals more susceptible to infection (Kaye & Shafer, 2011). Along with such comorbidities, the decreasing efficacy of the immune system with aging leads to even greater likelihoods of contracting infections. Add increasing frailty and the resulting higher odds of falls and injuries possibly followed by infections to this aging syndrome, and the elderly face difficult odds of remaining well with reasonable levels of functioning. And, here we are addressing effects of just aging. Combine these with being homeless and the accelerated aging effects noted earlier, and then the odds become even greater that such individuals will face major difficulties, including the likelihood of infections. See Salem et al. (2013) for an excellent literature review and an empirical study regarding frailty among homeless adults. See Table 7.1 (Wright & Tompkins, 2006) listing diseases found among homeless people.

Besides an increase in the likelihood of infections with aging, and especially the elderly homeless, there is the issue of infections in the elderly presenting in atypical ways (Kaye & Shafer, 2011). For example, there may not be fever or fever may not be prominent. Kaye and Shafer (2011) also note that, in the elderly, even changes in mental status might be a result of infection.

VIRAL INFECTIONS

Ashkan Vafadaran and Elham Faroughi
Viral infections are an important cause of morbidity and mortality in homeless elderly patients. Homelessness is associated with numerous behavioral,

TABLE 7.1 *Diseases Found Among Homeless People*

- Drug dependence syndrome: Most commonly heroin or cocaine
- Alcohol dependence syndrome
- Mental ill-health: Schizophrenia, depression and other affective disorders, psychosis, anxiety states, personality disorder, earlier onset of drug misuse, and severity of alcohol use
- Physical trauma
  - Injury
  - Foot trauma: Due to walking for long times in inappropriate shoes; standing or sitting for long periods leading to venous stasis, edema, and infection; frostbite, skin anesthesia due to alcoholic peripheral neuropathy, lack of hygiene due to overwearing of unwashed clothing, or overgrown toenails
  - Dental caries due to self-neglect
- Adverse effects of illicit drugs
  - Heroin-related death secondary to respiratory coma Cocaine: case reports of toxic inhalation leading to pulmonary inflammation and edema ("crack lung"), agitation, and paranoia due to acute toxicity and thromboembolic events. Adverse effects of alcohol overuse
  - Cardiological: Cardiomyopathy
  - Neurological: Peripheral neuropathy, erectile dysfunction, Wernicke's encephalopathy, Korsakoff's psychosis, amnesic syndrome, cerebellar degeneration, alcohol withdrawal seizures
  - Gastrointestinal and hepatobiliary: Hepatitis, liver cirrhosis, pancreatitis, gastritis, peptic ulceration, esophageal varices, carcinoma of the esophagus and oropharynx, cardiomyopathy
  - Metabolic: Vitamin deficiency (particularly thiamine), obesity
  - Psychosocial ill-health: Including depression and suicide, sexual dysfunction, alcoholic hallucinosis, marital, family, or employment breakdown
- Complications of injecting illicit drugs
  - Blood-borne virus infections (see next)
  - Skin commensals or pathogens causing septicemia, encephalitis, endocarditis, cellulitis, and abscesses or deep vein thrombosis (a combination of poor hygiene and repeated skin puncture)
  - Tetanus: Possibly secondary to injecting contaminated drugs
- Infections
  - Blood-borne virus: Hepatitis B, C, or HIV
  - Hepatitis A
  - Skin infections: Cutaneous diphtheria impetigo, viral warts
  - Secondary to louse infestations: Typhus (caused by *Rickettsia prowazekii*), trench fever (caused by *Bartonella quintana*), or relapsing fever (caused by *Borrelia recurrentis*)
  - Fungal: Most commonly tinea
- Inflammatory skin conditions
  - Erythromelalgia
  - Pediculosis
  - Seborrhoeic dermatitis
  - Acne rosacea
  - Eczematoid eruptions
  - Xerosis
  - Pruritus

(continued)

TABLE 7.1   *Diseases Found Among Homeless People (continued)*

- Skin infestations
  - ○ Body louse
  - ○ Scabies
- Respiratory illness
  - ○ Pneumonia: Common pathogens *Streptococcus pneumoniae*, *Haemophilus influenzae* type b, aspiration of anaerobes, or *Pneumocystis carinii* (the latter occurring almost exclusively in immunocompromised patients)
  - ○ Influenza
  - ○ Minor upper respiratory infections
  - ○ Tuberculosis (TB; often latent)

Source: Wright, N. M. J., & Tompkins, C. N. E. (2006). How can health services effectively meet the health needs of homeless people? *British Journal of General Practice, 56*(525), 286–293. Retrieved from https://www.ncbi.nlm.nih.gov/pmc/articles/PMC1832238

social, and environmental risks that expose persons to many communicable diseases, including viral infections, which may spread among the homeless, and aside from posing a threat to individuals' health can lead to outbreaks that can become serious public health concerns (Badiaga, Raoult, & Brouqui, 2008).

This situation can become even more serious in the homeless elderly, as older people experience enhanced susceptibility to viral and subsequent superimposed bacterial infections. Viral infections in the elderly may not only be more frequent and severe, but they also have distinct features with respect to clinical presentation, laboratory results, microbial epidemiology, treatment, and infection control. Management of viral infections in older adults is complicated by factors that include the infrequency or absence of common signs and symptoms of infection and adverse drug reactions (Bader & McKinsey, 2015; Gavazzi & Krause, 2002; Goldstein, 2010).

Other than the factors related to age, disease severity in the homeless elderly can be remarkably high because of additional factors such as extreme poverty, delays in seeking care, barriers that impair their access to healthcare, nonadherence to therapy, cognitive impairment, and the adverse health effects of homelessness itself (Hwang, 2001).

Evidence suggests that appropriate public health interventions can be effective in preventing and controlling the spread of numerous transmitted diseases among the homeless elderly, which is a public health concern both for the individuals and the larger population. These interventions should be tailored to the targeted populations (Badiaga, Raoult, & Brouqui, 2008).

HEPATITIS A

Hepatitis A is a viral infection of the liver caused by the hepatitis A virus (HAV) that may cause a short-term sickness, but generally does not cause prolonged liver disease. A person can only become infected once in his or her lifetime (Fantry, 2004a).

Epidemiology

Approximately 33% of the persons living in the United States have been infected with hepatitis A (Fantry, 2004a). Data from the Third National Health and Nutrition Examination Survey (NHANES III) indicates that 75% of those older than 70 years of age had serological evidence of prior HAV infection (Carrion & Martin, 2012).

Mode of Transmission

Hepatitis A virus is spread primarily by the fecal–oral route, either through person-to-person contact or ingestion of contaminated food or water. Transmission is often facilitated by poor personal hygiene, lack of sanitation, and oral–anal sexual contact (Fantry, 2004a). Urine and saliva do not transmit the hepatitis A virus. Stools of infected persons are infectious from approximately two weeks before until about one week after the appearance of yellow skin (jaundice). The most infectious period is before jaundice appears (Fantry, 2004a).

Signs, Symptoms, and Diagnosis

The early symptoms of hepatitis A are similar to many other diseases and are hard to recognize until jaundice appears. Symptoms usually develop within 15 to 50 days after exposure. Initial symptoms usually include fever, fatigue, poor appetite, nausea, and vomiting. Cough, sore throat, runny nose, and joint pain have been reported in some outbreaks. After several days to a week, the initial symptoms usually begin to diminish. At this point, the infected person may develop yellow skin and eyes, dark urine, light stools, itching, and abdominal pain. Jaundice may never arise in some cases. Weight loss may continue throughout the illness. In most cases, symptoms of hepatitis A resolve within one to two months (Fantry, 2004a).

Prevention and Control

Thorough hand washing is an essential part of preventing the spread of any infection, including hepatitis A. Hand washing is especially important before preparing or serving food and after diapering and using the bathroom. Persons with hepatitis A do not require any special type of isolation unless they are incontinent of stool. Infected people who regularly handle food should avoid tasks that require direct contact with food until one week after the appearance of jaundice (Fantry, 2004a).

Persons who are at increased risk for developing infection have increased risk of severe disease; those seeking long-term protection are recommended to receive the hepatitis A vaccination. Vaccines are given in two doses at least six months apart (Fantry, 2004a).

Special Considerations in Homeless Elderly

Homeless elderly, similar to other homeless people, are often at high risk for hepatitis A due to overcrowded and unsanitary living conditions (Badiaga, Raoult, & Brouqui, 2008); however, acute hepatitis A is often more clinically severe in older individuals. Elderly individuals with acute HAV are likely to have more profound hepatocellular dysfunction with frequent jaundice and a higher incidence of complications, leading to higher mortality rates, especially in individuals older than 75 years. Overall, the basis for worse outcomes in the elderly is thought to be multifactorial and influenced by higher prevalence of comorbid conditions, decline in immune function, and reduced regenerative capacity of the liver with advanced age (Carrion & Martin, 2012).

HEPATITIS A

Hepatitis A outbreaks are reported by the CDC (CDC, 2018). Throughout 2017, an outbreak of hepatitis A affected the homeless population across multiple states and resulted in the CDC releasing interim outbreak specific guidance on post exposure prophylaxis for hepatitis A. It is important to follow the CDC for up-to-date guidance when caring for homeless adults, as many infections can spread rapidly among homeless groups.

HEPATITIS B

Hepatitis B is a viral infection that primarily affects the liver caused by the hepatitis B virus (HBV). Those infected with HBV may show no symptoms, have a self-limited acute illness, progress to acute liver failure, or develop chronic liver disease (Fantry, 2004b).

Epidemiology

It is estimated that 19,200 acute hepatitis B cases occurred in 2014. An estimated 850,000 to 2.2 million persons in the United States have chronic HBV infection. Chronic infection is an even greater problem globally, affecting approximately 240 million persons (CDC, 2017b).

Mode of Transmission

The spread of hepatitis B depends on the contact of blood, semen, or saliva with open skin or mucous membranes (mouth, eyes, vagina, or rectum). This can happen through sexual contact; sharing needles, syringes, or other drug-injection equipment; needlesticks; sharing items such as razors or toothbrushes with an infected person; or from mother to baby at birth. Blood has the highest concentration of HBV. Researchers have found HBV in almost every other body fluid as well. However, their roles in the transmission of the virus are not clearly known. The most common modes of transmission in the United States are through injection drug use and sexual contact (CDC, 2017b; Fantry, 2004b).

Signs, Symptoms, and Diagnosis

The symptoms may start from 50 to 180 days after being infected. Cold- or flu-like symptoms characterize the first stages of the acute illness, which include headache, runny nose, cough, weakness, fatigue, mild fever, poor appetite, nausea, vomiting, sore throat, and aches in the muscles and joints. Some people lose their taste for cigarettes or coffee. This early phase lasts between 1 and 28 days. The second stage of the acute illness, the "icteric" phase, is characterized by yellow skin (jaundice) and eyes, dark urine, and light or tan stools. Nausea and vomiting can continue and grow worse, while other symptoms found in the first stage usually diminish. Some people complain of mild right-sided abdominal pain or itching. Infection without symptoms can happen at any age (Fantry, 2004b). An infected person may become a "chronic carrier." Although chronic carriers may show no symptoms of the disease, they can infect others with the virus for the rest of their lives. Chronic carriers can also develop chronic hepatitis, cirrhosis, and liver cancer (CDC, 2017b).

The diagnosis of acute hepatitis B is made by finding the hepatitis B surface antigen (HBsAg) and IgM anti-hepatitis B core antibody (anti-HBc) in the blood of an infected person. Other blood tests can determine whether a person is immune to hepatitis B or a chronic carrier (Fantry, 2004b).

Prevention and Control

Active hepatitis B vaccine, which allows the body to make antibodies against hepatitis B, offers the best method of prevention. The vaccine is given intramuscularly in the deltoid muscle in a series of three shots, with the second and third given at one- and six-month intervals after the first. Vaccination against HBV is recommended in elderly individuals at risk for infection (Fantry, 2004a).

Special Considerations in Homeless Elderly

Homeless people who inject drugs or have frequent sexual contacts are at high risk for hepatitis B if they are not vaccinated (Fantry, 2004a).

The natural course of chronic HBV infection is determined by multiple variables, including age. Clinical manifestations of acute hepatitis B in the elderly may be different than in younger adults. The rate of progression to chronic hepatitis B is higher in elderly individuals than in younger adults (Carrion & Martin, 2012). Liver cancer linked to HBV has a higher prevalence and a different presentation in the elderly. Its treatment is the same as in younger people, but is less often possible (Loustaud-Ratti, Jacques, Debette-Gratien, & Carrier, 2016). Older age is a predictor for development of liver cancer in patients with chronic hepatitis B. Therefore, age is a factor in determining initiation of surveillance for liver cancer in patients with chronic HBV infection (Carrion & Martin, 2012).

The prevalence of HBV is paradoxically more important in the elderly in areas having vaccination programs because of a loosening of the prevention in older patients. Vaccination in the elderly may be less efficient, as in immunocompromised patients, and needs specific protocols. Liver transplantation is contraindicated after 70 years (Loustaud-Ratti et al., 2016).

HEPATITIS C

Hepatitis C is a leading cause of chronic liver disease. After infection with the hepatitis C virus (HCV), 75% to 85% of individuals fail to clear the virus and develop chronic hepatitis C infection. This disease is usually indolent and often asymptomatic, yet can have dire consequences and can lead to progressive hepatic fibrosis, cirrhosis, and liver cancer (hepatocellular carcinoma) (CDC, 2017b; Greer, 2004).

Epidemiology

HCV is now the most common blood-borne infection in the United States and a leading cause of chronic liver disease. Almost four million Americans have been infected with HCV, and 2.7 million are chronically infected. Many of those who are chronically infected are unaware because they have no signs or symptoms (Greer, 2004).

Rates of HCV infection are disproportionately higher in older patients. In fact, patients born between 1945 and 1965 represent the highest proportion (70%) of HCV-infected individuals in the United States (Rheem, Sundaram, & Saab, 2015).

In studies involving homeless persons in the United States, the prevalence of HCV was found to range from 19% (among homeless caregivers) to 69.1%. Two studies that involved homeless veterans found prevalences of 41% and 44%. Homeless persons infected with HIV had the highest prevalences of HCV (65% and 69.1%) (Chak, Talal, Sherman, Schiff, & Saab, 2011).

Mode of Transmission

HCV is transmitted primarily through percutaneous (i.e., passage through the skin) exposures to infectious blood.

Risk factors for HCV infection in older individuals include blood product transfusions or solid organ transplants before 1992, injection drug use (current or former users, including those who injected only once many years ago), sex with infected person, tattooing with contaminated needles or ink, extensive body piercing, and hemodialysis (Carrion & Martin, 2012; CDC, 2017b; Greer, 2004).

Currently, the most common means of HCV transmission in the United States is injection drug use. HCV is infrequently transmitted through sex with an HCV-infected person, or sharing personal items such as razors or toothbrushes contaminated with infectious blood (inefficient means of transmission; CDC, 2017b).

Signs, Symptoms, and Diagnosis

Individuals with acute HCV infection usually are asymptomatic or have mild nonspecific symptoms. Approximately 20% to 30% of those newly infected with HCV experience fatigue, abdominal pain, poor appetite, or jaundice. Most persons with chronic HCV infection are also asymptomatic, but may have slowly progressing chronic liver disease (CDC, 2017b).

Adults older than 65 years of age, compared with younger individuals, more often present with complications of cirrhosis, particularly hepatic failure and cancer as initial manifestations of HCV infection (Carrion & Martin, 2012).

Chronic HCV infection could be associated with cognitive impairment. The prevalence of cognitive impairment among older patients, who may have a higher susceptibility to this complication, has not been studied (Hepatitis C Association, n.d.).

An initial blood test can detect the presence of anti-HCV antibody, which is present from 6 to 16 weeks after the acute infection. Another type of blood test determining the viral load provides important information on the likelihood of response to antiviral treatment, although it should be noted that disease severity is not correlated with the level of the viral load. The viral load is measured regularly during and after treatment to determine success or failure. The goal is to maintain a sustained viral response (SVR) after treatment (Greer, 2004).

Prevention and Control

Currently, there is no vaccine to prevent hepatitis C. The primary prevention of illegal drug injecting will eliminate the greatest risk factor for HCV infection in the United States. Testing for HCV infection should be routinely performed for persons at high risk for infection (Alter, 2002).

The emergence of direct-acting antiviral (DAA) agents has revolutionized the treatment schema for hepatitis C. From cure rates to tolerability, especially in the elderly, DAA agents have shown outstanding profiles compared with the prior therapies (Rheem, Sundaram, & Saab, 2015).

Special Considerations in Homeless Elderly

The prevalence of HCV is estimated to be 10 to 20 times higher in some subgroups of the homeless population than in the general population. The prevalence increases with age among homeless people (Fantry, 2004a). Beyond drug-use behaviors, over 70% of the homeless adults report unprotected sex with multiple partners, which may increase their risk for HCV infection. In addition, many homeless individuals have histories of mental illness and incarceration, which have been demonstrated to be important considerations in evaluating risk for HCV infection (Nyamathi et al., 2002).

Most of the older adults with chronic HCV infection acquired the disease earlier in life. Elderly patients are more likely than younger patients to have advanced liver disease (likely related to concomitant liver conditions), increased duration of infection, and an increased rate of disease progression (Rheem, Sundaram, & Saab, 2015; Vespasiani-Gentilucci et al., 2015). Among HCV-infected individuals, liver cirrhosis becomes more prevalent with age (High, Marcus, & Tur-Kaspa, 2005).

Recently, attention has been directed to other symptoms associated with chronic HCV infection, including cognitive impairment. Because depression, fatigue, and cognitive impairment are common among the general elderly population, they may be overlooked in those with HCV infection or may not be attributed to the disease (High, Marcus, & Tur-Kaspa, 2005).

HIV/AIDS

HIV can severely damage a person's immune system and impede the body's ability to fight certain infections, cancers, and other diseases. When this virus progresses and causes enough damage, the person develops AIDS, or acquired immunodeficiency syndrome. At this stage, the immune system has been compromised and can no longer fight off life-threatening infections and cancers (Hohl, Pulaski, & Avery, 2004).

Epidemiology

At the end of 2014, an estimated 1.1 million persons aged 13 and older were living with HIV infection in the United States. People aged 55 and older accounted for 26% of all Americans living with diagnosed or undiagnosed HIV infection in 2013. They have the same HIV risk factors as younger people, but may be less aware of their HIV risk factors. Older Americans are more likely to be diagnosed with HIV infection later in the course of their disease (CDC, 2017a). Previous research has shown that HIV is three to nine times more prevalent among homeless individuals than among individuals in stable housing situations (Kidder, Wolitski, Campsmith, & Nakamura, 2007).

Mode of Transmission

HIV is transmitted through person-to-person contact with blood or other body fluids such as semen, vaginal secretions, and breast milk. Common ways to transmit the virus include: sexual contact; sharing needles or other drug paraphernalia; and mother to child during pregnancy, birth, or breast-feeding. Cocaine users who share contaminated drug paraphernalia can transmit the virus through the breakdown in the lining of the nose. HIV is not transmitted through casual or household contact. Neither is HIV transmitted through sweat, tears, urine, or feces. While HIV can be found in saliva, scientists have found no evidence of transmission through saliva (Hohl, Pulaski, & Avery, 2004).

Signs, Symptoms, and Diagnosis

"Acute HIV infection" is a syndrome that develops a few days to a few weeks after exposure to the virus and is typically a "flu-like illness" accompanied by fevers, headache, sore throat, and enlarged lymph nodes. Persons with acute HIV syndrome are highly infectious and have a large burden of virus in the bloodstream. After the initial infection, the person with HIV may have no signs or symptoms for months or years. More serious infections can ensue as the CD4 count falls, and the immune system becomes more compromised. As HIV progresses, people can develop many infections caused by viruses, bacteria, and parasites. They are also at greater risk of developing some cancers, such as lymphoma (cancer of the lymph nodes), Kaposi's sarcoma, and cervical and anal cancer (Hohl et al., 2004).

The diagnosis of HIV infection is made by testing antibodies to HIV in the blood or oral fluid. Rapid testing can be more efficient in outreach settings, including shelters. The diagnosis of AIDS in a person with HIV infection is made when the CD4 count has dropped below 200 or when the individual has developed one of the infections or cancers associated with HIV infection (Hohl et al., 2004).

Prevention and Control

Prevention is the key to control of HIV/AIDS and includes safer sex and safer use of needles and other drug paraphernalia. No sexual contact is completely safe even with the use of condoms and other barriers. Even oral sex has some risk of spreading the HIV virus. Condoms can break or fall off. For these reasons, HIV counselors use the term "safer sex" rather than "safe sex." Any person with "acute HIV infection" who has a history of recent high-risk behavior, such as injection drug use or unsafe sex, should immediately receive a thorough medical evaluation (Hohl et al., 2004).

Special Considerations in Homeless Elderly

The prevalence of HIV/AIDS is dramatically higher among homeless people than in the general population. Homelessness and HIV/AIDS are widespread and intersecting problems that occur in both urban and rural populations throughout the United States. Conditions associated with homelessness make HIV prevention and control especially difficult (Clinician's Health Care for the Homeless Network, 1998; National Health Care for the Homeless Council, 2012; Song, 1999).

Housing status can be a significant predictor of health status, healthcare and emergency department use, use of HIV medications, and HIV medication adherence (Kidder et al., 2007).

Preventive measures commonly used in other populations at increased risk for HIV infection are often unavailable to homeless people. Homeless people with HIV/AIDS are particularly susceptible to a number of other medical conditions, which, if untreated, may exacerbate their illness and even threaten their survival. Crowded, unsanitary living conditions increase their risk of exposure to communicable diseases and parasites. Limited resources result in unmet subsistence needs, reducing their natural resistance to disease (Song, 1999).

As the HIV population ages and the rate of newly detected infections in the elderly rises, clinicians should be aware of the increasing need to balance HIV care and the management of comorbid conditions commonly associated with aging and medication side effects or interactions (CDC, 2017a; Nguyen & Holodniy, 2008).

Because changes in the immune system are very similar to aging effects, progression of HIV infection in the elderly may be more pronounced. Studies have demonstrated that age is an independent predictor of clinical progression in HIV (Nguyen & Holodniy, 2008). Older people in the United States are more likely than younger people to be diagnosed with HIV infection late in the course of the infection, which results in their starting treatment late and possibly suffering more immune system damage. Late diagnoses can occur because healthcare providers may not always test older people for HIV infection, and older people may not consider themselves to be at risk of HIV infection or may mistake HIV symptoms for those of normal aging and not consider HIV as a cause.

Stigma is a particular concern among older people because they may already face isolation due to illness or loss of family and friends. Stigma negatively affects people's quality of life, self-image, and behaviors and may prevent them from seeking HIV care and disclosing their HIV status (CDC, 2017a).

Complete sexual histories may not be routinely obtained from older patients by practitioners as a result of discomfort regarding their own sexuality, the sexual orientation of the patient, or the lack of recognition that continued sexual activity is important in overall wellness of patients. In addition, older patients may not be comfortable with disclosing information that they feel they should be discrete about (Nguyen & Holodniy, 2008).

The presence of both psychiatric disorders and cognitive decline can be a significant morbidity in the aging HIV-infected patient. While some studies suggest that medication adherence may be improved in the older HIV-infected patient, substance abuse and cognitive dysfunction may contribute to poor adherence (Nguyen & Holodniy, 2008).

INFLUENZA

Influenza is a contagious respiratory illness caused by either influenza A or influenza B viruses that occurs primarily during the winter months in temperate climates. Influenza is usually a self-limited illness; however, elderly persons and people with chronic medical conditions are at higher risk for developing severe complications from influenza (Rogers, Gordon Wright, & Levy, 2004).

Epidemiology

Outbreaks of influenza often occur in unvaccinated populations. The rates of infection are highest in children, but elderly persons and persons with certain medical conditions that predispose them to complications from influenza have the highest rates of serious morbidity and mortality (Rogers et al., 2004).

Mode of Transmission

Influenza virus is primarily spread from person to person through coughing and sneezing of virus particles in respiratory secretions. The period of infectivity for adults begins about one day prior to the development of symptoms and typically lasts for three to five days after the onset of symptoms (Rogers et al., 2004).

Signs, Symptoms, and Diagnosis

The spectrum of clinical presentations of influenza is extremely broad. Classic symptoms include high-grade fever, myalgia, chills, headache, sore throat, dry cough, and malaise, with sudden onset after an incubation period of one or two days. The clinical presentation of influenza in the elderly is not well characterized and might be atypical. Elderly patients may present with only lassitude, fever, and confusion. Influenza can result in falls and greater dependency in activities of daily living. Elderly patients may also present with complications of influenza, such as bacterial pneumonia, or exacerbation of underlying conditions, such as chronic obstructive pulmonary disease or congestive heart failure (Bader & McKinsey, 2015).

Rapid antigen tests have become widely used to diagnose influenza in outpatient clinics because results can be obtained within 30 minutes or less. When interpreting the results of rapid tests, one should take into account the community prevalence of influenza and the pre-test probability of the disease (Rogers et al., 2004).

Prevention and Control

Vaccination is the best way to prevent influenza and is indicated for persons at increased risk of complications from influenza, as well as close contacts of those at increased risk (Rogers et al., 2004). The primary goal of influenza vaccination is prevention of the serious consequences of the disease, not prevention of influenza epidemics (Bader & McKinsey, 2015). Vaccine effectiveness depends on the match between the vaccine and circulating virus, as well as the age and immune status of the host. Most influenza infections occur in late December through March. Peak antibody protection occurs two weeks after vaccination. The antibody levels begin to fall in the elderly within four months, but data are not available to support a second administration of the vaccine to boost immunity (Rogers et al., 2004). Education, cleaning and disinfection, facemasks, and respirators can decrease the risk of transmission of influenza viruses (Scott, 2009).

Special Considerations in the Homeless Elderly

The crowded living conditions and poor ventilation in many shelters, as well as the high incidence of chronic medical conditions, may place homeless persons at increased risk for contracting influenza (Rogers et al., 2004). On the other hand, influenza causes substantial morbidity and mortality in older adults. It has a significant negative impact on the functional capacity of frail elderly patients. Older adults account for over 90% of the deaths attributed to pneumonia and influenza (Bader & McKinsey, 2015).

Vaccines fail to provide as high a level of protection for older people as for younger people, likely caused by age-induced alterations in the immune system (Goldstein, 2010). When infected, most elderly patients seek medical attention beyond 48 hours, when the benefits of antiviral treatment of influenza remain unproved (Nicholson, Kent, Hammersley, & Cancio, 1997).

Although homeless shelters are likely sites for transmission of influenza, at the same time, they offer a unique opportunity to administer influenza vaccines to both residents and staff. Vaccination may be provided to all residents and staff who do not have specific contraindications. Because homeless populations are often mobile, a coordinated effort to vaccinate all staff and residents during the same day or week in a particular area may be attempted. This effort should include outreach efforts to vaccinate homeless populations not living in shelters to maximize coverage (Rogers et al., 2004).

West Nile Virus and Other Mosquito-Borne Infections

West Nile virus (WNV) can cause serious and sometimes fatal illness. This virus is most often spread through the bite of an infected mosquito. Other mosquito-borne viral infections in the United States include: St. Louis encephalitis (SLE), Eastern and Western equine encephalitis (EEE and WEE), and La Crosse (LAC) encephalitis. Human illness due to these other viruses is less common than WNV, though occasional large outbreaks can occur (Zielinski-Gutiérrez, 2004).

Epidemiology

WNV is established as a seasonal epidemic in North America that flares up in the summer and continues into the fall. Most people are infected from June through September. The risk of infection is highest for people who are homeless, work outside, or participate in outdoor activities because of greater exposure to mosquitoes (CDC, 2017c).

Mode of Transmission

The most important route of WNV transmission is through the bite of an infected mosquito. Mosquitoes become infected with WNV when they feed on infected birds (Zielinski-Gutiérrez, 2004). Additional routes of human infection have also been documented. It is important to note that these methods of transmission represent a very small proportion of cases and may include blood transfusions, organ transplants, and from mother to baby during pregnancy, delivery, or breastfeeding. WNV is not transmitted from person-to-person or from animal-to-person through casual contact (CDC, 2017c).

Signs, Symptoms, and Diagnosis

About 80% of human WNV infections do not result in any symptoms or illness. About 20% of the infected individuals develop West Nile fever (WNF), which can be difficult to distinguish from other viral infections (fever, headache, body aches, skin rash, and swollen lymph nodes). Only one in 150 infected persons develops severe disease such as encephalitis (inflammation of the brain) or meningitis (inflammation of the lining of the brain and spinal cord). Recovery from severe disease may take several weeks or months. Some of the neurologic effects may be permanent. About 10% of the people who develop neurologic infection due to WNV will die. Serious illness can occur in people of any age. However, advanced age is, by far, the most significant risk factor for developing severe disease after infection. People with certain medical conditions, such as cancer, diabetes, hypertension, kidney disease, and people who have received organ transplants, are also at greater risk for serious illness (CDC, 2017c; Zielinski-Gutiérrez, 2004).

Diagnosis is based on a combination of clinical signs and symptoms and specialized laboratory tests of blood or spinal fluid (CDC, 2017c).

Prevention and Control

There are no medications to treat or vaccines to prevent WNV infection. The most effective way for individuals to avoid infection is to prevent mosquito bites. This can be accomplished with regular use of insect repellent on exposed skin and clothing when outdoors. Mosquitoes may bite through thin clothing, so spraying clothes with proper repellent will give extra protection. Wearing long sleeves and pants from dusk through dawn when many mosquitoes are most active and getting rid of mosquito breeding sites by emptying standing water are also recommended (CDC, 2017c).

Special Considerations in the Homeless Elderly

Homeless populations may be at higher risk for WNV and other mosquito-borne diseases due to their increased exposure to the outdoors and their limited access to preventive measures. Healthcare providers should vigorously promote the use of insect repellents, especially for homeless persons over the age of 50. Advanced age is the most important risk factor for death, with patients older than 70 years of age at highest risk.

WNV and other mosquito-borne viral diseases, while relatively low in incidence, pose a significant risk to homeless elderly populations due to their potential for mosquito bites and extensive exposure to the outdoors. All persons over the age of 50 are at higher risk for severe disease, which typically results in hospitalization (Zielinski-Gutiérrez, 2004).

The studies that have evaluated risk factors for infection in the United States found that increased time outdoors (spending greater than six hours outside per day during the summer and fall), inconsistent use of mosquito repellant, and age were predictors for infection. Being homeless greater than one year was highly associated with increased time spent outdoors, and also predicted infection (Meyer et al., 2007).

REFERENCES

Alter, M. J. (2002). Prevention of spread of hepatitis C. *Hepatology, 36*(Suppl. S1), S93–S98. doi:10.1002/hep.1840360712
Bader, M. S., & McKinsey, D. S. (2015). Viral infections in the elderly: The challenges of managing herpes zoster, influenza, and RSV. *Journal of Postgraduate Medicine, 118*(5), 45–54. doi:10.3810/pgm.2005.11.1687

Badiaga, S., Raoult, D., & Brouqui, P. (2008). Preventing and controlling emerging and reemerging transmissible diseases in the homeless. *Emerging Infectious Diseases, 14*(9), 1353–1359. doi:10.3201/eid1409.082042

Brown, R. T., Hemati, K., Riley, E. D., Lee, C. T., Ponath, C., Tieu. L., Guzman, D., & Kushel, M. B. (2017). Geriatric conditions in a population-based sample of older homeless adults. *Gerontologist, 57*(4), 757–766. doi:10.1093/geront/gnw011

Cahill, S., & Valadéz, R. (2013). Growing older with HIV/AIDS: New public health challenges. *American Journal of Public Health, 103*(3), e7–e15. doi:10.2105/AJPH.2012.301161

Carrion, A. F., & Martin, P. (2012). Viral hepatitis in the elderly. *The American Journal of Gastroenterology, 107*, 691–697. doi:10.1038/ajg.2012.7

Centers for Disease Control and Prevention. (2017a). HIV/AIDS. Retrieved from https://www.cdc.gov/hiv

Centers for Disease Control and Prevention. (2017b). Viral hepatitis. Retrieved from https://www.cdc.gov/hepatitis

Centers for Disease Control and Prevention. (2017c). West Nile virus. Retrieved from https://www.cdc.gov/westnile

Centers for Disease Control and Prevention. (2018). Viral hepatitis: Hepatitis A outbreaks. Retrieved from https://www.cdc.gov/hepatitis/outbreaks/index.htm

Chak, E., Talal, A. H., Sherman, K. E., Schiff, E. R., & Saab, S. (2011). Hepatitis C virus infection in USA: An estimate of true prevalence. *Liver International, 31*(8), 1090–1101. doi:10.1111/j.1478-3231.2011.02494.x

Clinician's Health Care for the Homeless Network. (1998). Network to study HIV and homelessness. *Healing Hands, 2*(5), 1–4. Retrieved from https://www.nhchc.org/wp-content/uploads/2012/02/hh.09_98.pdf

Fantry, L. (2004a). Hepatitis A. In J. J. O'Connell (Ed.), *The health care of homeless persons: A manual of communicable diseases & common problems in shelters & on the streets* (pp. 30–33). Boston, MA: The Boston Health Care for the Homeless Program. Retrieved from http://www.bhchp.org/health-care-homeless-persons

Fantry, L. (2004b). Hepatitis B. In J. J. O'Connell (Ed.), *The health care of homeless persons: A manual of communicable diseases & common problems in shelters & on the streets.* (pp. 35–39). Boston, MA: The Boston Health Care for the Homeless Program. Retrieved from http://www.bhchp.org/health-care-homeless-persons

Garibaldi, B., Conde-Martel, A., & O'Toole, T. P. (2005). Self-reported comorbidities, perceived needs, and sources for usual care for older and younger homeless adults. *Journal of General Internal Medicine, 20*(8), 726–730. doi:10.1111/j.1525-1497.2005.0142.x

Gavazzi, G., & Krause, K.-H. (2002). Ageing and infection. *The Lancet: Infectious Disease, 2*(11), 659–666. doi:10.1016/S1473-3099(02)00437-1

Goldstein, D. R. (2010). Aging, imbalanced inflammation and viral infection. *Virulence, 1*(4), 295–298. doi:10.4161/viru.1.4.12009

Greer, P. J. (2004). Hepatitis C. In J. J. O'Connell (Ed.), *The health care of homeless persons: A manual of communicable diseases & common problems in shelters & on the streets* (pp. 41–46). Boston, MA: The Boston Health Care for the Homeless Program. Retrieved from http://www.bhchp.org/health-care-homeless-persons

Hepatitis C Association. (n.d.). Chronic hepatitis C in the elderly. Retrieved from https://hepcassoc.org/news/article121.html

High, K. P., Marcus, E.-L., & Tur-Kaspa, R. (2005). Chronic hepatitis C virus infection in older adults. *Clinical Infectious Diseases, 41*(11), 1606–1612. doi:10.1086/497597

Hohl, C., Pulaski, P. E., & Avery, R. K. (2004). HIV/AIDS. In J. J. O'Connell (Ed.), *The health care of homeless persons: A manual of communicable diseases & common problems in shelters & on the streets* (pp. 53–61). Boston, MA: The Boston Health Care for the Homeless Program. Retrieved from http://www.bhchp.org/health-care-homeless-persons

Hwang, S. W. (2001). Homelessness and health. *Canadian Medical Association Journal, 164*(2), 229–233. Retrieved from http://www.cmaj.ca/content/cmaj/164/2/229.full.pdf

Inouye, S. K., Studenski, S., Tinetti, M. E., & Kuchel, G. A. (2007). Geriatric syndromes: Clinical, research, and policy implications of a core geriatric concept. *Journal of the American Geriatrics Society, 55*, 780–791. doi:10.1111/j.1532-5415.2007.01156.x

Kaye, K. S., & Shafer, E. (2011, September). Comorbidities, metabolic changes in elderly more susceptible to infection. *Infections Disease News.* Retrieved from https://www.healio.com/infectious-disease/news/print/infectious-disease-news/%7Ba029cda7-ca04-4b1e-98ae-677d27670ceb%7D/comorbidities-metabolic-changes-make-elderly-more-susceptible-to-infection

Kidder, D. P., Wolitski, R. J., Campsmith, M. L., & Nakamura, G. V. (2007). Health status, health care use, medication use, and medication adherence among homeless and housed people living with HIV/AIDS. *American Journal of Public Health, 97*(12), 2238–2245. doi:10.2105/AJPH.2006.090209

Knopf-Amelung, S. (2013, September). Aging and housing instability: Homelessness among older and elderly adults. In *Focus: A Quarterly Research Review of the National HCH Council, 2*(1). Nashville, TN: National Health Care for the Homeless Council. Retrieved from http://www.nhchc.org/wp-content/uploads/2011/09/infocus_september2013.pdf

Loustaud-Ratti, V., Jacques, J., Debette-Gratien, M., & Carrier, P. (2016). Hepatitis B and elders: An underestimated issue. *Hepatology Research, 46*(1), 22–28. doi:10.1111/hepr.1249

Martens, W. H. (2009). Vulnerable categories of homeless patients in Western societies: Experience serious barriers to health care access. *Medicine Law, 28*(2), 221–239.

Meyer, T. E., Bull, L. M., Holmes, K. C., Pascua, R. F., Travassos da Rosa, A. P., Gutierrez, C. R., . . . Murray, K. O. (2007). West Nile virus infection among the homeless, Houston, Texas. *Emerging Infectious Diseases, 13*(10), 1500–1503. doi:10.3201/eid1310.070442

National Health Care for the Homeless Council. (2012, December). HIV/AIDS among persons experiencing homelessness: Risk factors, predictors of testing, and promising testing strategies. *In Focus.* Retrieved from http://www.nhchc.org/wp-content/uploads/2011/09/InFocus_Dec2012.pdf

Nguyen, N., & Holodniy, M. (2008). HIV infection in the elderly. *Clinical Interventions in Aging, 3*(3), 453–472. Retrieved from https://www.ncbi.nlm.nih.gov/pmc/articles/PMC2682378/

Nicholson, K. G., Kent, J., Hammersley, V., & Cancio, E. (1997). Acute viral infections of upper respiratory tract in elderly people living in the community: Comparative, prospective, population based study of disease Burden. *British Medical Journal, 315*(7115), 1060–1064. doi:10.1136/bmj.315.7115.1060

Nyamathi, A. M., Dixon, E. L., Robbins, W., Smith, C., Wiley, D., Leake, B., . . . Gelberg, L. (2002). Risk factors for hepatitis C virus infection among homeless adults. *Journal of General Internal Medicine, 17*(2), 134–143. doi:10.1046/j.1525-1497.2002.10415.x

Rheem, J., Sundaram, V., & Saab, S. (2015). Antiviral therapy in elderly patients with hepatitis C virus infection. *Gastroenterology & Hepatology, 11*(5), 294–346. Retrieved from https://www.ncbi.nlm.nih.gov/pmc/articles/PMC4962680/

Rogers, M. A., Gordon Wright, J., & Levy, B. D. (2004). Influenza. In J. J. O'Connell (Ed.), *The health care of homeless persons: A manual of communicable diseases & common pProblems in shelters & on the streets* (pp. 67–71). Boston, MA: The Boston Health Care for the Homeless Program. Retrieved from www.bhchp.org/health-care-homeless-persons

Salem, B. E., Nyamathi, A. M., Brecht, M.-L., Phillips, L. R., Mentes. J. C., Sarkisian, C., & Leake, B. (2013). Correlates of frailty among homeless adults. *Western Journal of Nursing Research, 35,* 1128–1152. doi:10.1177/0193945913487608

Scott, M. (2009). Pandemic influenza guidance for homeless shelters and homeless service providers. Nashville, TN: National Health Care for the Homeless Council. Retrieved from http://www.nhchc.org/wp-content/uploads/2011/10/flumanual.pdf

Sermons, M. W., & Henry, M. (2010). *Demographics of Homelessness Series: The rising elderly population.* Washington, DC: Homelessness Research Institute. Retrieved from https://endhomelessness.org/resource/the-rising-elderly-population

Seto, J., Wada, T., Suzuki, Y., Ikeda, T., Mizuta, K., Yamamoto, T., & Ahiko, T. (2017). Mycobacterium tuberculosis transmission among elderly persons, Yamagata Prefecture, Japan, 2009–2015. *Emerging Infectious Diseases, 23*(3), 448–455. doi:10.3201/eid2303.161571

Song, J. (1999). HIV/AIDS & homelessness: Recommendations for clinical practice and public policy. Nashville, TN: National Health Care for the Homeless Council. Retrieved from http://www.nhchc.org/wp-content/uploads/2011/10/AIDS-Homelessness.pdf

Strausbaugh, L, J. (2001). Emerging health care-associated infections in the geriatric population. *Emerging Infectious Diseases, 7*(2). Retrieved from https://wwwnc.cdc.gov/eid/article/7/2/pdfs/70-0268.pdf

Vespasiani-Gentilucci, U., Galati, G., Gallo, P., De Vincentis, A., Riva, E., & Picardi, A. (2015). Hepatitis C treatment in the elderly: New possibilities and controversies towards interferon-free regimens. *World Journal of Gastroenterology, 21*(24), 7412–7426. doi:10.3748/wjg.v21.i24.7412

Wood, S. P. (2012). Vaccination programs among urban homeless populations: A literature review. *Journal of Vaccines & Vaccination, 3*(6). doi:10.4172/2157-7560.1000156

Wright, N. M. J., & Tompkins, C. N. E. (2006). How can health services effectively meet the health needs of homeless people? *British Journal of General Practice, 56*(525), 286–293. Retrieved from https://www.ncbi.nlm.nih.gov/pmc/articles/PMC1832238

Zielinski-Gutiérrez, E. (2004). Mosquito-borne infections. In J. J. O'Connell (Ed.), *The health care of homeless persons: A manual of communicable diseases & common problems in shelters & on the streets.* The Boston Health Care for the Homeless Program, Mosquito-borne Infections, (pp. 181–186). Boston, MA: The Boston Health Care for the Homeless Program. Retrieved from www.bhchp.org/health-care-homeless-persons

Infectious Diseases in Homeless Geriatrics Population: Part II: Bacterial Infections, Tuberculosis, and Arthropods Infestation

Roxana Aminbakhsh, Therese Gibson, Diane Chau, Ashlyn Melvin, Marilee Nebelsick-Tagg, Ashkan Vafadaran, and Elham Faroughi

BACTERIAL INFECTIONS

Therese Gibson

Urinary tract infection (UTI), pneumonia, and foot infections are three of the most commonly diagnosed bacterial infections in the elderly and the elderly homeless population. They are at a much higher risk for complications and even death. As our population ages, the burden of UTI in older adults increases the need for early diagnosis (Rowe & Juthani-Mehta, 2013). Early diagnosis and treatment can be difficult due to the social issues the elderly homeless face such as overcrowded shelters, poor hygiene, lack of medical care, and multiple comorbidities.

The incidence of UTI is higher in women than men across all age groups (Rowe & Juthani-Mehta, 2013). However there are 30% more elderly homeless men than women. Over 10% of women and 0.5% of men older than 65 years of age reported having a UTI within the past 12 months. In both men and women over the age of 85 years, the incidence of UTI increases substantially (Rowe & Juthani-Mehta, 2013).

There are very few studies addressing elderly homeless and bacterial infections. Many of the studies only address the elderly and not the elderly homeless. With the growing number of elderly homeless, the burden of UTI in the elderly grows, creating a need for improvement in diagnostic, management, and prevention strategies critical to improving the care of the elderly

(Rowe & Juthani-Mehta, 2013). The elderly homeless are at a higher risk for severe infection with higher morbidity and mortality.

Urinary Tract Infections

UTIs are the most common cause for hospitalization in adults 65 years or older according to current literature. Changes caused by infection in the elderly are subtle, and nonspecific complaints may be the only indications. They are much harder to diagnose in this age group, leading to multiple hospitalizations or even death according to Stevenson (2015).

Diagnosis of infection in older adults is more challenging because of the atypical presentation of symptoms, yet early diagnosis and treatment is imperative because of the higher incidence of morbidity and mortality (Mouton, Bazaldua, Pierce, & Espino, 2001). Nonspecific symptoms, such as loss of appetite, decline in functioning, mental status changes, incontinence, and falls, may be the presenting signs of infection (University of Maryland Medical Center [UMMC], n.d.). Other research states that elderly patients with infections commonly present with cognitive impairment or a change in mental status; frank delirium occurs in 50% of the older adults with infections. Furthermore, anorexia, functional decline, falls, weight loss, or a slight increase in respiratory rate may be the only signs of infection in older patients (Muirhead, Roberson, & Secrest, 2009).

Many signs and symptoms of infection seen in younger patients, such as fever and leukocytosis, are present less frequently or not at all in older adults according to current studies on the elderly. While 60% of the older adults with serious infections develop leukocytosis, its absence does not rule out an infectious process. Because frail older adults tend to have poorer body temperature response, elevations in body temperature of 2°F from their normal baseline temperature should be considered a febrile response. Fevers higher than 101°F often indicate severe, life-threatening infections in older adults, and hospitalizations should be considered for these patients (UMMC, n.d.).

Contributing factors specific to gender include prostate enlargement in men, and an increase in vaginal pH, vaginal atrophy that is due to postmenopausal estrogen depletion, and incomplete emptying of the bladder in women. These factors provide the opportunity for bacterial colonization and are likely to contribute to the higher rates of asymptomatic bacteriuria and UTIs in the elderly (Metersky, Masterton, Lode, File Jr., & Babinchak, 2012).

The most common organism responsible for causing UTIs is *Escherichia coli*, followed by other enterobacteriaceae, such as *Proteus mirabilis*, *Klebsiella*, and *Providentia* species. Gram-positive organisms, such as methicillin-resistant *Staphylococcus aureus* and Enterococcus, are less common overall, but are seen with increasing frequency due to overuse of antibiotics in the elderly population (Rowe & Juthani-Mehta, 2013).

According to current literature, overtreatment with antibiotics for suspected UTI remains a significant problem and leads to a variety of negative consequences, including the development of multidrug-resistant organisms (Metersky et al., 2012).

Despite advances in antibiotic therapy, infectious diseases continue to be a major cause of mortality in older adults (Mouton et al., 2001).

Treatment of asymptomatic bacteriuria does not appear to reduce morbidity or mortality and may increase the likelihood of development of drug-resistant microorganisms and adverse reactions to antibiotics (Stevenson, 2015).

One of the most common organisms that cause UTIs is enterococci. Over the past two decades, most enterococci have become resistant to beta-lactam antibiotics, and recently, resistance to aminoglycosides has become widespread according to recent studies.

Antibiotic treatment does not appear to be efficacious (Metersky et al., 2012). The recent rise of antibiotic-resistant bacteria (e.g., methicillin-resistant *Staphylococcus aureus* (MRSA) and vancomycin-resistant enterococcus) is a particular problem in the elderly because they are exposed to infections at higher rates in hospital and institutional settings (White, Ellis Jr, & Simpson, 2014). Treatment of colonization and active infection is problematic; strict adherence to hygiene practices is necessary to prevent the spread of resistant organisms (Mouton et al., 2001). However, the elderly homeless often do not have the ability to maintain good hygiene, proper shelter, or healthy diet for a variety of reasons, including multiple comorbidities.

Bacterial Pneumonia

While the incidence of pneumonia is declining, it continues to be a national healthcare issue, especially among the elderly homeless. The aging population, antibiotic resistance, and increasing healthcare costs make this a particularly challenging problem (UMMC, n.d.). The growing population of elderly homeless only adds to this widespread and significant healthcare issue.

Both hospital-acquired pneumonia (HAP) and community-acquired pneumonia (CAP) continue to be the most common bacterial infections among the elderly. Pneumonia is the most common hospital-acquired infection (UMMC, n.d.). The causes are Streptococcus pneumonia, Haemophilus influenza, Mycoplasma pneumonia, and Chlamydia pneumonia (UMMC, n.d.).

Streptococcus pneumonia is the most common cause of bacterial pneumonia, bacteremia, and meningitis in adults and is a major cause of morbidity and mortality in the general population according to Plevneshi et al. (2009). Homeless adults may be at greater risk than other adults both because of underlying medical conditions that increase their risk of infection such as chronic obstructive pulmonary disease (COPD), chronic liver disease, or HIV infection and because communal living in shelters may be associated with transmission of pathogenic strains (Plevneshi et al., 2009).

More than 60% of the seniors over 65 years get admitted to hospitals due to pneumonia, according to experts. Seniors are at greater risk for pneumonia for a variety of reasons, including changes in lung capacity, increased exposure to disease in community settings, and increased susceptibility due to other conditions like cardiopulmonary disease or diabetes. Classic symptoms like fever, chills, and cough are less frequent in the elderly; they often present to the emergency department (ED) in advanced stages of the infection, as per the infectious disease clinics of North America. One can only keep an eye out for nonrespiratory symptoms like weakness, confusion, or delirium to aid in the diagnosis (Stevenson, 2015).

Pneumonia and influenza combined are the sixth leading cause of death in the United States. And, about 90% of these deaths occur in adults 65 years and older. In fact, more than 60% of people 65 years and older are admitted to hospitals because of pneumonia. Changes in pulmonary reserve, decreased cough reflex, decreased elasticity of alveoli, and poor ventilation, all of which lead to diminished cough and airway patency, cause older adults to be more susceptible to pneumonia (Mouton et al., 2001). Other risk factors are tobacco and alcohol use, as well as cognitive decline of the elderly homeless.

Homelessness is an important and growing problem in the developed world. Previous studies have documented a significant burden of illness among homeless persons due to underlying chronic medical conditions, TB, HIV infection, trauma, and mental illnesses and addictions. This burden of chronic illness, and crowded living conditions in shelters, would be expected to be associated with an increased incidence of invasive pneumococcal disease (Plevneshi et al., 2009).

The very high proportion of smokers (95%) among homeless persons with invasive pneumococcal disease may also explain the fact that the rates of invasive infection in homeless persons do not decrease during the summer months in parallel to decreases in invasive infection in other adults per recent studies. If homeless persons have higher carriage rates of *S. pneumonia* and the high carriage rate persists in the summer, transmission might also explain the relative excess of summer disease. However, one would expect crowding to be greater in winter months when shelters are used more often (Mouton et al., 2001).

Pneumonia is prevalent among the elderly homeless year round. It is a source of high morbidity and mortality, creating the need for early diagnosis and improved community living centers. This could improve the spread and treatment outcomes of the elderly suffering from CAP.

Foot Infections

Foot conditions are an important concern among homeless individuals. Risk factors are history of diabetes, hypertension, and peripheral vascular disease. The condition of shoes, socks, and foot odor was identified by participants as a major deterrent to using foot care services (Muirhead et al., 2009).

Foot problems are prevalent among the homeless and are often attributed to extended exposure to moisture, poor footwear, prolonged standing and walking, poor foot hygiene, and repetitive trauma. Foot infections may be complicated by peripheral neuropathy associated with alcoholism and diabetes, as well as peripheral arterial disease (Muirhead et al., 2009).

Cellulitis is an inflammatory condition of the skin and subcutaneous tissue, characterized by erythema, swelling, warmth, and pain. The etiologic agents are most often *Streptococcus pyogenes* and *Staphylococcus aureus*, followed by nongroup A B-hemolytic streptococci and gram-negative bacilli (Plevneshi et al., 2009).

Toe webs that are colonized by or infected with potential bacterial pathogens are significant sites of entry for the causative organisms. Risk factors are obesity, h/o cellulitis, chronic leg edema, disruption of the cutaneous barrier, and toe web dermatophytosis (Bjornsdottir et al., 2005).

Bacterial infections are widespread and significant in the homeless adult. Poor foot hygiene, unsanitary living conditions, long periods of standing and walking, repetitive trauma from ill-fitting shoes, and macerated skin from wet socks and shoes predispose patients to abrasions, abscesses, and cellulitis. Prolonged standing leads to edema and venous stasis, which may lead to ulcerations and cellulitis requiring subsequent hospitalizations (Muirhead et al., 2009).

Research is needed to determine the effectiveness of foot protocols and foot care models that are designed to improve use of health services, increase positive health outcomes, and reduce health risk and consequences in the homeless population (Bjornsdottir et al., 2005).

According to past studies, compared with the general U.S. population, homeless persons are three to six times more likely to become ill, their hospitalization rates are four times higher, and they are three to four times more likely to die at a younger age (White et al., 2014).

Homeless persons tend to have the same medical conditions as the general population. They differ from the general population, however, in that they experience long-term exposure to the disease agents according to Maness and Khan (2014). Their distrust can affect their ability to respond appropriately to these adverse conditions and manage their medical problems. Based on these factors, homeless persons tend to present with advanced disease, and the approach to therapy is different depending on each person's situation (Maness & Khan, 2014).

In the homeless person, the association of one or more chronic illnesses with substance abuse or mental illness appears to increase the risk of early death. Compared to the general U.S. population, homeless persons are three to six times more likely to become ill, their hospitalization rates are four times higher, and they are three to four times more likely to die at a younger age (Maness & Khan, 2014).

Many homeless adults have multiple hospitalizations with complications due to lack of regular primary care. Homeless patients rely heavily on emergency departments (EDs) for healthcare services for conditions that are manageable with timely and appropriate primary care (White et al., 2014). Access to healthcare, lack of trust in the system, lack of clean environment, and the increasing elderly homeless population make treating pneumonia very challenging, according to the experts.

Many homeless individuals experience difficulties retaining a usual source of care due to a lack of health insurance. Consequently, many homeless individuals have worse health outcomes for preventable conditions than the general population (White et al., 2014). Future studies are needed to identify the direction needed to improve our national homeless healthcare due to the cost of caring for this population. There is very little research on the elderly homeless and bacterial infections. The three most common infections are UTIs, bacterial pneumonia, and skin infections. Elderly homeless are particularly vulnerable to these infections and often have very poor treatment outcomes. Improvement of access to care is paramount in contributing to the needs of this overlooked population.

TUBERCULOSIS

Marilee Nebelsick-Tagg

TB is one of the top 10 causes of death worldwide. In 2015, 10.4 million people were infected with TB and 1.8 million died as the result. Of these deaths, over 95% occurred in low- and middle-income countries largely due to the limitation in resources to treat these individuals. Six countries account for 60% of the new TB cases, with India leading, followed by Indonesia, China, Nigeria, Pakistan, and South Africa (World Health Organization, 2017).

Worldwide, TB affects all age groups. Most studies and reports put the highest rates globally among those 45 to 55 years old. But, many reports also indicate that the rate of TB is increasing in those over the age of 65 years. This increase in the older adults is likely to pose major challenges to control and treatment of this disease globally.

This increase in the geriatric population can be related to several factors. The elderly living now would have been alive when TB was prevalent. This makes it likely that they have been exposed or infected with the tubercle bacillus at some point. The natural weakening of the immune system with aging predisposes them to reactivation of the disease. This is largely the result of the biological changes associated with the disruption of the protective barriers and impaired microbial clearance mechanisms. The greatest percentage of the cases of TB in this age group is reactivation of the endogenous infection. Acute and chronic disease such as diabetes, along with malnutrition and smoking, increase the risk of development of active infection in the geriatric population.

Living arrangements also contribute to this increase. Many of the elderly throughout the world live in a communal type of arrangement. This living style encompasses those who live with family, friends, or in some type of facility such as nursing homes or assisted-living communities. Another increase is seen in the homeless population because of the close contact associated with this type of lifestyle. In addition, the comorbidities associated with the homeless, malnutrition, poverty, and lack of access to adequate healthcare contribute to this increase (Centers for Disease Control and Prevention [CDC], 1992; Thomas & Rajagopalan, 2001).

Estimates of the world's homeless population plus those living in poor housing are approaching 1 billion. In 2015, 564,708 people were experiencing homelessness in the United States (World Health Organization, n.d.). Homelessness encompasses all age groups. Specific figures for the elderly homeless are lacking. In addition, the overall incidence of active TB and the prevalence of latent TB infection among the homeless are unknown. The prevalence of clinical active disease ranges from 1.6% to 6.8%, and the prevalence of latent TB infection ranges from 18% to 51% (CDC, 1992).

Because TB is a major problem among the homeless, recommendations to prevent and control TB in this population are important. The highest priority should focus on detecting, evaluating, and reporting homeless individuals with TB and completing the appropriate course of therapy for those with active disease. Additional priorities should address screening and preventing therapy for those with or likely to have HIV, developing treatment plans for those who were inadequately treated, and screening and treating those exposed to infection and those with known medical conditions that increase the risk of TB such as diabetes, smoking, and malnutrition (CDC, 1992).

Once a homeless person is diagnosed with TB, the focus should be on developing a treatment plan that is appropriate for the individual. Efforts are made to actively engage the person in the plan of care. It is essential that rapport between all healthcare providers and the patient is established and maintained.

All providers need to remember that the patient's priorities may not be on TB treatment, but rather on shelter, food, and safety.

To help assure a successful treatment outcome, the patient must be carefully monitored. Failure of the individual to take all the medications as prescribed can result in relapses, drug resistance, increased transmission to others, and even death. Research supports the use of direct observation treatment plans to help increase adherence to therapy. ʼ

TB clinics for the homeless should be located close to shelters or other places that provide services to this population. If that cannot be done, then transportation to the clinic needs to be arranged. The hours of operation need to match what is appropriate for the homeless in the area. Incentives and rewards are also shown to encourage adherence to the plan of care. These rewards can include food, vouchers, cash, lodging, clothing, priority in getting food or a place to sleep, and assistance in filing needed paperwork for other benefits. Treatment outcomes are likely to be more successful if the patient has a reliable source of food and shelter for the duration of therapy.

Regardless of the risk factors for TB or the characteristic of the individual, the pathogenesis of TB involves a well-integrated disease mechanism. The primary route of entry for the bacteria and organ of the disease is the lung. Bronchial airflow allows the tubercle bacilli to enter the basal segments of the lower, middle lingual, or anterior segments of the upper lobe, all of which are the usual segments that are infected. With the elderly, however, several studies reveal that, for this age group, the middle or lower lobes are involved (Byng-Maddick & Norsadeghi, 2016; Negin, Abinbola, & Marais, 2015; Thomas & Rajagopalan, 2001).

TB bacteria persist in the air and spread more easily in dark, poorly ventilated, and overcrowded areas. This fact increases the risk of infection for those who are living in homeless shelters, as well as slums, shanty towns, and other make-shift arrangements. The immune stresses associated with homelessness such as rough sleeping, cold, malnutrition, drinking, and drug abuse further increase the chances of exposure and development of infection.

With the elderly, these immune stresses and the normal dysregulation that occurs with aging may play a role in the recurrence of the disease in those who were never exposed, those with reactivated latent and dormant infection, and those who are no longer infected, but are at risk for reinfection (CDC, 1992).

TB in the geriatric and homeless population is harder to diagnose. One of the reasons for this is the atypical presenting symptoms. Many do not have the classical symptoms of cough, hemoptysis, fever, night sweats, and weight loss. Instead, they may present with a decline in their functional status, chronic fatigue, cognitive impairment, anorexia, or unexplained low-grade fever. Practitioners should be alerted to these nonspecific symptoms in this population and suspect TB, especially if productive cough and fever are present for more than one to three weeks. With the homeless elderly, healthcare providers should also look for disseminated or military TB, TB meningitis, and skeletal or genitourinary TB (Byng-Maddick & Norsadeghi, 2016; Negin, Abinbola, & Marais, 2015; Thomas & Rajagopalan, 2001).

Sputum examination and x-rays must be pursued. The smear and culture examination should be done for all those individuals with pulmonary symptoms and/or radiographic evidence of disease or those who have not been previously treated for TB. If sputum samples cannot be obtained, then a more aggressive test should be considered for sputum sample collection. To help with diagnosis, tests such as the nucleic acid amplification, or other rapid diagnostic procedures, should be considered for this population.

Treatment issues with the homeless and elderly also play a role in the control of this infection. Many studies report the increased likelihood of adverse drug effects with these individuals. The results of these studies need to be carefully reviewed to assure that important factors that could affect serum concentration are adequately addressed. Hepatotoxicity and acute kidney injury remain at higher risk with this population (Byng-Maddick & Norsadeghi, 2016; Negin, Abinbola, & Marais, 2015; Thomas & Rajagopalan, 2001).

The standard regimen for treating TB in the homeless and elderly is the same as the general population. This regimen includes use of the following medications: isoniazid (INH), rifampicin, ethambutol, and pyrazinamide. The drug combination used and duration of treatment varies depending on the bacterial sensitivities, epidemiology of the area, type of infection—active or latent, and overall health of the individual being treated. Recent studies have supported the use of fewer drugs and shorter time frames with positive results. One such treatment regimen is for weekly dosing of the medications for 12 weeks. Currently, the shorter time frames and decreased medications have been used for younger adults. Studies on the effectiveness of these types of regimens will need to be considered for the geriatric population in the future. Newer drugs, bedaquiline, delamanid, and linezolid, have been tried as add-on therapy for those with multidrug-resistant infection.

The drugs used to treat TB need to be modified based on what is available in the area. Because of the cost, fewer options are available worldwide. All treatment plans need to be tailored to the individual's overall health, medications available, support systems, and cost. A strong recommendation for all treatment options is the use of a combination of medications. Monotherapy is not advised secondary to the increased risk of the development of drug resistance if this option is used (Nahid et al., 2016).

TB is a treatable and curable disease. The clear majority of TB cases can be cured when medicines are provided and taken properly. Between 2000 and 2015, an estimated 49 million lives were saved through TB diagnosis and treatment (World Health Organization, 2016).

ARTHROPODS INFESTATION

Ashkan Vafadaran and Elham Faroughi

The majority of arthropods (joint-legged invertebrates) are not harmful to humans. A number of species are considered medically important because they may affect human health by direct exposure or indirectly (allergy, disease transmission, fear of insects, or infestation) (Telford, 2011).

Homeless people suffer infestations at a rate three times higher than the general adult population. The higher prevalence of skin infections in the homeless people mainly results from the body louse infestation, scabies, and bacterial super-infection of skin surfaces that have been breached by frequent scratching (Badiaga, Menard, et al., 2005). The environments in which they live, from crowded shelters to outdoor camps, lack of hygiene, and their overall poor physical and mental health place homeless people at risk for secondary infections and serious illnesses (Hale et al., 2005).

Many functional, demographic, and immunologic changes associated with aging are responsible for increasing the incidence and severity of infectious diseases in the elderly. One must be aware that the geriatric population can present with certain challenges with regard to diagnosis of these diseases because history taking may be more difficult, and patients often already have a set of other medical problems, which may overshadow the skin lesions. In addition, the clinical manifestations of these infections may not appear classical and may be altered. Management is complicated by age-related organ system changes. Because many of the elderly are on multiple medications for underlying illnesses, antimicrobial therapy needs to be chosen, keeping drug interactions and adverse events in mind. Dosages of drugs used to treat these infections, even topical agents, may require adjustments in this population. In addition, stigma attached to such infestations may affect the type of care homeless people receive (Htwe, Mushtaq, Robinson, Rosher, & Khardori, 2007; Tan & Goh, 2001).

In this chapter, the focus will be the arthropods of medical importance encountered in the United States. These include lice, scabies mites, and bed bugs, with lesser emphasis on ticks, fleas, and other arthropods.

Lice

Pediculosis is an infestation of human lice, which include *Pediculus humanus* (head lice and body lice) and *Phthirus pubis* (pubic "crab" lice). Body lice have three forms: the egg (also called a nit), the nymph, and the adult. All species produce oval eggs (**nits**), usually yellow to white in color, that are attached firmly to the base of a hair shaft (head and pubic lice) or to clothing (body lice). A **nymph** is an immature louse that hatches from the nit. The **adult** body louse is about the size of a sesame seed, has six legs, and is tan to grayish-white. Adult body and head lice are morphologically indistinguishable by the unaided human eye. Pubic lice are 1 to 2 mm in length and have a "crab"-like appearance. Lice do not jump or fly (Bonilla, Kabeya, Henn, Kramer, & Kosoy, 2009; Buchanan, Cleary, Williams, & May, 2004b; CDC, n.d.).

Epidemiology

Infestations occur in essentially every area of the world inhabited by humans. Major epidemics have occurred during times of war, overcrowding, or widespread inattention to personal hygiene. **Head lice** infestation occurs worldwide, with a reported incidence of 12 million cases per year in the United States. It affects all socioeconomic and ethnic groups. It occurs most often in school children and may also occur in the homeless population where the lice may be transferred by pillow cases, hats, and combs. Of note, hair length is not an important risk factor for infestation. **Body lice** infestations occur primarily in settings with low income, poor hygiene, and overcrowded living conditions (as seen with homeless individuals). Epidemics of diseases transmitted by body lice have been seen typically in areas where climate, poverty, war, and social upheaval prevent regular changes and laundering of clothing. **Pubic lice** infestations primarily affect sexually active individuals, particularly teenagers and young adults, and often exist concurrently with other sexually transmitted infections (Bonilla et al., 2009; Buchanan et al., 2004b; CDC, n.d.; Faith-Fernandez & Tomecki, 2012).

Transmission of all forms of human lice requires close contact. **Head lice** are transmitted via close personal (head-to-head) contact and sharing of hats, grooming implements (e.g., combs, brushes), and towels. It is transmitted less often by fomites. **Body lice** are transmitted by contact with infested persons, who usually live in close, crowded conditions and cannot bathe or change clothes regularly. **Pubic lice** are transmitted primarily via sexual or skin contact. Dogs, cats, and other pets do not play a role in the transmission of human lice (Bonilla et al., 2009; Buchanan et al., 2004b; CDC, n.d.).

Signs, Symptoms, and Diagnosis

Intense itching ("pruritus") is the hallmark of all forms of lice infestation. Eczematous changes and secondary bacterial infection can follow a patient's scratching. **Head lice** nits initially attach to the base of the hair shaft. The presence of head lice or nits establishes the diagnosis. The presence of nits alone can simply indicate past infestation. Brushing with a fine-toothed comb can enhance detection of head lice. **Body lice** are usually not seen until a person has been heavily infested. Numerous nits are typically found in clothing seams. **Pubic lice** most commonly infect the pubis and usually do not move far from the initial site of contact. Up to one-third of those with pubic lice may have another sexually transmitted infection (Bonilla et al., 2009; Buchanan et al., 2004b; CDC, n.d.).

Body lice are known to transmit disease. The body louse is an efficient vector for *Bartonella quintana* (trench fever), *Rickettsia prowazekii* (Epidemic typhus), and *Borrelia recurrentis* (louse-borne relapsing fever). *Bartonella quintana* is the most common louse-borne disease reported in the urban homeless (Badiaga, Raoult, & Brouqui, 2008). Since 1992, *B. quintana* has been recognized as a reemerging infection in homeless populations in the United States and Europe, as well as an opportunistic pathogen in patients with AIDS (Bonilla et al., 2009). It causes a wide range of diseases, some of which occur more frequently in the homeless population, including trench fever, chronic bacteremia, endocarditis, and bacillary angiomatosis (Badiaga, Raoult, & Brouqui, 2008). It has been shown that, in homeless individuals with cutaneous parasitic infestations, increasing age of the individual and number of years of homelessness are both independently associated with a positive *B. quintana* serology (Buchanan et al., 2004b).

Scabies Mites

The scabies mite is a parasite that completes its entire life cycle on humans. Only female mites burrow into the skin. About 5 to 15 female mites live on a host infected with classic scabies, but the number can reach hundreds or even millions in cases of crusted scabies. The skin eruption of classic scabies is considered a consequence of both infestation and a hypersensitivity reaction to the mite (Chosidow, 2006).

Epidemiology

The worldwide prevalence of scabies is uncertain. The prevalence undergoes cyclical fluctuations on a worldwide basis. The estimated prevalence ranges from 0.2% to 71% (lowest in Europe and the Middle East and highest in the Pacific and Latin American regions), with as many as 100 million people affected worldwide (no data available for North America) (Romani, Steer, Whitfeld, & Kaldor, 2015). Scabies occurs in both sexes, at all ages, in all ethnic groups, and at all socioeconomic levels. Crowded conditions increase the prevalence of scabies in the population (Chosidow, 2006).

Scabies is more prevalent in the homeless than in the general population. The reported prevalence of scabies varies from 3.8% in shelter-based investigations to 56.5% among hospitalized homeless persons (Badiaga, Raoult, & Brouqui, 2008). The risk of severe outbreaks and complicated scabies is particularly high in institutions (including nursing homes and hospitals) and among socially disadvantaged populations and immune-compromised hosts (Chosidow, 2006).

Signs, Symptoms, and Diagnosis

Classically, scabies presents as a pruritic skin eruption. Classic manifestations of scabies include generalized and intense itching, usually sparing the face and head. Pruritus is worse at night. Physical examination typically reveals the presence of the burrows (thread-like, wavy lesions terminating in small vesicles that harbor the female mites) (Chosidow, 2006; Wilson, Philpott, & Breer, 2001). Although pathognomonic for scabies, they are not always easily identified. Typical skin disease is erythematous papules and vesicles in the interdigital spaces, flexural surface of the wrists and elbows, axillae, areolae, and genitals. Secondary changes, such as excoriations, eczema, and secondary infection, often follow and may occur anywhere, especially if disease is persistent. Atypical papular scabies occurs in the elderly, localized or generalized crusted scabies in immunocompromised patients, and impetigo in patients whose scabies is superinfected. Pruritus may be mild or absent (i.e., scabies incognito).

Diagnosis of scabies is based on clinical presentation and demonstration of the mite or eggs (or both) microscopically. It rests largely on the history and examination of the patient, as well as on the history of the family and close contacts (Buchanan et al., 2004c; Chosidow, 2006; Faith-Fernandez & Tomecki, 2012).

Special Considerations in the Elderly

Host factors are a determinant of the clinical manifestation of scabies; therefore, the clinical presentation of scabies may vary in older or cognitively impaired persons. The itch–scratch cycle in scabies may also be affected by aging. The onset of pruritus in scabies coincides with the development of the immune response. Reduced hypersensitivity due to altered lymphocyte function in elderly persons may suppress itching. The coexistence of cognitive or functional disability in the older adult may impair the ability to scratch, and thus prevent effective elimination of the mite. These factors, acting in concert, may explain the tendency for scabies to assume a more generalized distribution in older adults. The absence of epidermal undulations in aging skin may reduce impedance and allow the adult mite to travel further as it seeks a site to burrow. An increase in skin renewal time and reduction in shedding are other age-related skin changes. These changes may reduce the rate of scabies transmission from an infested older adult and have some bearing on the absence of reported scabies among the staff in the facility. Often, secondary infection is already present, complicating the picture and delaying the diagnosis. The elderly patient may experience toxicity from local or systemic scabicidal treatment.

Elderly and immunocompromised hosts are at risk for a severe "crusted" form of scabies. Crusted scabies, also known as Norwegian scabies, is a hyperinfestation with thousands of mites that results from the host's inability to mount an immune response to control the infestation. The load of parasite is much higher (generally thousands of mites as opposed to 5 to 10 mites in more classic scabies), and the disease is, therefore, much more contagious (Buchanan et al., 2004c; Faith-Fernandez & Tomecki, 2012; Tjioe & Vissers, 2008; Wilson et al., 2001; Wooltorton, 2003).

Prevention and Control

Scabies can be transmitted by direct and prolonged skin-to-skin contact with a person who has scabies. Scabies can also be transmitted by sharing bedding or clothing (fomites). The disease spreads easily to household members, roommates, and sexual partners of a person with scabies. Scabies can spread more easily in crowded settings like hospitals, nursing homes, and homeless shelters (Buchanan et al., 2004c). Persons who have prolonged skin-to-skin contact with the infested person, but not those with more casual contact, should be treated. Prescriptions should be provided for all household members and any sexual contacts, even if they are asymptomatic. In institutional settings, patient care staff and support staff (e.g., cleaning staff and laundry employees) should be considered to have been exposed to infested persons.

The spread of classic scabies without direct person-to-person contact is rare. Ideally, clothes and bed linens should be machine washed at 60°C and machine dried the day after the first treatment; insecticide powder or aerosolized insecticide is generally reserved for materials that cannot be laundered. Items may also be kept in a sealed plastic bag for at least 48 to 72 hours. On the basis of the survival of mites, only clothes and linens that were in contact with the patient during the previous 48 to 72 hours warrant these cleaning procedures (Buchanan et al., 2004c; Chosidow, 2006).

Bed Bugs

Common bed bugs (*Cimex lectularius*) are small but easily visible (approximately 5 mm), flat, and wingless parasitic insects that cannot fly or jump and feed solely on the blood of people while they sleep. A bed bug is light brown as a nymph and reddish-brown in color as it matures to adulthood. Adults may survive for long periods of time without feeding (up to a year). *Cimex hemipterus*, the tropical bedbug, is occasionally found in Florida and is distinguished by a longer pointed body (Buchanan et al., 2004a; CDC, n.d.).

Bed bugs hide in cracks and crevices in beds, wooden furniture, floors, and walls during the daytime and emerge at night to feed on their preferred host, humans. Bed bugs cannot fly and are transferred from place to place in luggage, bedding, and used furniture. Dispersal of human-associated bed bugs generally depends on their human hosts for movement from one location to another. Given the constant turnover of shelter residents, bed bugs could potentially affect a large number of homeless people over the course of a year. Their population can increase dramatically in a short period of time if the issue is overlooked or ignored. Bed bugs have not been shown to transmit diseases, despite their evolution as a blood-feeding pest of humans (Buchanan et al., 2004a; Goddard & deShazo, 2009; Hwang, Svoboda, De Jong, Kabasele, & Gogosis, 2005).

Epidemiology

The common bed bug has re-emerged as a significant pest of humans in the United States, Canada, Europe, Australia, and other developed countries after a 40-year period of near absence. Bed bug infestations have been reported increasingly in the United States since 1980. For example, reports of bed bug infestations in San Francisco doubled between 2004 and 2006. The resurgence affects other countries as well (Buchanan et al., 2004a; Goddard & deShazo, 2009).

Bed bugs are an increasingly common cause of pruritic rashes among homeless people in shelters. The appearance of bed bugs in homeless shelters is becoming increasingly problematic. The transient lifestyle of the homeless population makes them particularly vulnerable to bed bugs due to potential exposure to bed bug infestations in emergency shelters, transitional housing, and so on. After being exposed, they can inadvertently move bed bugs from place to place, including into homeless shelters (Michigan Department of Community Health & Michigan Bed Bug Working Group, 2010).

Signs, Symptoms, and Diagnosis

Medical issues associated with bed bugs include multiple itchy bites and inflammation, secondary skin infection, a minor potential for anemia from blood loss, minor risk of anaphylaxis, stress, anxiety, sleeplessness, asthma exacerbations, or other systemic responses, and the potential for overexposure to pesticides used in their control. Anemia has been reported in the elderly and very young in cases where homes are heavily infested.

Bites occur in clusters or lines, in open areas of the skin, and where clothing is not tight, usually on exposed areas of the face, neck, and extremities, and generally spare the intertrigenous regions and areas under tight clothing that are commonly affected by scabies. Lesions are often arranged in a linear fashion in groups of three, known as the "breakfast, lunch, dinner" pattern. An itchy night-time dermatitis, especially grouped papules, should suggest bed bug bites. Patients typically present with multiple pruritic bites that are usually noticed when arising in the morning. Skin manifestations of the bites present in a variety of ways, depending on the degree of immunological response.

The diagnosis of bed bug bites is suggested by the history and physical exam and is confirmed by characteristic findings in the living space or by a positive identification of the offending bug. Bites are usually the early warning sign of a bed bug infestation. Skin reactions to bites vary widely from practically no reaction, to small itchy red or white bumps, to blisters or pustules. Not every person in a household will react the same way, and many times, only one person will show signs of bites, leading others to believe it cannot be bed bugs. It is difficult, if not impossible, to distinguish bed bug bites from those of other biting pests without other circumstantial evidence that will link to a specific pest. It is critical to confirm bed bugs in the sleeping or living area through inspection to be sure that bites are caused by bed bugs. Bed bug bites can resemble mosquito and flea bites (Buchanan et al., 2004a; Faith-Fernandez & Tomecki, 2012; Gangloff-Kaufmann & Pichler, 2008).

Other Arthropods

There are other causes of bites and lesions aside from lice, scabies mites, and bed bugs. Spiders, mosquitoes, ticks, fleas, and ants also pose risks for homeless people, particularly those who live outdoors. Homeless people can have a difficult time avoiding bites from mosquitoes and ticks, which can carry diseases. They often are outside during the peak hours of mosquito activity, from dusk to dawn, and they may have no access to insect repellent. While bites can vary, the activities of the person bitten may help determine the cause.

- Fleas—Flea bites are usually associated with the presence of animals serving as flea hosts, such as pets and occasionally wildlife. Fleas tend to leave multiple bites on the arms and legs. Fleas can transmit disease.
- Spiders—Spiders leave behind one or two puncture wounds when they bite. Bites are usually associated with some localized pain. The venom of the brown recluse spider is toxic to human cells and tissues and may cause significant necrosis (tissue death). However, such bites are rare, and most necrotic wounds diagnosed as brown recluse bites are something else. One of the problems in diagnosing a brown recluse spider bite, even in the Midwestern and Southeastern states where they are found, is locating the spider to make a definitive diagnosis. Misdiagnosis of a spider bite can delay the needed treatment for serious conditions. Particularly in urban homeless populations, providers should consider that what appears to be a spider bite may be a case of community-acquired MRSA (Hale et al., 2005; Gangloff-Kaufmann & Pichler, 2008).
- Fire ants include the red fire ant and the black fire ant. They are well established in the southeastern United States after their importation from South America in the early 20th century. Approximately 30% to 60% of the residents in that area are stung every year. Fire ants are aggressive critters,

attacking in groups when the anthill is disturbed. The initial bite or sting has a burning sensation followed by an erythematous wheal-and-flare reaction. Within hours, sterile pustules form at the sites of the stings. The pustules are commonly arranged in a rosette or ring pattern, because the ants bite, then pivot and sting in a circular fashion. Anaphylactic reactions occur in 1% of the affected persons, usually within hours of the sting. Local reactions deserve symptomatic treatment with compresses, elevation of the affected extremity, and topical corticosteroids. For anaphylactic reactions, immunotherapy with imported fire ant whole body extract has been effective in selected cases (Faith-Fernandez & Tomecki, 2012).

Delusional Parasitosis

Delusional (delusory) parasitosis (DP) or mystery bites, also known as Ekbom's syndrome, is the feeling or fear that one is being infested with parasitic organisms, which may be accompanied by a physical sensation of itching or crawling on the skin. Sufferers may scratch, injure themselves, apply pesticides to their skin or surroundings, and often compulsively gather evidence of the infestation. Evidence may be in the form of marks on the skin, particles of cloth, fibers, and other debris, and carefully recorded observations of the parasite behaviors. Often, sufferers seek insect- or mite-related causes, and they may have unshakable beliefs that their bodies or surroundings are infested with bed bugs, mites, fleas, and other real and imaginary organisms.

Sufferers commonly compulsively gather such "evidence" and then present it to medical professionals when seeking help. This presentation of "evidence" is known as "the matchbox sign" because the "evidence" is frequently presented in a small container, such as a matchbox. DP is seen more commonly in women, and the frequency is much higher past the age of 40 (https://en.wikipedia.org/wiki/Delusional_parasitosis - cite_note-Ekbom-3).

It is critical to determine whether an insect or mite is present in the living area before considering treatments, especially pesticide use, which may exacerbate itching or other medical conditions. If no arthropod can be identified in the living environment, yet the individual insists that his or herr symptoms are real, or if the individual has inflicted damage upon himself or herself as a result of a perceived infestation, other causes must be explored. Commonly, DP sufferers have medical or psychogenic causes of itching and prickly sensations. Symptoms of DP may be caused by a wide variety of conditions including, but not limited to:

- Diabetes, hyperthyroidism
- Medications

- Drug abuse (including but not limited to cocaine and methamphetamine)
- Hormonal changes
- Mild allergies to environmental stimuli, such as detergents
- Dementia, anxiety, depression, paranoia
- Nutritional deficiencies
- Central nervous system infections

It appears that many of these physiological factors, as well as environmental factors such as airborne irritants, are capable of inducing a "crawling" sensation in otherwise healthy individuals.

Treatment of DP is addressed by treating the primary associated psychological or physical condition. However, it is also characteristic that sufferers will reject the diagnosis of DP by medical professionals, and very few are willing to be treated, despite demonstrable efficacy of treatment (Gangloff-Kaufmann & Pichler, 2008; Hinkle, 2000, 2011; Webb, 1993).

CONCLUSION

Roxana Aminbakhsh

As discussed earlier in the past two chapters, homelessness is a rising healthcare problem. Secondary to poor living situations and limited access to healthcare services, homeless people are at increased risk for exposure to various communicable diseases, including viral and bacterial infections, TB, and arthropod carried diseases. As a result, the homeless population has a higher prevalence of many infectious diseases. On the other hand, many functional and immunologic changes associated with aging are responsible for increasing the incidence and severity of infectious diseases in the elderly. Attention to these important facts is needed for implementing appropriate preventive and curative plans to decrease the incidence and prevalence of infectious diseases among the homeless geriatrics population.

REFERENCES

Badiaga, S., Menard, A., Tissot-Dupont, H., Ravaux, I., Chouquet, D., Graveriau, C., . . . Brouqui, P. (2005). Prevalence of skin infections in sheltered homeless of Marseilles (France). *European Journal of Dermatology*, 15(5), 382–386. Retrieved from http://www.jle.com/fr/revues/ejd/e-docs/prevalence_of_skin_infections_in_sheltered_homeless_of_marseilles_france__266408/article.phtml

Badiaga, S., Raoult, D., & Brouqui, P. (2008). Preventing and controlling emerging and reemerging transmissible diseases in the homeless: Interventions for scabies, body louse infestations, and louse-borne diseases. *Emerging Infectious Diseases*, 14(9), 1353–1359. Retrieved from https://www.ncbi.nlm.nih.gov/pmc/articles/PMC2603102/

Bjornsdottir, S., Gottfredsson, M., Thorisdottir, A. S., Gunnarsson, G. B., Rikardsddottir, H., Kristjansson, M., & Hilmarsddotir, I. (2005). Risk factors for acute cellulitis of the lower limb: A prospective case-control study. *Clinical Infectious Diseases. 41*(10), 1416–1422. Retrieved from https://academic.oup.com/cid/article/41/10/1416/346054

Bonilla, D. L., Kabeya, H., Henn, J., Kramer, V. L., & Kosoy, M. Y. (2009). *Bartonella quintana* in body lice and head lice from homeless persons, San Francisco, California, USA. *CDC Emerging Infectious Diseases, 15*(6), 912–915. Retrieved from https://wwwnc.cdc.gov/eid/articles/issue/15/6/table-of-contents

Buchanan, D., Cleary, C., Williams, K., & May, A. (2004a). Bed bugs. In J. J. O'Connell (Ed.), *The health care of homeless persons: A manual of communicable diseases & common problems in shelters & on the streets* (pp. 3–4). Boston, MA: The Boston Health Care for the Homeless Program. Retrieved from http://www.bhchp.org/health-care-homeless-persons

Buchanan, D., Cleary, C., Williams, K., & May, A. (2004b). Lice. In J. J. O'Connell (Ed.), *The health care of homeless persons: A manual of communicable diseases & common problems in shelters & on the streets* (pp. 73–79). Boston, MA: The Boston Health Care for the Homeless Program. Retrieved from http://www.bhchp.org/health-care-homeless-persons

Buchanan, D., Cleary, C., Williams, K., & May, A. (2004c). Scabies. In J. J. O'Connell (Ed.), *The health care of homeless persons: A manual of communicable diseases & common problems in shelters & on the streets* (pp. 113–116). Boston, MA: The Boston Health Care for the Homeless Program. Retrieved from http://www.bhchp.org/health-care-homeless-persons

Byng-Maddick, R., & Norsadeghi, M. (2016). Does tuberculosis threaten our ageing populations? *BMC Infectious Diseases, 16*(119). doi:10.1186/s12879-016-1451-0

Centers for Disease Control and Prevention. (n.d.). Parasites. Retrieved from https://www.cdc.gov/parasites/index.html

Centers for Disease Control and Prevention. (1992). Prevention and control of tuberculosis among homeless of persons recommendations of the Advisory Council for the Elimination of Tuberculosis. *MMWR Recommendations and Reports, 41*(RR-5), 13–23. Retrieved from https://www.cdc.gov/mmwr/preview/mmwrhtml/00019922.htm

Chosidow, O. (2006). Scabies. *New England Journal of Medicine, 354*(16), 1718–1727.

Faith-Fernandez, E., & Tomecki, K. J. (2012). Bugs, bites, and stings. *Current Clinical Medicine*, 329–333. Retrieved from http://www.clevelandclinicmeded.com/medical-pubs/diseasemanagement/dermatology/bugs-bites-and-stings

Gangloff-Kaufmann, J. L., & Pichler, C. (2008). *Guidelines for prevention and management of bed bugs in shelters and group living facilities*. Geneva: New York State Integrated Pest Management Program. Retrieved from https://ecommons.cornell.edu/bitstream/handle/1813/43862/guidelines-bed-bugs-group-NYSIPM.pdf?sequence=1

Goddard, J., & deShazo, R. (2009). Bed bugs (*Cimex lectularius*) and clinical consequences of their bites. *Journal of the American Medical Association, 301*(13), 1358–1366. Retrieved from https://www.ncbi.nlm.nih.gov/pubmed/19336711

Hale, A., Allen, J., Caughlan, J., Harrison, F., Hartford, L., Hines, L., . . . Post P. (2005). Bugs that bite: Helping homeless people and shelter staff cope. *Healing Hands, 9*(1), 1–4. Retrieved from https://www.nhchc.org/wp-content/uploads/2012/03/Feb2005HealingHands.pdf

Hinkle, N. C. (2000). Delusory parasitosis. *American Entomologist, 46*(1), 17–25. Retrieved from https://academic.oup.com/ae/article/46/1/17/2389588

Hinkle, N. C. (2011). Ekbom syndrome: A delusional condition of "bugs in the skin." *Current Psychiatry Reports, 13*(3), 178–186. Retrieved from http://entnemdept.ifas.ufl.edu/sepmc/HANDOUTS2015/Hinkle_HO_SEPMC2015.pdf

Htwe, T. H., Mushtaq, A., Robinson, S. B., Rosher, R. B., & Khardori, N. (2007). Infection in the elderly. *Infectious Disease Clinics of North America, 21*(3), 711–743. Retrieved from https://www.sciencedirect.com/journal/infectious-disease-clinics-of-north-america/vol/21/issue/3

Hwang, S. W., Svoboda, T. J., De Jong, I. J., Kabasele, K. J., & Gogosis, E. (2005). Bed bug infestations in an urban environment. *Emerging Infectious Diseases, 11*(4), 533–538. Retrieved from https://www.ncbi.nlm.nih.gov/pmc/articles/PMC3320350/

Maness, D. L., & Khan, M. (2014). Care of the homeless: An overview. *American Family Physician, 89*(8), 634–640. Retrieved from http://www.aafp.org/afp/2014/0415/p634. html

Metersky, M. L., Masterton, R. G., Lode, H., File Jr., T. M., & Babinchak, T. (2012). Epidemiology, microbiology, and treatment considerations for bacterial pneumonia complicating influenza. *International Journal of Infectious Diseases.* doi:10.1016/j. ijid.2012.01.003

Michigan Department of Community Health & Michigan Bed Bug Working Group. (2010, September). *Michigan manual for the prevention and control of bed bugs: Comprehensive guidance to identify, treat, manage and prevent bed bugs* (Version 1.01). Retrieved from http://www.michigan.gov/documents/emergingdiseases/Bed_Bug_Manual_v1_full_reduce_326605_7.pdf

Mouton, C. P., Bazaldua, O. V., Pierce, B., & Espino, D. V. (2001). Common infections in older adults. *American Family Physician, 63,* 257–268. Retrieved from www.aafp.org/afp

Muirhead, L., Roberson, A. J., & Secrest, J. (2009). Utilization of foot care services among homeless adults: Implications for advanced practice nurses. *Journal of the American Academy of Nurse Practitioners, 23,* 209–215. doi:10.1111/j.1745-7599.2011.00598.x

Nahid, P., Dorman, S. E., Alipanah, N., Barry, P. M., Brozek, J. L., Cattamanchi, A., . . . Vernon, A. (2016). Official American Thoracic Society/Centers for Disease Control and Prevention/Infectious Disease Society of America clinical practice guideline: Treatment of drug–susceptible tuberculosis. *Clinical Infectious Diseases, 63*(7), e147–e195. Retrieved from https://academic.oup.com/cid/article/63/7/e147/2196792

Negin, J., Abinbola, S., & Marais, B. J. (2015). Tuberculosis among older adults—time to take notice. *International Journal of Infectious Disease, 32,* 135–137. Retrieved from https://www.sciencedirect.com/journal/international-journal-of-infectious-diseases/vol/32

Plevneshi, A., Svoboda, T., Armstrong, I., Tyrrell, G. J., Miranda, A., Green, K., . . . McGeer, A. (2009). Population-based surveillance for invasive pneumococcal disease in homeless adults in Toronto [Entire issue]. *PLOS ONE, 4*(9). Retrieved from www.plosone. org

Romani, L., Steer, A. C., Whitfield, M. J., & Kaldor, J. M. (2015). Prevalence of scabies and impetigo worldwide: A systematic review. *The Lancet Infectious Diseases, 15*(8), 960–967. Retrieved from http://www.thelancet.com/journals/laninf/article/PIIS1473-3099(17)30469-3/fulltext

Rowe, T. A., & Juthani-Mehta, M. (2013). Urinary tract infection in older adults. *Aging Health, 9*(5), 519–528. doi:10.2217/ahe.13.38. Retrieved from https://www.future medicine.com/toc/ahe/9/5

Stevenson, S. (2015). The 5 most common infections in the elderly. *Senior Living.* Retrieved from http://www.aplaceformom.com/blog/2013-10-22-common-elderly-infections

Tan, H. H., & Goh, C.-L. (2001). Parasitic skin infections in the elderly—recognition and drug treatment. *Drugs and Aging, 18*(3), 165–176. Retrieved from https://www.ncbi .nlm.nih.gov/pubmed/11302284

Telford, S. (2011). Arthropods of medical importance. In J. Versalovic, K. Carroll, G. Funke, J. Jorgensen, M. Landry, & D. Warnock (Eds.), *Manual of clinical microbiology* (10th ed., pp. 2255–2274). Washington, DC: ASM Press.

Thomas, T. Y., & Rajagopalan, S. (2001). Tuberculosis and aging: A global health problem. *Clinical Infectious Disease, 33*(7), 1034–1039. doi:10.1086/322671. Retrieved from https://academic.oup.com/cid/article/33/7/1034/429393

Tjioe, M., & Vissers, W. H. (2008). Scabies outbreaks in nursing homes for the elderly, recognition, treatment options and control of reinfestation. *Drugs and Aging, 25*(4), 299–306.

University of Maryland Medical Center. (2017). Pneumonia. Retrieved from https://umm.edu/health/medical/reports/articles/pneumonia

Webb, J. P., Jr. (1993). Case histories of individuals with delusions of parasitosis in Southern California and a proposed protocol for initiating effective medical assistance. *Bulletin of the Society of Vector Ecologists, 18*(1), 16–24. Retrieved from https://academic.oup.com/cid/article/33/7/1034/429393

White, B. M., Ellis, Jr, C., & Simpson, K. N. (2014). Preventable hospital admissions among the homeless in California: A retrospective analysis of care for ambulatory care sensitive conditions. *BMC Health Services Research, 14*(1). doi:10.1186/s12913-014-0511-7

Wilson, M. G., Philpott, C. D., & Breer, W. A. (2001). Atypical presentation of scabies among nursing home residents. *Journal of Gerontology, 56A*(7), M424–M427. Retrieved from https://academic.oup.com/biomedgerontology/subscribe

Wooltorton, E. (2003). Concerns over lindane treatment for scabies and lice. *Canadian Medical Association Journal, 168*(11), 1447–1448. Retrieved from https://www.ncbi.nlm.nih.gov/pmc/journals/188/

World Health Organization. (2016). *Global tuberculosis report 2016.* Geneva, Switzerland: Author. World Health Organization. (n.d.). Ending Global TB 2035. Retrieved from https://www.ncbi.nlm.nih.gov/pmc/journals/188/

World Health Organization. (2017). Tuberculosis fact sheet. Retrieved from http://www.who.int/mediacentre/factsheets/fs104/en

9

Cardiovascular Disease in Homeless Older Adults

Beth Palmer, Amin Sabet, Dianne M. McGuirk, and Shannon Slama

CASE STUDY

J.G., a 59-year-old chronically homeless African American man, was brought to a Veterans Affairs (VA) homeless clinic by a VA outreach social worker. Several years earlier, the VA had identified him as a vulnerable person, but because he had no address or phone number, he was difficult to find and engage. Eventually, the outreach staff found him sleeping in front of a church downtown. The church staff allowed the outreach workers to leave messages for J.G. The social workers were then successful at getting him registered for VA healthcare and placed him in temporary housing at a local shelter.

Social History: J.G. was born and raised in Illinois. He served honorably in the U.S. Marine Corps, but became homeless shortly after his military discharge in 1975. A review of the records indicated he was diagnosed with schizophrenia while on active duty, but was not receiving a service-connected compensation for this illness. He was unable to obtain gainful employment post-discharge and became homeless. He then began to use illicit substances, including cocaine, heroin, methamphetamines, and alcohol. At the time of his presentation to the homeless outreach clinic, J.G. had been homeless most of the prior 40 years He was addicted to methamphetamines, estranged from his family, and was collecting cans for a living.

Past Medical History: J.G carried diagnoses of hypertension, hyperlipidemia, chronic hepatitis C, and schizophrenia. Approximately one year prior to his presentation at the VA homeless clinic, J.G. was diagnosed with heart failure with reduced ejection fraction (EF 20%). In the prior year, he had been seen in the emergency department (ED) more than 30 times and was hospitalized 20 times for decompensated heart failure. The records indicated that he continued to abuse methamphetamines and was non-compliant with his heart failure medications.

Multiple studies suggest that mortality rates in the adult homeless are higher than the general population (Baggett, Hwang, et al., 2013; Beijer, Andreasson, Ågren, & Fugelstad, 2011; Kasprow & Rosenheck, 2000; LePage, Bradshaw, Cipher, Crawford, & Hoosyhar, 2014; Schinka, Bossarte, Curtiss, Lapcevic, & Casey, 2016). Homeless mortality ratios vary between countries, but are typically 2 to 5 times those of the age-adjusted general population (Fazel, Geddes, & Kushel, 2014). Older homeless people in the United States die from similar causes as older people in the general population, but on an average of 10 to 15 years earlier (Baggett, Hwang, et al., 2013).

According to the Centers for Disease Control and Prevention (CDC, 2015b), cardiovascular disease (CVD) continues to be the leading cause of death in the United States. Recent estimates are that 92.1 million U.S. adults have CVDs, accounting for over 800,000 deaths in 2014. Homeless people experience chronic stress, malnutrition, and failure to engage in protective health behaviors and preventative medical care. These conditions are associated with an increased prevalence of CVD (Curtis & O'Keefe, 2002; Schinka, Curtis, et al., 2016). Baggett, Hwang, et al. (2015) suggested that CVD has been reduced to the second leading cause of homeless mortality in the United States, with drug overdose being the primary cause. However, the study further indicates that cancer and heart disease remain the leading causes of death in homeless adults over age 45. Nonetheless, chronic disease rates, including CVD, are expected to rise along with the increasing rate of older adult homelessness in the United States (Hahn, Kushel, Bangsberg, Riley, & Moss, 2006). This chapter will examine the risk factors, barriers to prevention, and treatment, and provide care recommendations for older adult homeless persons with CVD.

RISK FACTORS

Increased cardiovascular (CV) morbidity and mortality rates in the homeless are attributable to a complex interaction between traditional and less-traditional CV risk factors. Traditional CV risk factors are hypertension, diabetes, smoking, and hyperlipidemia. Less-traditional risk factors include substance abuse; the psychological stress of fulfilling survival needs, including food, shelter, and safety; and a decrease in diagnostic and preventative medical care. These less-traditional risk factors result in an increased prevalence of and/or poorer control of the traditional risk factors (Jones et al., 2009).

Hypertension

Hypertension is the most common condition seen in primary care. If not detected early, and treated appropriately, hypertension leads to myocardial infarction, heart failure, stroke, renal failure, and death (James et al., 2014). The CDC (2016) estimates that 75 million Americans (32%) have hypertension. The rates of uncontrolled blood pressure among U.S. hypertensive persons aged 40 to 59 years and 60 to 79 years are 19.6% and 24.8%, respectively (Bernstein, Meurer, Plumb, & Jackson, 2015). Several studies between 1990 and 2002 suggested that homeless adults were more likely to have hypertension at younger ages than the general population (Burt, 1999; Gelberg, Linn, & Mayer-Oakes, 1990; Kinchen & Wright, 1991; Kleinman, Freeman, Perlman, & Gelberg 1996; Szerlip & Szerlip, 2002; Wright, 1990). Although a recent meta-analysis by Bernstein et al. (2015) suggested no difference in hypertension prevalence between the homeless and general population, a recent study by Asgary (2016) found a greater than 40% rate of uncontrolled blood pressure among homeless adults using New York City shelter-based clinics.

A high prevalence of smoking, substance abuse, chronic stress, and lack of healthy food may play a role in higher rates of uncontrolled blood pressure in homeless adults (Bernstein et al., 2015; Szerlip & Szerlip, 2002). Additionally, it has been suggested that a lack of health insurance is a strong predictor of uncontrolled blood pressure among hypertensive homeless adults (Hwang, Orav, O'Connell, Lebow, & Brennan, 1997).

Diabetes

Diabetes is the seventh leading cause of death in the United States and is a major contributor to CVD. Although a recent meta-analysis by Bernstein et al. (2015) suggested no difference in diabetes prevalence between the homeless and general populations, the CDC has consistently identified socioeconomic disparities in the increasing prevalence rate of diabetes in the United States (CDC, 2013). Homeless diabetics typically suffer from poor glycemic control. The most commonly reported challenges are related to diet, access to healthcare, medications and supplies, and the coordination of medications with meals (Zlotnick & Zerger, 2009).

Tobacco Dependence

Tobacco dependence is a major risk factor for CVD (CDC, 2017b). In comparison, cigarette smoking is more prevalent in homeless persons than in the general population (Szerlip & Szerlip, 2002). A large Canadian study reported double the rate of smoking-related deaths among the homeless when compared with stably housed people (Hwang, Wilkins, Tjepkema, O'Campo, & Dunn, 2009). Multiple factors create challenges for cessation or reducing tobacco use in this population. Homeless smokers have a high burden of nicotine dependence, psychiatric symptoms, and coexisting substance-use disorders (Arnsten, Reid, Bierer, & Rigotti, 2004). In addition, homeless smokers are more likely than nonsmokers to have experienced physical or sexual trauma.

High Cholesterol

People with high cholesterol have about twice the risk of heart disease when compared with people with normal cholesterol levels. It has been reported that 12.1% of U.S. adults age 20 years and over have high cholesterol (greater than or equal to 240 mg/dL) (CDC, 2017a). Gelberg et al. (1990) found that 36% of homeless adults under age 50 and 55% age 50 and older had elevated cholesterol levels. Homeless people often eat foods prepared by charity shelters, churches, fast-food restaurants, 24-hour convenience stores, and from garbage cans. Studies have shown that homeless people's diets are frequently high in saturated fats and cholesterol and inadequate in essential nutrients, contributing to hyperlipidemia (Hu & Willett, 2002; Luder, Boey, Buchalter, & Martinez-Weber, 1989). In addition, there is evidence of inadequate diagnosis and treatment of high cholesterol in this population (Lee et al., 2005). The National Coalition for the Homeless (2009a) found that use of prescription cholesterol-lowering medication was three times greater among adults who had health insurance when compared with those without health insurance. The majority of homeless adults lack health insurance, making them less likely to take prescription cholesterol-lowering medication, and thus more likely to suffer the effects of untreated hyperlipidemia (Baggett, O'Connell, Singer, & Rigotti, 2010).

Alcohol and Illicit Substance Use

Alcohol and substance abuse both cause and are a consequence of homelessness. Since 2002, substance use in adults over the age of 50 has doubled (Substance Abuse and Mental Health Services Administration, 2013). The "Baby Boomers," those born between 1946 and 1964, account for this increase in substance dependence in aging adults. Unfortunately, homeless individuals have an even higher prevalence of substance-use disorders than the general population (Culhane, Metraux, & Bainbridge, 2010).

Alcohol and illicit substance use represent prevalent and potent less-traditional CDC risk factors (Rehm, Sempos, & Trevisan, 2003; Lange & Hillis,

2001). Alcohol use dependency (AUD), which is more common than illicit substance dependence in the older homeless population, often leads to serious CV problems (Stringfellow et al., 2016). Excessive drinking can cause stroke, cardiomyopathy, cardiac arrhythmia, and sudden cardiac death (American Heart Association, 2015). Most illicit substances have the potential for adverse effects on the CV system. In particular, cocaine, amphetamines, and MDMA (ecstasy and molly) exacerbate hypertension and coronary vasoconstriction. If left untreated, chronic substance use can lead to CV complications, such as acute myocardial ischemia and infarction, arrhythmias, cardiomyopathy, aortic dissection, or endocarditis (Maraj, Figueredo, & Morris, 2010).

Mental Illness

According to the Substance Abuse and Mental Health Services Administration, 20% to 25% of the homeless population in the United States suffers from some form of severe mental illness. In comparison, only 4% of all Americans are diagnosed with severe mental illness (National Institute of Mental Health, 2015).

Mental illness is frequently considered to be a CVD risk factor (Stansfeld, Fuhrer, Shipley, & Marmot, 2002). In one study, participants with severe mental illness had significantly lower high-density lipoprotein-cholesterol (HDL-cholesterol) levels, higher total cholesterol/HDL-cholesterol ratios, were more likely to smoke, were more likely to have diabetes, and had elevated overall coronary heart disease risk scores for their age and gender (Osborn, Nazareth, & King, 2006). Depression can accelerate atherosclerosis, increase the risk of an unhealthy lifestyle, and increase cortisol levels, leading to increased blood sugar and blood pressure. There is evidence that anxiety, anger, and stress may increase CV risk (Chaddha, Robinson, Kline-Rogers, Alexandris-Souphis, & Rubenfire, 2016). Additionally, common metabolic side effects of the medications used to treat severe mental illness, such as weight gain and increased insulin resistance, can contribute to CV risk (Mangurian, Newcomer, Modlin, & Schillinger, 2016).

Psychosocial Factors

Homeless people experience a daily battle for the necessities of life, including food, shelter, and safety. They also experience an increased risk of a multitude of social problems, including victimization and violence (CDC, 2010). These factors lead to significantly higher levels of stress than that experienced by the general population. Chronic stress, both early in life and in adulthood, has been associated with an approximately 40% to 60% excess risk of coronary heart disease (Steptoe & Kivimäki, 2012). Along with a lack of informational support networks, isolation and loneliness are common among people who are homeless. A meta-analysis by Steptoe and Kivimäki (2012) indicated that patients with coronary heart disease or other chronic conditions have a significantly worse prognosis if they experience social isolation.

Hyperhomocysteinemia

Homocysteine levels greater than 15 mol/L have been correlated with an elevated risk of coronary artery disease (Clarke et al., 1991). In a study by Malinow, Bostom, and Krauss (1999), 7% of the homeless population were in this range. The vitamin and mineral deficiencies commonly found in homeless people can also indirectly increase the CVD risk through elevation of homocysteine levels.

BARRIERS TO PREVENTION AND TREATMENT

CV health requires prevention, as well as prompt intervention, and close follow-up when a CV event occurs. Prevention of CVD involves eating a healthy diet, maintaining a normal weight, regular exercise, and smoking cessation. Treatment of elevated blood pressure and/or cholesterol is vital to the prevention of CV events. Prompt intervention for a CV event mandates patient knowledge of emergent symptoms and what to do when these occur. After a cardiac event, close medical follow-up and medication compliance are necessary to prevent further events. Barriers to CV health for homeless individuals include their environment, lack of access to care, difficulty obtaining healthy food, substance dependence, mental health comorbidities, and issues surrounding medication access, storage, and adherence.

Environment

Many of the barriers to CV health faced by homeless people are inherent in being without a home or regular shelter. Sleep deprivation due to sleeping outdoors or in a crowded shelter is a common occurrence. Fear for personal safety and/or having one's belongings stolen contribute to a lack of or inadequate sleep. For those with peripheral vascular disease or heart failure, sleeping in a sitting position contributes to lower extremity edema. Limited access to basic hygiene, including lack of access to showers, clean clothes, and a need to keep shoes on for long periods of time, also contribute to poor health. Communal eating, bathing, and sleeping in shelters facilitate the transmission of communicable disease. Exposure to the elements when living outdoors increases the risk for sunstroke, sunburn, frostbite, and hypothermia. When a homeless person becomes ill, there is no place for him/her to rest (McMurray-Avila, 2001).

In addition, researchers have noted that the location of medical services can be a barrier to seeking healthcare. Homeless people may be less willing to go to a clinic if it is located in an area they are unfamiliar with or feel uncomfortable in because of the potential for greater public and/or police surveillance (Campbell, O'Neill, Gibson, & Thurston, 2015). The need to carry all of one's personal belongings for fear of theft if they are left behind is an additional environmental barrier to seeking healthcare.

Access to Care

Among the homeless, access to healthcare is limited by social, economic, and behavioral barriers, and competing needs (O'Toole, Johnson, Aiello, Kane, & Pape, 2016; National Coalition for the Homeless, 2009a). Social issues include stigmatization and marginalization of the homeless by healthcare providers (Gerber, 2013). Homeless adults report experiencing unmet health needs due in part to perceived discrimination in healthcare settings (Kushel, Vittinghoff, & Haas, 2001). Social behaviors such as an episodic lifestyle, attempts at invisibility to stay safe, and living one day at a time also play a role (Gerber, 2013). Economic issues that limit access to care include lack of or limited finances to pay for healthcare, lack of a telephone, and no mailing address. Behavioral barriers consist of poor medical follow-up, high-risk behaviors, substance dependence, non-compliance, and health illiteracy (Gerber, 2013; National Coalition for the Homeless, 2009a; O'Toole, Johnson, Aiello, Kane, & Pape, 2016). Competing needs, such as food, shelter, safety, and substance abuse, also impact the ability of homeless people to access traditional primary care.

These access-to-care barriers often lead the homeless to seek only crisis-oriented or convenient healthcare (Homeless Veteran Patient Aligned Care Team. Update, 2013; O'Toole, Johnson, Aiello, Kane, & Pape, 2016). Due to their ease and 24-hour accessibility, many homeless individuals use emergency departments (ED) when they are ill or injured (Doran, Raven, & Rosenheck, 2013; O'Toole, Johnson, Aiello, Kane, & Pape, 2016). Utilization of EDs for non-urgent healthcare issues leads to fragmented care; illness prevention and ongoing medical and mental health needs are not typically addressed in the ED (Baggett et al., 2010; Doran, Raven, & Rosenheck, 2013; O'Toole, Johnson, Kane, & Pape, 2016; Tsai & Rosenheck, 2013; White & Newman, 2014). Delays in seeking care make it more likely that homeless people will be hospitalized. In fact, the rates of hospitalization of homeless individuals are 2 to 3 times higher than those who are housed. In addition, on average, the homeless spend three to four more days as inpatients (Baggett et al., 2010; Doran, Raven, & Rosenheck, 2013; O'Toole, Johnson, Kane, & Pape, 2016; White & Newman, 2014).

Substance Dependence

Substance users are less likely to seek healthcare and are at increased risk for non-adherence to medical treatment. For many homeless persons, illicit substances, which include alcohol and drugs, are used as a means to cope with their undesirable circumstances (National Coalition for the Homeless, 2009b).

Substance dependence creates barriers to the prevention and treatment of CVD, especially for the homeless. Competing needs, such as finding food and shelter, take priority over drug counseling. Many homeless people are estranged from family and friends, and therefore do not have the social support network that is vital to recovery from substance dependence. Even when successful, remaining clean and sober is difficult while living on the street where illicit substances are frequently used and easily available (National Coalition for the Homeless, 2009b).

Substance dependence programs are traditionally structured toward younger clients and may be unprepared to deliver treatment to older adults with comorbidities such as CVD (Spinelli et al., 2016). Furthermore, many shelters, medical clinics, or rehab programs will not admit or provide care to an individual who is actively using illicit drugs.

Mental Illness

As previously mentioned, mental illness is inordinately prevalent among the homeless. Barriers to CV health in people with mental illness include inadequate self-management, lack of social support, and unhealthy behaviors (Correll et al., 2017). Characteristics of mental illness, such as lack of initiative and lack of energy and motivation, are additional barriers to CV prevention and treatment (Blomqvist, Sandgren, Carlsson, & Jormfeldt, 2017).

Mental illness often co-occurs with substance dependence. Homeless persons with untreated mental illness may inappropriately turn to illicit drugs or alcohol to treat their symptoms. Unfortunately, many treatment programs for persons with mental illnesses do not accept those with substance dependence disorders (National Coalition for the Homeless, 2009b).

Food Insecurity

A healthy diet is fundamental for the prevention and management of CVD (American Heart Associations Diet and Lifestyle Recommendations, 2017). Dietary modifications for preventing and managing CVD are: decreasing portion size, decreasing foods high in saturated fats, and increasing intake of whole grains, fruits, and vegetables (American Heart Associations Diet and Lifestyle Recommendations, 2017). Following a heart-healthy diet has been shown to reduce heart disease risk by lowering blood pressure, decreasing body weight, and maintaining healthy glycemic levels (American Heart Associations Diet and Lifestyle Recommendations, 2017).

According to Feeding America, one out of eight people do not get enough food, including five million senior citizens over the age of 60 (Weinfield, Mills, Borger, Gearing, Macaluso, Montaquila, & Zedlewski, 2014). It is estimated that 12% of Americans have limited access to basic nutritious foods, or are "food insecure" (Coleman-Jensen, Rabbitt, Gregory, & Singh, September, 2016). Due to limited financial resources, and physical and psychological barriers, food insecurity is especially prevalent among homeless persons. The chronically homeless are particularly vulnerable (Coleman-Jensen, Rabbitt, Gregory, & Singh, September 2016).

Many homeless shelters provide meals. However, foods served in these facilities lack variety, are high in saturated fats and carbohydrates, and provide limited or no fresh fruits and vegetables (Richards & Smith, 2006; Seale, Fallaize, & Lovegrove, 2016). Some homeless people scavenge for food, sell belongings, ask strangers for food, or use food stamps. Nonetheless, barriers to accessing heart-healthy foods exist (Richards & Smith, 2006; Seale, Fallaize, & Lovegrove, 2016).

Physiological barriers, including infectious diseases, injury, and degenerative diseases, make it difficult for homeless people to access food (Lee & Greif, 2008). Homeless people with mental health and/or substance abuse issues may isolate and avoid social situations, thus reducing their likelihood of seeking out food at a shelter or church. Lack of cooking facilities and lack of places for food storage are added physical barriers to eating a heart-healthy diet (Lee & Greif, 2008; Richards & Smith, 2006; Seale, Fallaize, & Lovegrove, 2016).

RECOMMENDATIONS

It is evident that CVD is very prevalent in older homeless persons. Unfortunately, significant barriers to CVD prevention and treatment in this population exist. Research suggests that integrating social support and social determinants of health into clinical care is an effective way to manage the healthcare of people who are homeless (O'Toole, Johnson, Aiello, Kane, & Pape, 2016). Suggested interventions for improving non-ED care access are case management, integration of primary care, social and mental health services, fixed or mobile outreach, orientation of services available at primary care clinics, and supportive housing services (Health Quality Ontario, 2016).

Housing

Environmental barriers to CV health/healthcare include sleep deprivation, fear for personal safety, limited access to basic hygiene, communicable disease exposure, exposure to the elements, and lack of storage for belongings. Studies of homeless adults and older adults have consistently supported the benefits of housing in reducing hospital visits, admissions, and lengths of stay (Larimer et al., 2009; Sadowski, Kee, VanderWeele, & Buchanan, 2009). A 2016 study of homeless veterans found that permanent supportive housing significantly increased treatment for chronic and acute physical illness, mental illness, and substance-use disorders (O'Connell, Kasprow, & Rosenheck, 2012). Permanent housing may improve CV health in particular, by decreasing chronic psychological stress and allowing for healthier food choices.

Access to Care

Access to healthcare for homeless persons is limited by perceived discrimination, isolation, economic concerns, and competing needs. Research indicates that increased access occurs with street outreach, "Housing First" models, and utilization of multidisciplinary teams of clinicians working together to integrate the various components of the healthcare system (O'Toole et al., 2016; Sadowski et al., 2009).

When providing care to homeless clients, it is imperative that providers examine their personal feelings about homeless people. A non-judgmental clinician, who upholds the dignity of the homeless individual by showing genuine caring and respect, can engender the trust and engagement that is critical for continuous care and adherence to the treatment plan. Admittedly, this can be difficult when hygiene is poor, infestation is suspected, and/or the patient presents with all of his or her earthly belongings. However, clinicians who work with and are able to establish trust with homeless individuals find that most are "normal" people who have experienced serious adversity in their lives and who are extremely appreciative of any assistance/care provided.

The episodic lifestyle of homeless persons mandates that their healthcare be open-access, with walk-in capacity and flexible scheduling. Street or shelter outreach and availability of clinics with multidisciplinary staff in areas where there are large numbers of homeless people enhances access to care. Having food, toiletries, clothing, and bus passes available allows homeless clients to focus on their social and health needs, rather than where they will get their next meal, or how they will get back to their shelter or usual sleeping location. In-clinic shower facilities are a definite benefit. A list of homeless services in the area (including free meals, showers, laundry, mailboxes, storage for belongings) should also be available.

A Multidisciplinary Team

A cohesive team, including at minimum a medical provider, nurse, social worker, and mental health provider who are available on-site, will prevent the need for referrals that, for a variety of reasons, may not be scheduled or attended. A nurse who understands the unique needs of homeless clients can monitor vital signs, weight, and blood glucose, as well as provide CVD lifestyle education and medication teaching. Using prepared handouts with pictures and real packaged foods, clients can be taught to read labels and make better food choices. A nurse can address medication issues such as storage, scheduling, compliance, theft, and side effects. Homeless clients who carry their medications in a backpack find that the compartments in medication organizers can inadvertently open and spill their contents. Additionally, having no place to leave medications out and visible makes remembering to take them difficult. Something as simple as teaching a client to set an alarm on his or her cell phone (yes, homeless clients often have cell phones) can increase medication compliance. In fact, a recent study suggested that cell phones might be a feasible method for communicating medication and appointment information to homeless persons (Moczygemba et al., 2016).

A social worker who has experience working with homeless people and who is knowledgeable about available homeless resources in the community can assist the homeless client to find temporary or permanent housing. A social worker can also assist the homeless person to apply for food stamps, pharmaceutical patient assistance programs, Medicaid, Supplemental Security Income (SSI), Supplemental Security Disability Income (SSDI), or veterans benefits. Homeless social work case management programs have been shown to decrease hospitalizations, length of stay, ED visits, and have a positive impact on housing stability (O'Toole et al., 2016; Sadowski et al., 2009). Ideally, a social work case management program provides monthly client visits and includes coordination with hospital discharge planning, assistance with permanent or temporary housing, coordination of medical and mental healthcare, and substance-abuse treatment referral.

Due to the extremely high rate of mental illness among homeless individuals, a mental health provider is a priority for an effective multidisciplinary homeless care team. Collaboration between the mental health and medical care provider can lead to improved client outcomes. For example, a medical provider could advocate for an antidepressant that also treats chronic pain. A mental health provider might request the medical providers' assistance with treatment of erectile dysfunction related to an antidepressant or ask that a beta-blocker be discontinued due to worsening depression. With regard to CVD, treatment of depression may decrease stress hormone levels and increase motivation to engage in lifestyle changes that promote CV health. Treatment for anxiety may help with blood pressure reduction, as well as increase the likelihood of medical and mental healthcare follow-up.

When a homeless client is hospitalized, a visit from one or more of the care team members is extremely beneficial. Homeless patients often isolate, and therefore may have no visitors during their hospitalization. Seeing a familiar face while in a strange and unfamiliar environment is reassuring. In addition, the outpatient care team can provide invaluable insight and pertinent medical/mental health history to the inpatient care providers. Finally, and most importantly, post-hospitalization follow-up can be arranged prior to discharge. This is particularly important when the homeless person has no address or phone number.

Medical Treatment for Cardiovascular Disease

When working with homeless clients, evidence-based treatment guidelines for CVD (hypertension, hyperlipidemia, coronary artery disease, heart failure, etc.) should be followed whenever possible. However, certain adaptations must be considered. The information presented here is an amalgamation of the practice adaptation recommendations of the Strehlow, Robertshaw, Louison, Lopez, Colangelo, Silver, & Post (2009) with those of the authors of this chapter, who have extensive experience in caring for homeless clients with CVD.

Obtaining the medical history of a homeless person is similar to that of permanently housed clients, with a few exceptions. Living conditions must be addressed at each visit. Clients should be asked where they sleep, where they spend their time and with whom, where they get their food, where they store their medications, and if they feel safe. It is essential that contact information be updated at each encounter. If the client has no address or phone, it is inherent that a place and time for future contact be arranged.

The physical exam can be a challenge. Homeless people often wear multiple layers of clothing and can be very sensitive and embarrassed about their poor hygiene. The provider must be empathetic to these feelings and may need to defer all or part of the physical exam until trust is established. If infestation is suspected, care must be taken to prevent the client from feeling like a pariah, while at the same time preventing its spread.

When providing care to homeless persons, there is no substitute for longer clinic appointments and more frequent follow-up. Gaining the trust of homeless clients, assisting them to select and set realistic goals, and monitoring their progress toward goal achievement takes time. CVDs such as hypertension and hyperlipidemia are often asymptomatic. Education about the adverse health effects of these morbidities and the benefits of treatment takes time. Additional time is necessary to allow for and to answer client questions.

Homeless people often have multiple comorbidities and may not have received medical care for "years." The medical provider must prioritize the problem list and address the most urgent issues first. The tendency of medical providers to tackle too many problems at one visit can lead to an overwhelmed client who does not follow through on any of the provider recommendations. Referrals to specialists should be minimized whenever possible. The e-consultation process provided by the Veterans Administration Healthcare System allows primary care providers to seek specialist opinions/recommendations without the specialist having to see the client. At a minimum, multiple visits to a specialist can be avoided if the primary care provider orders any necessary testing or labs prior to the initial specialty consultation.

Because lifestyle modification is difficult at best, initiation of CV medications may need to occur sooner with homeless clients. Availability of bathroom facilities and the ability to have follow-up labs should be ascertained prior to ordering diuretic therapy. Beta-blockers and clonidine should be prescribed with care, as sudden discontinuation can result in rebound hypertension.

Simplification of the drug regimen through the use of once-daily dosing regimens and combination drugs will help improve adherence. Prescribing small amounts of medication may encourage follow-up visits and decrease the risk of theft, loss, or misuse. Limiting the amount of medication dispensed should definitely be considered in clients who are determined to be at high risk for suicide.

Thorough medication reconciliation by the provider at each encounter is imperative. Homeless clients should be advised to bring all of their medications to each and every visit. It is not uncommon to find duplicate or missing medications in this transient population. Inconsistent adherence is common.

While maintaining a non-judgmental attitude, an exploration of barriers to adherence and an exploration of ways to address these barriers should then be undertaken. Medications, **other than** opioids or those known to react with EtOH (Ethanol) or other illicit drugs, should not be withheld due to substance dependence. Active amphetamine users, in particular, tend to be very hypertensive and should be treated with anti-hypertensive medication(s).

Providing home blood pressure monitors or weight scales to homeless clients (even those living in shelters) is not advised. These pieces of equipment are difficult to carry and are frequently lost or stolen. It is preferable to offer anytime, no-wait, walk-in opportunities for clients who need frequent blood pressure or weight monitoring. Glucometers are small and easy to carry and hide, and can thus be provided to diabetic homeless persons in most instances.

Tobacco Cessation

Although medical treatment for CVD is extremely important, smoking cessation is critical to reducing CV risk. Studies suggest that psychosocial stressors and the physical hazards of daily living diminish the perceived benefits of smoking cessation for homeless persons (Baggett & Rigotti, 2010; Baggett, Tobey, & Rigotti, 2013). There is, however, evidence that many homeless smokers want to quit (Arnsten et al., 2004). Baggett, Tobey, and Rigotti (2013) suggest the following: (a) pair smoking cessation pharmacotherapy with behavioral counseling located near shelters or walk-in clinics, (b) emphasize the immediate symptom relief and financial benefit of cessation, and (c) address smoking cessation at every clinical encounter. In addition, for male smokers, emphasizing that tobacco use causes erectile dysfunction may convince them to attempt cessation!

Substance Dependence

Homeless clients often lack understanding about the adverse effects of illicit substances and alcohol on their CV system. The relationship between excessive alcohol intake and stroke, enlarged heart, heart rhythm disturbances, and sudden cardiac death should be stressed. Those dependent on cocaine, stimulants, and/or ecstasy should be educated that these substances can cause high blood pressure, heart attack, irregular heart rhythms, and/or heart failure. Motivational interviewing can be used to promote substance-dependence treatment. If a team member ascertains readiness for treatment, both inpatient and outpatient referral resources must be readily available.

Geriatric adults are more susceptible to adverse reactions between illicit drugs and their medications (Lindsey, Stewart, & Childress, 2012). If substance dependence or alcohol use is known or suspected, stern warnings about these interactions should be provided. Certain hypertensive medications (e.g., clonidine) have been known to increase and prolong the psychoactive effects of heroin and are sold on the streets to reduce the withdrawal symptoms of opioid addiction (Maness & Khan, 2014).

CASE STUDY CONTINUED

At the time of his presentation to the VA homeless clinic, J.G. was living in a homeless shelter. He was greeted warmly and thanked for his service to our country. He was offered donated toiletries, socks, food, and water. An echocardiogram was arranged. It revealed worsening heart failure with an ejection fraction (EF) of 13%. At his discharge from the hospital two weeks prior, he had been prescribed aspirin, atorvastatin, furosemide, lisinopril, metoprolol SA, olanzapine, ranitidine, tamsulosin, and spironolactone. He had been clean and sober for 90 days. Fortunately, J.G. brought his medications with him to the clinic. A complete medication reconciliation was completed. He was educated about heart failure in simple terms. J.G. was strongly advised to take his medications as prescribed and to avoid illicit substances. He was provided with a computer print-out of his medication list.

Between this initial visit and his next presentation to the clinic five months later, J.G. was hospitalized with a left middle cerebral artery stroke. He was discharged on his prior medications, except furosemide was changed to bumetanide, and warfarin and aspirin were added. He admitted to taking his medications only intermittently. He was again living on the street. The homeless clinic primary care provider (PCP) made the difficult decision to discontinue the warfarin due to safety concerns (inconsistent adherence and inability to have frequent laboratory monitoring). As an alternative, his aspirin dose was increased to 325 mg daily. Medication reconciliation at this visit revealed two containers of spironolactone and no bumetanide. He was 10 lbs. above his dry weight. Duplicate medications were combined and obsolete medications were discarded. Arrangements were made to obtain a supply of bumetanide at a nearby pharmacy. A medication list was provided.

During follow-up two weeks later by the homeless clinic nurse, his weight was down by only 1 lb. Medication counts did, however, reveal adherence. His bumetanide dose was increased, and he was provided with a $5 coupon book to spend at the VA store or cafeteria. He was given a bus pass so that he could return for labs in one week.

Several days later, J.G. walked-in to the homeless clinic with new-onset slurred speech. He was taken immediately to the ED and admitted to the hospital. Discharge documentation indicated a "re-expression" of the old stroke. He was discharged on his pre-hospitalization medications with dabigatran added for anticoagulation (aspirin was discontinued). Social work was unable to arrange temporary or transitional housing; J.G. was discharged to the street. However, the homeless clinic team was able to visit him while he was hospitalized to provide insight to the inpatient medical team, and they provided J.G. with a primary care follow-up appointment.

J.G. was seen in the homeless clinic one week post-discharge. Medication reconciliation revealed dabigatran AND aspirin in the client's possession. Aspirin was discarded. The clinic PCP was nervous about the dabigatran, as although it does not require laboratory monitoring, missing doses of this anticoagulant can cause hypercoagulation. It was stressed to the client that he MUST take this medication daily to prevent another stroke. J.G. was very frustrated about his dysphasia that consisted of word salad and difficulty with word finding. A speech therapy consult was entered, but he never scheduled the appointment. J.G. reported he did not like taking too many medications at one time and refused a medication organizer ("too bulky, and the containers open and spill into my backpack"). The PCP separated the daily medication containers into morning and evening. She placed a blue colored sticker on each morning medication and a red sticker on each evening medication. She placed both blue and red stickers on carvedilol (a twice-daily medication).

Unfortunately, three weeks later, J.G. was admitted to the hospital with another heart failure exacerbation. His urine toxicology screen was positive for amphetamines. An echocardiogram indicated his EF had decreased to 8%. He was diuresed, provided with donated clothing, and discharged to the street with scheduled primary care and social work case manager follow-up appointments. With each hospital discharge, he adamantly declined skilled nursing facility placement.

Subsequently, J.G. was seen monthly by the PCP with in-between registered nurse visits for weight and medication reconciliation. He was ultimately assigned to a VA supportive housing (VASH) social work case manager who arranged admission to a supervised transitional living program for physical and mental health stabilization. She assisted J.G. to apply for a VA pension, and he was ultimately housed in an apartment downtown. The social worker also assisted J.G. to locate members of his family. He was in contact with them by phone.

Unfortunately, two weeks after he was permanently housed, J.G. was admitted to the hospital again. His EF was only 3%. He died several days later. The homeless clinic team members were sad, but took comfort knowing that J.G died, not as a nameless, homeless, drug-addicted statistic. He died as a veteran of the U.S. Marine Corps and was buried with honor at the local veterans cemetery.

CONCLUSION

CVD remains the leading cause of death in older homeless people. Traditional CV risk factors, such as hypertension, diabetes, smoking, and hyperlipidemia, and nontraditional CV risk factors, such as substance abuse, psychological stress, and lack of diagnostic and preventative medical care, contribute to CVD in this population. Barriers to CV prevention and treatment in homeless individuals include their environment, lack of access to care, substance dependence, mental illness, food insecurity, and medication non-adherence. Healthcare models that provide Housing First and just-in-time care by non-judgmental multidisciplinary teams have been shown to improve the CV health of people who are homeless. CV healthcare practice adaptations for homeless clients include ascertaining living conditions, improvising the physical exam, scheduling longer clinic appointments with frequent follow-up, prioritization of the plan of care, and simplification of the medication regimen.

REFERENCES

American Heart Association. (2017a). Correction to: Heart disease and stroke statistics—2017 update. *Circulation, 135*(10). doi:10.1161/cir.0000000000000491

American Heart Association. (2017b, January 31). Heart failure projected to increase dramatically, according to new statistics. Retrieved from http://news.heart.org/heart-failure-projected-to-increase-dramatically-according-to-new-statistics

American Heart Association. (2015). Alcohol and heart health. Retrieved from http://www.heart.org/HEARTORG/HealthyLiving/HealthyEating/Nutrition/Alcohol-and-Heart-Health_UCM_305173_Article.jsp#

American Heart Associations Diet and Lifestyle Recommendations. (2017). Retrieved from https://www.heart.org/HEARTORG/HealthyLiving/HealthyEating/Nutrition/The-American-Heart-Associations-Diet-and-Lifestyle-Recommendations_UCM_305855_Article.jsp

Arnsten, J. H., Reid, K., Bierer, M., & Rigotti, N. (2004). Smoking behavior and interest in quitting among homeless smokers. *Addictive Behaviors, 29*(6),1155–1161. doi:10.1016/j.addbeh.2004.03.010

Asgary, R., Sckell, B., Alcabes, A., Naderi, R., Schoenthaler, A., Ogedegbe, G. (2016). Rates and predictors of uncontrolled hypertension among hypertensive homeless adults using New York City shelter-based clinics. *Annals of Family Medicine, 14*(1), 41–46. doi:10.1370/afm.1882

Baggett, T. P., Hwang, S. W., O'Connell, J. J., Porneala, B. C., Stringfellow, E. J., Orav, E. J., ... Rigotti, N. A. (2013). Mortality among homeless adults in Boston: Shifts in causes of death over a 15-year period. *JAMA Internal Medicine, 173*(3), 189–195. doi:10.1001/jamainternmed.2013.1604

Baggett, T. P., O'Connell, J. J., Singer, D. E., & Rigotti, N. A. (2010). The unmet health care needs of homeless adults: A national study. *American Journal of Public Health, 100*(7), 1326–1333. doi:10.2105/AJPH.2009.180109

Baggett, T. P., & Rigotti, N. A. (2010). Cigarette smoking and advice to quit in a national sample of homeless adults. *American Journal of Preventive Medicine, 39*(2), 164–172. doi:10.1016/j.amepre.2010.03.024

Baggett, T. P., Tobey, M. L., & Rigotti, N. A. (2013). Tobacco use among homeless people—Addressing the neglected addiction. *New England Journal of Medicine, 369*(3), 201–204. doi:10.1056/nejmp1301935

Beijer, U., Andreasson, S., Ågren, G., & Fugelstad, A. (2011). Mortality and causes of death among homeless women and men in Stockholm. *Scandinavian Journal of Public Health, 39*(2), 121–127. doi:10.1177/1403494810393554

Bernstein, R. S., Meurer, L. N., Plumb, E. J., & Jackson, J. L. (2015). Diabetes and hypertension prevalence in homeless adults in the United States: A systematic review and meta-analysis. *American Journal of Public Health, 105*(2). doi:10.2105/ajph.2014.302330

Blomqvist, M., Sandgren, A., Carlsson, I.-M., & Jormfeldt, H. (2017). Enabling healthy living: Experiences of people with severe mental illness in psychiatric outpatient services. *International Journal of Mental Health Nursing.* Advance online publication. doi:10.1111/inm.12313

Burt, M. R., Aron, L. Y., Douglas, T., Valente, J., Lee, E., & Iwen, B. (1999). *Homelessness: Programs and the people they serve.* Washington, DC: U.S. Interagency Council on Homelessness. Retrieved from https://www.urban.org/research/publication/homelessness-programs-and-people-they-serve-findings-national-survey-home-less-assistance-providers-and-clients/view/full_report

Campbell, D. J., O'Neill, B. G., Gibson, K., & Thurston, W. E. (2015). Primary healthcare needs and barriers to care among Calgary's homeless populations. *BMC Family Practice, 16*, 139. doi:10.1186/s12875-015-0361-3

Centers for Disease Control and Prevention. (2010, November). Homelessness and health [Audio podcast]. Retrieved from https://www2c.cdc.gov/podcasts/player.asp?f=4097507

Centers for Disease Control and Prevention. (2013). *CDC Health Disparities and Inequalities Report—United States, 2013.* Retrieved from https://www.cdc.gov/mmwr/pdf/other/su6203.pdf

Centers for Disease Control and Prevention. (2015a, September 10). *CDC health disparities & inequalities report (CHDIR).* Retrieved from https://www.cdc.gov/minorityhealth/chdireport.html

Centers for Disease Control and Prevention. (2015b, August 10). Conditions that increase risk for heart disease. Retrieved from https://www.cdc.gov/heartdisease/conditions.htm

Centers for Disease Control and Prevention. (2016, November 30). High blood pressure facts. Retrieved from https://www.cdc.gov/bloodpressure/facts.htm

Centers for Disease Control and Prevention. (2017a, January 19). Cholesterol. Retrieved from https://www.cdc.gov/nchs/fastats/cholesterol.htm

Centers for Disease Control and Prevention. (2017b, January 19). Heart disease. Retrieved from https://www.cdc.gov/nchs/fastats/heart-disease.htm

Centers for Disease Control and Prevention. (2017c, January 20). Leading causes of death. Retrieved from https://www.cdc.gov/nchs/fastats/leading-causes-of-death.htm

Chaddha, A., Robinson, E. A., Kline-Rogers, E., Alexandris-Souphis, T., & Rubenfire, M. (2016). Mental health and cardiovascular disease. *The American Journal of Medicine, 129*(11), 1145–1148. doi:10.1016/j.amjmed.2016.05.018

Clarke, R., Daly, L., Robinson, K., Naughten, E., Cahalane, S., Fowler, B., & Graham, I. (1991). Hyperhomocysteinemia: An independent risk factor for vascular disease. *New England Journal of Medicine, 324*, 1149–1155. doi:10.1056/NEJM199104253241701

Coleman-Jensen, A., Rabbitt, M., Gregory, C., & Singh, A. (2016). USDA household food security in the United States in 2016. Retrieved from https://www.ers.usda.gov/publications/pub-details/?pubid

Correll, C. U., Solmi, M., Veronese, N., Bortolato, B., Rosson, S., Santonastaso, P., . . . Stubbs, B. (2017). Prevalence, incidence and mortality from cardiovascular disease in patients with pooled and specific severe mental illness: a large-scale meta-analysis of 3,211,768 patients and 113,383,368 controls. *World Psychiatry, 16*, 163–180. doi:10.1002/wps.20420

Culhane, D. P., Metraux, S., & Bainbridge, J. (2010). *The age structure of contemporary homelessness: Risk period or cohort effect?* Penn School of Social Policy and Practice Working Paper. Retrieved from https://repository.upenn.edu/spp_papers/140

Curtis, B. M., & O'Keefe, J. H., Jr. (2002). Autonomic tone as a cardiovascular risk factor: The dangers of chronic fight or flight. *Mayo Clinic Proceedings, 77*(1), 45–54. doi:10.4065/77.1.45

Doran, K., Raven, M., & Rosenheck, R. (2013). What drives frequent emergency department use in an integrated health system? National Data from the Veterans Health Administration. *Annals of Emergency Medicine, 62*(2), 151–159.

Fazel, S., Geddes, J. R., & Kushel, M. (2014). The health of homeless people in high-income countries: Descriptive epidemiology, health consequences, and clinical and policy recommendations. *The Lancet, 384*(9953), 1529–1540. doi:10.1016/S0140-6736(14)61132-6

Gelberg, L., Linn, L. S., & Mayer-Oakes, S. A. (1990). Differences in health status between older and younger homeless adults. *Journal of the American Geriatrics Society, 38*(11), 1220–1229. doi:10.1111/j.1532-5415.1990.tb01503.x

Gerber, L. (2013). Bringing home effective nursing care for the homeless. *Nursing 2013 43*(3), 32–38. doi: 10.1097/01.NURSE.0000426620.51507.0c

Hahn, J. A., Kushel, M. B., Bangsberg, D. R., Riley, E., & Moss, A. R. (2006). Brief report: The aging of the homeless population: Fourteen-year trends in San Francisco. *Journal of General Internal Medicine, 21*, 775–778. doi:10.1111/j.1525-1497.2006.00493.x

Health Quality Ontario. (2016). Interventions to improve access to primary care for people who are homeless: A systematic review. *Ontario Health Technology Assessment Series, 16*(9), 1–50. Retrieved from https://www.ncbi.nlm.nih.gov/pmc/articles/PMC4832090

Hu, F. B., & Willett, W. C. (2002). Optimal diets for prevention of coronary heart disease. *Journal of the American Medical Association, 288*(20), 2569–2578. doi:10.1001/jama.288.20.2569

Hwang, S. W., Orav, E. J., O'Connell, J. J., Lebow, J. M., & Brennan, T. A. (1997). Causes of death in homeless adults in Boston. *Annals of Internal Medicine, 126*(8), 625–628. doi:10.7326/0003-4819-126-8-199704150-00007

Hwang, S. W., Wilkins, R., Tjepkema, M., O'Campo, P. J., & Dunn, J. R. (2009). Mortality among residents of shelters, rooming houses, and hotels in Canada: 11 year follow-up study. *British Medical Journal, 339*, b4036. Retrieved from http://www.bmj.com/content/339/bmj.b4036

James, P. A., Oparil, S., Carter, B. L., Cushman, W. C., Dennison-Himmelfarb, C., Handler, J., . . . Ortiz, E. (2014). Evidence-based guideline for the management of high blood pressure in adults. Report from the panel members appointed to the Eighth Joint National Committee. *Journal of the American Medical Association, 311*(5), 507–520. doi:10.1001/jama.2013.284427

Jones, C., Perera, A., Chow, M., Ho, I., Nguyen, J., & Davachi, S. (2009). Cardiovascular disease risk among the poor and homeless—What we know so far. *Current Cardiology Reviews, 5*(1), 69–77. doi:10.2174/157340309787048086

Kasprow, W. J., & Rosenheck, R. (2000). Mortality among homeless and nonhomeless mentally ill veterans. *The Journal of Nervous and Mental Disease, 188*(3), 141–147. doi:10.1097/00005053-200003000-00003

Kinchen, K., & Wright, J. D. (1991). Hypertension management in health care for the homeless clinics: Results from a survey. *American Journal of Public Health, 81*(9), 1163–1165. doi:10.2105/AJPH.81.9.1163

Kleinman, L. C., Freeman, H., Perlman, J., & Gelberg, L. (1996). Homing in on the homeless: Assessing the physical health of homeless adults in Los Angeles County using an original method to obtain physical examination data in a survey. *Health Services Research, 31*(5), 533–549. Retrieved from https://www.ncbi.nlm.nih.gov/pubmed/8943989

Kushel, M. B., Vittinghoff, E., & Haas, J. S. (2001). Factors associated with the health care utilization of homeless persons. *Journal of the American Medical Association, 285*(2), 200–206. doi:10.1001/jama.285.2.200

Lange, R. A., & Hillis, L. D. (2001). Cardiovascular complications of cocaine use. *New England Journal of Medicine, 345*(5), 351–358. doi:10.1056/nejm200108023450507

Larimer, M. E., Malone, D. K., Garner, M. D., Atkins, D. C., & Burlingham, B., Lonczak, H. S., . . . Marlatt, G. A. (2009). Health care and public service use and costs before and after provision of housing for chronically homeless persons with severe alcohol problems. *Journal of the American Medical Association, 301*(13), 1349–1357. doi:10.1001/jama.2009.414

Lee, B., & Greif, M. (2008). Homelessness and hunger. *Journal of Health and Social Behavior, 49*(1), 3–19. doi:10.1177/002214650804900102

Lee, T. C., Hanlon, J. G., Ben-David, J., Booth, G. L., Cantor, W. J., Connelly, P. W., & Wang, S. W. (2005). Risk factors for cardiovascular disease in homeless adults. *Circulation, 111*(20), 2629–2635. doi:10.1161/circulationaha.104.510826

LePage, J., Bradshaw, L., Cipher, D., Crawford, A., & Hoosyhar, D. (2014). The effects of homelessness on veterans' health care service use: An evaluation of independence from comorbidities. *Public Health, 128*(11), 985–992. doi:10.1016/j.puhe.2014.07.004

Lindsey, W. T., Stewart, D., & Childress, D. (2012). Drug interactions between common illicit drugs and prescription therapies. *The American Journal of Drug and Alcohol Abuse, 38*(4), 334–343. doi:10.3109/00952990.2011.643997

Luder, E., Boey, E., Buchalter, B., & Martinez-Weber, C. (1989). Assessment of the nutritional status of urban homeless adults. *Public Health Reports, 104*(5), 451–457. Retrieved from http://www.jstor.org/stable/4628702

Malinow, M. R., Bostom, A. G., & Krauss, R. M. (1999). Homocyst(e)ine, diet, and cardiovascular diseases: A statement for healthcare professionals from the Nutrition Committee, American Heart Association. *Circulation, 99*, 178–182. doi:10.1161/01.CIR.99.1.178

Maness, D. L., & Khan, M. (2014). Care of the homeless: An overview. *American Family Physician, 89*(8), 634–640. Retrieved from http://www.aafp.org/afp/2014/0415/p634.html

Mangurian, C., Newcomer, J. W., Modlin, C., & Schillinger, D. (2016). Diabetes and cardiovascular care among people with severe mental illness: A literature review. *Journal of General Internal Medicine, 31*(9), 1083–1091. doi:10.1007/s11606-016-3712-4

Maraj, S., Figueredo, V. M., & Morris, D. L. (2010). Cocaine and the heart. *Clinical Cardiology, 33*(5), 264–269. doi:10.1002/clc.20746

McMurray-Avila, M. (2001). *Organizing health services for homeless people: A practical guide* (2nd ed.). Nashville, TN: National Health Care for the Homeless Council.

Moczygemba, L. R., Cox, L. S., Marks, S. A., Robinson, M. A., Goode, J.-V. R., & Jafari, N. (2016). Homeless patients' perceptions about using cell phones to manage medications and attend appointments. *International Journal of Pharmacy Practice, 25*(3), 220–230.

National Coalition for the Homeless. (2009a). Health care and homelessness. Retrieved from http://www.nationalhomeless.org/factsheets/health.html

National Coalition for the Homeless. (2009b). Substance abuse and homelessness. Retrieved from http://www.nationalhomeless.org/factsheets/addiction.pdf

National Institute of Mental Health. (2015). Serious mental illness. Retrieved from https://www.nimh.nih.gov/health/statistics/mental-illness.shtml

Osborn, D. P. J., Nazareth, I., & King, M. B. (2006). Risk for coronary heart disease in people with severe mental illness. *British Journal of Psychiatry, 188*, 271–277. doi:10.1192/bjp.bp.104.008060

O'Connell, M. J., Kasprow, W. J., & Rosenheck, R. A. (2012). Differential impact of supported housing on selected subgroups of homeless veterans with substance abuse histories. *Psychiatric Services, 63*(12), 1195–1205.

O'Toole, T. P., Johnson, E. E., Aiello, R., Kane, V., & Pape, L. (2016). Tailoring care to vulnerable populations by incorporating social determinants of health: The Veterans Health Administration's "Homeless Patient Aligned Care Team" program. *Preventing Chronic Disease, 13*, E44. doi:10.5888/pcd13.150567

Rehm, J., Sempos, C. T., & Trevisan, M. (2003). Average volume of alcohol consumption, patterns of drinking and risk of coronary heart disease: A review. *European Journal of Cardiovascular Prevention & Rehabilitation, 10*(1), 15–20. doi:10.1177/174182670301000104

Richards, R., & Smith, C. (2006). The impact of homeless shelters on food access and choice among homeless families in Minnesota. *Journal of Nutrition Education Behavior, 38*, 96–105.

Sadowski, L. S., Kee, R. A., VanderWeele, T. J., & Buchanan, D. (2009). Effect of a housing and case management program on emergency department visits and hospitalizations among chronically ill homeless adults. *Journal of the American Medical Association, 301*(17), 1771–1778. doi:10.1001/jama.2009.561

Schinka, J. A., Bossarte, R. M., Curtiss, G., Lapcevic, W. A., & Casey, R. J. (2016). Increased mortality among older veterans admitted to VA homelessness programs. *Psychiatric Services, 67*(4), 465–468. doi:10.1176/appi.ps.201500095

Schinka, J. A., Curtis, B., Leventhal, K., Bossarte, R. M., Lapcevic, W., & Casey, R. (2016). Predictors of mortality in older homeless veterans. *The Journals of Gerontology: Series B, 72*(6), 1103–1109. doi:10.1093/geronb/gbw042

Seale, J., Fallaize, R., & Lovegrove, J. (2016). Nutrition and the homeless: The underestimated challenge. *Nutrition Research Reviews, 29*(2), 143–151.

Spinelli, M. A., Ponath, C., Tieu, L., Hurstak, E. E., Guzman, D., & Kushel, M. (2016). Factors associated with substance use in older homeless adults: Results from the HOPE HOME study. *Substance Abuse, 38*(1), 88–94. doi:10.1080/08897077.2016.1264534

Stansfeld, S. A., Fuhrer, R., Shipley, M. J., & Marmot, M. G. (2002). Psychological distress as a risk factor for coronary heart disease in the Whitehall II Study. *International Journal of Epidemiology, 31*(1), 248–255. doi:10.1093/ije/31.1.248

Steptoe, A., & Kivimäki, M. (2012). Stress and cardiovascular disease. *Nature Reviews Cardiology, 9*, 360–370. doi:10.1038/nrcardio.2012.45

Strehlow, A., Robertshaw, D., Louison, A., Lopez, M., Colangelo, B., Silver, K., & Post, P. (2009). Adapting your practice: Treatment and recommendations for homeless patients with hypertension, hyperlipidemia, & heart failure. Retrieved from http://www.nhchc.org/wp-content/uploads/2011/09/CardioDiseases.pdf

Stringfellow, E. J., Kim, T. W., Gordon, A. J., Pollio, D. E., Grucza, R. A., Austin, E. L., . . . Kertesz, S. G. (2016). Substance use among persons with homeless experience in primary care. *Substance Abuse, 37*(4), 534–541. doi:10.1080/08897077.2016.1145616

Substance Abuse and Mental Health Services Administration. (2013). Results from the 2012 National Survey on Drug Use and Health (NSDUH): Summary of national findings. Retrieved from https://store.samhsa.gov/product/Results-from-the-2012-National-Survey-on-Drug-Use-and-Health-NSDUH-/SMA13-4795

Szerlip, M. I., & Szerlip, H. M. (2002). Identification of cardiovascular risk factors in homeless adults. *The American Journal of the Medical Sciences, 324*(5), 243–246. doi:10.1097/00000441-200211000-00002

Tsai, J., & Rosenheck, R. (2013). Risk factors for ED use among homeless veterans. *American Journal of Emergency Medicine, 31*(5), 855–858.

Weinfield, N., Mills, G., Borger, C., Gearing, M., Macaluso, T., Montaquila, J., & Zedlewski, S. (2014). Hunger in America 2014 National Report. Retrieved from http://help.feedingamerica.org/HungerInAmerica/hunger-in-america-2014-full-report.pdf?s_src=W182REFER&s_referrer=https%3A%2F%2Fwww.bing.com%2F&s_subsrc=http%3A%2F%2Fwww.feedingamerica.org%2Fresearch%2Fhunger-in-america%2F&_ga=2.101309640.877281802.1518627144-2142594713.1518627144

White, B., & Newman, S. (2015). Access to primary care services among the homeless: A synthesis of the literature using the equity of access to medical care framework. *Journal of Primary Care and Community Health, 6*(2), 77–87.

Wright, J. D. (1990). Poor people, poor health: The health status of the homeless. *Journal of Social Issues, 46*(4), 49–64. doi:10.1111/j.1540-4560.1990.tb01798.x

Zlotnick, C., & Zerger, S. (2009). Survey findings on characteristics and health status of clients treated by the federally funded (US) Health Care for the Homeless Programs. *Health & Social Care in the Community, 17*(1), 18–26. doi:10.1111/j.1365-2524.2008.00793.x

10

Geriatric Diabetic Homeless Patients and Their Care

Stephanie Diana Garcia, Ian Curtis Neel, Veronica Gonzalez,
Marlina Mansour, and Jairo Romero

Diabetes mellitus is one of the most common chronic conditions in older, homeless adults. Self-reported prevalence of diabetes is 8% (95% confidence interval = 6.8%, 9.2% n = 39 (Bernstein, Meurer, Plumb, & Jackson, 2015; Egede, 2015). Adverse clinical outcomes for this special population include hospitalization and decreased life expectancy; average life expectancy is 42 to 52 years old (Maness & Khan, 2014). The prevalence of diabetes in hospitalized adults aged 65 to 75 years and over 80 years of age, is estimated to be 20% and 40%, respectively (Umpierrez, 2017). To prevent hospitalizations, mortality, and success in reaching patient-derived glycemic range goals of VA/DoD *Clinical Practice Guideline for the Management of Type 2 Diabetes Mellitus in Primary Care,* high-quality, individualized education to make informed decisions is essential. Diabetic care and management begins with the relationship building between a provider and patient to ensure medication adherence. For many homeless persons, survival requires a great deal of patience and resilience. Empathetic, nonjudgmental interview styles have been shown to be more effective than confrontational approaches. Providers can begin by recognizing these strengths in their patient to empower them by identifying that they already have the necessary tools to control their condition.

DESCRIPTION

There are more than two types of diabetes mellitus, but the most classic are type 1 and type 2. Diabetes can be caused by genetic defects in the B-cell function or insulin action, disease of the exocrine pancreas, or induced by drugs or chemicals. Type 1 diabetes mellitus is defined as islet cell destruction or absolute insulin deficiency, and these patients are dependent on exogenous insulin. This special population is at highest risk of the acute presentation of diabetic ketoacidosis (DKA). The onset of this subtype is usually in younger patients, but can occur throughout adulthood. In a previously asymptomatic, undiagnosed individual, DKA may be a person's initial debut with diabetes (Vellanki & Umpierrez, 2017). Type 2 diabetes mellitus, the most common type of diabetes, is characterized by insulin resistance and is most commonly associated with obesity. However, in older adults, 30% of lean body mass is lost, making body habitus an unreliable marker of risk. Type 2 diabetes mellitus is characterized as relative insulin deficiency. Providers must also consider the various other causes of diabetes that are significant and prevalent in geriatric homeless patients: chronic use of steroids, pancreatic insufficiency (both acute and chronic), hemochromatosis, cystic fibrosis, and intestinal resection. The provider must also consider drugs that can induce diabetes such as protease inhibitors or atypical antipsychotics.

PREDIABETES

As diabetes mellitus (DM) rises in incidence, more vigilance must be paid to appropriate screening in asymptomatic older adults, especially if BMI is greater than 25 kg/m^2. Screening constitutes the use of HbA1c, fasting plasma glucose, or OGTT. A single elevated fasting plasma glucose does not constitute as screening for DM. These tests should be repeated at three-year intervals in homeless older patients, which is a recommendation no different than for appropriately housed populations.

POST-HOSPITAL ADMISSION

Prevalence of diabetes in hospitalized adults aged 65 to 75 years and over 80 years of age is estimated to be 20% and 40% (Umpierrez, 2017), respectively. The homeless elderly patient is particularly prone to noncompliance with discharge medications, and thus discharge planning is essential to be performed to maximize the chance of these patients having successful control of diabetes in the long term. Many health factors can compound in the older adult to make it difficult to follow through with even the best planned discharge diabetic regimen. For example, patients who are homeless with cognitive impairment are particularly at risk, and care must be taken to ensure appropriate aftercare planning is arranged for these individuals.

The best strategy for discharge planning is to use an interdisciplinary team approach, involving all members of the inpatient healthcare team, including social work and case management, physical and/or occupational therapy, nursing, the medical team, the patient, and, if available, their family. Upon discharge from the hospital setting, key to their improvement and readmission is follow-up with a primary care physician (PCP). Many cities have long-standing free clinics that may be more comfortable for a patient to go to than a typical outpatient clinic. Use the shared decision-making approach to identify factors that lead to lack of adherence for follow-up after previous hospitalizations. The case study at the end of this chapter will highlight how appropriate care of a dementia patient with diabetes should be managed post discharge.

Referral options may vary depending on the structure of the hospital. However, the PCP should make it his or her duty to refer for follow-up in a timely manner. If within the Veterans Affairs (VA) and DoD healthcare system, high-quality care includes timely referral to an endocrinologist and other specialist as appropriate.

CLINICAL MANIFESTATIONS

Homeless populations face an uphill battle with social determinants of health (education level, financial well-being, food security, safe and secure housing) stacked against them and commonly have a history of erratic glycemic levels. Geriatrics problems such as polypharmacy, cognitive impairment, pain, and fall risks are further compounded by higher rates of depression, substance use, and physical disability (Mehta & Wolfsdorf, 2010).

History gathering is key; however, it is important to note that record keeping, such as asking for a log of blood sugars to be tracked outpatient, is especially difficult for the homeless older adult. Provide your patient with a small notebook and pen to keep track of hypoglycemic episodes and symptoms to look out for, and ask them if they think they can record them. A provider can help set a daily alarm on patients' phones to remind them, if they have one. Patients may or may not be able to keep documentation, but one cannot underestimate preventative strategies or the individuals' motivation to adhere to a recommendation as they see fit.

Clinical manifestations of diabetes include macrovascular and microvascular complications, but often the disease initially may present with polyuria, polydipsia, or polyphagia. It is important, however, to take into account less-usual initial presentations of diabetes, especially in the older adult, which include unexplained weight loss, or no symptoms at all. If the patient appears intoxicated (a more common issue among the homeless population), it is important to keep hypoglycemia on the differential and prepare for alcohol withdrawal symptoms. Eliciting information to assess for complications, such as cardiovascular signs and symptoms, vision changes, numbness, paresthesias, skin changes such as hyperpigmentation, venous status, and ulcers, must be thoroughly carried out.

Patients may or may not have a regular general practitioner they visit for follow-up appointments. If the patient is new, establish how long ago he or she was first diagnosed (Kalinowski, Tinker, Wismer, & Meinbresse, 2013). Be knowledgeable of the local free clinic, homeless population-directed care, and sources for corroborative information, such as investigating for a social worker or case worker. Careful and deliberate data gathering must take place to understand current health behaviors. Importantly, the patient's health literacy, memory, and performance of activities of daily living (ADLs) and instrumental activities of daily living (iADLs) will help assess functional status.

NUTRITION STATUS AND FOOD SECURITY

Screening for food insecurity and access is pivotal in a diabetic older adult. Importantly, in resource-restricted settings, a dietitian may not be available. Providers should gather information about nutrition status, eating habits (timing of meals), weight changes, and food sources (e.g., soup kitchens) (Kalinowski et al., 2013). Some soup kitchens have modified menus for diabetic patients.

FALL RISK ASSESSMENT

Fall risk assessment is especially important. Gather information about use of assistive mobility devices, such as a wheelchair or cane, use of eyeglasses if they are prescribed, appropriate footwear, and last appointment with an eye doctor. The etiology of causes of falls should be carefully addressed. Weakness in individuals' legs, psychomotor agitation, impulsivity, vascular compromise, or changes in their vision can increase their risk of falls.

DEPRESSION

Depression in a homeless person should not be overlooked. Use a Patient Health Questionnaire (PHQ), but if the patient finds it difficult to follow along use the Geriatric Depression Scale. Geriatric patients, especially those who are homeless, are vulnerable to depression and should be adequately managed beginning with a selective serotonin reuptake inhibitor (SSRI). Appropriate management of depression can help stabilize the patient back into permanent housing and living within an environment where appropriate diabetic self-care can exist.

COGNITIVE IMPAIRMENT

Administration of one of the various cognitive impairment assessment tools (Montreal Cognitive Assessment, Mini Mental Status Exam, or St. Louis University Mental Status Exam) can help a provider delineate if dementia may be underlying a patient's diabetes. Most commonly vascular dementia is associated with diabetes.

VISION

Severe eye pain, sensitivity to light, blurring or loss of vision, double vision, floaters, or light flashes should be specifically asked about. Diabetic retinopathy is one of the first microvascular complications of diabetes. It is the leading cause of blindness in the United States, but early detection and treatment can decrease vision loss by 50%. Treatment includes laser photocoagulation. Homeless persons have a two-fold risk of cataract and a three-fold risk of glaucoma (Mohamed, Gillies, & Wong, 2007). Risk factors for the progression of retinopathy include poor diabetic control, insulin use, the presence of microvascular disease, chronic disease, hyperlipidemia, and poor control of systolic blood pressure (systolic greater than 160 mmHg); these should motivate a provider to recommend eye exams at least every two years.

SOCIAL HISTORY

Lack of access to transportation and overall poor health make keeping previously scheduled appointments difficult. Calling ahead of time to cancel appointments is difficult, as access to shelter phones can be limited. A patient will likely return to the clinic when it is most convenient for him or her, when his or her health has improved, or when his or her symptoms become unbearable. Clinics that serve homeless individuals should anticipate walk-ins for this reason. Also, providers should be aware of pharmacy cards made available for the purchase of medication and supplies.

POLYPHARMACY

In addition to medication reconciliation, a treatment team must take the time to call the patient's pharmacy to confirm the date of last refill and last pick-up to confirm medication adherence. Providers should identify community-based lancet strips sales and exchanges. They are becoming a readily profitable sale item online and are regularly on local advertisements. Discourage your patient from engaging in this activity.

PHYSICAL EXAM

Besides vital signs, at each visit, obtain a full physical exam with focus on the cardiovascular, pulmonary, neurologic, musculoskeletal, and dermatologic systems. Point of care management of symptoms is key during a diabetic follow-up appointment.

A comprehensive foot exam, including vibration and monofilament sensation, should be performed at least annually. A patient should never leave your office without you looking at his or her feet at every visit. Ulcers or other worrisome skin changes are particularly common due to constant ambulation, exposure to harsh weather, and poor hygiene.

Evaluate any insulin injection sites for signs of infection.

DIAGNOSTIC TESTS

A series of diagnostic tests should be ordered at an initial visit of a person with diabetic symptoms, such as a urinalysis and HbA1c (point of care testing). To assess kidney status, the best test is albumin to creatinine. A 24-hour urine test is not recommended for many homeless patients because it is not practical (Department of Veterans Affairs, 2017). This supports the importance of understanding whether a patient's homeless status is chronic, acute, temporary, or long term.

Lipid status should be evaluated with a fasting lipid panel; however, if the patient has not been fasting, his or her low-density lipoprotein (LDL) cholesterol can still be accurately measured. Fasting may not be realistic or appropriate if the patient acquires his or her meals from soup kitchens within set time frames.

Criteria for Diagnosis—One or More of the Following (Reuben et al., 2017):

- Symptoms of polyuria, polydipsia, unexplained weight loss plus casual plasma glucose concentration greater than or equal to 200 mg/dL
- Fasting (no caloric intake for greater than or equal to 8 h) plasma glucose greater than or equal to 126 mg/dL
  - Two-hour plasma glucose greater than or equal to 200 mg/dL during an oral glucose tolerance test (OGTT)

- Unless hyperglycemia is unequivocal, diagnosis should be confirmed by repeat testing.
- HbA1c greater than 6.5

Prediabetes—Any of the Following (Reuben et al., 2017):

- Impaired fasting glucose: defined as fasting plasma glucose greater than or equal to 100 and less than 126 mg/dL
- Impaired glucose tolerance: Two-hour plasma glucose 140–199 mg/dL
- HbA1c 5.7% to 6.4%

FURTHER WORK-UP

A retinal exam is used to detect retinopathy; if acute changes in vision or a change in ocular function is found, the patient should receive prompt, urgent referral to an eye care provider.

PATIENT EDUCATION AND SELF-MANAGEMENT

Literature, peer interaction, and support groups are particularly successful approaches to self-management that involve patients in the learning process. A motivational interview is a good approach to reduce the risk of complications from conditions that necessitate behavioral change. Simply assessing a patient's readiness to quit substance use can move the patient in the right direction. Programs such as Alcoholics Anonymous and/or Narcotics Anonymous are available most hours of the day, including 5 a.m. and late night hours; encouragement to find a group that fits the patient's personality and needs may be of great benefit. Group treatment can help the patient find support and community depending on the patient's readiness for seeking sobriety.

PREVENTION

Patients should carry out a daily foot inspection on themselves. A provider can recommend patients always encourage foot exams by future providers at subsequent visits (Handelsman & Jellinger, 2011). It is okay to acknowledge the difficulties of following-up with a steady provider. Take time to show them how to identify problematic skin breakdown, callus, erythema, and tinea pedis. Use of mirrors, leg elevation at night, and nightly washing of their socks can be greatly beneficial. Encourage patients to take off their shoes and socks at night. Remind them that pain may or may not be present with even severe infection. In fact, as a provider, fever and white blood cell counts may or may not be present even with limb-threatening infections. Consider that nonadherence may stem from the risk of shoes being stolen or one's inability to remove shoes.

TREATMENT

End-organ complications of diabetes can be delayed or prevented if hyperglycemic states are minimized and treated in an appropriate and timely manner. In homeless older populations, self-monitoring blood glucose is difficult and complicated by monitoring with home glucometers and lancet strips, which can be expensive. Providers can inform their patients that these supplies can be obtained at no cost from companies as samples or at reduced prices. If the patient is unable or unwilling to monitor blood glucose, focusing on blood pressure management is appropriate, as tight glycemic control might be dangerous for patients on insulin or sulfonylureas who cannot predict the number or timing of meals.

HbA1c is strongly predictive of microvascular complications, such as retinopathy, neuropathy, and nephropathy, but the benefits of tight glycemic control may not outweigh the risks of hypoglycemic events, which can be life threatening. Goal setting using colorful charts that indicate seriously concerning HbA1c levels and their attributable average glucose indication may facilitate understanding. Glycemic goals, as stated in the American Diabetes Association (2013) guidelines and European Association for the Study of Diabetes, recommend HbA1c of eight in particularly vulnerable populations, as opposed to seven in healthy older adults with longer life expectancy. Furthermore, the American Geriatrics Society and Veterans Affairs and Department of Defense recommend an A1c target of 8% to 9% (Department of Veterans Affairs, 2017; Williams et al., 2014). Furthermore, in more diverse communities, it is important to consider racial differences between estimated average glucose and HbA1c values in patients with T2DM based on seven-point glucose testing (Department of Veterans Affairs, 2017). Ethnic differences in glycemic markers in patients with type 2 diabetes usually involve hemoglobinopathy such as sickle cell disease; G6PD deficiency, which is more common in Black populations, can be associated with falsely lowered HbA1c (English et al., 2015). African Americans have about a 0.4% higher HbA1c level than White individuals; the difference cannot be explained by measured differences in glycemia or sociodemographic factors, clinical factors, access to care, or quality of care (Viberti et al., 2006). Keeping these things in mind can help inform analysis of results, although no differences in management are recommended at this time. This is also why HbA1c ranges versus levels above or below a specific target are recommended;t the strongest evidence supports patients with T2DM. A level of 7% to 8.5% is appropriate for most individuals with established microvascular or macrovascular disease, comorbid conditions, or 5 to 10 years of life expectancy (Department of Veterans Affairs, 2017). Providers are tasked with helping the patient understand that, by reducing hyperglycemia, symptoms of acute fatigue will be lessened; however, a major goal is to avoid hypoglycemia (California Healthcare Foundation/American Geriatrics Society Panel on Improving Care for Elders With Diabetes, 2003; Department of Veterans Affairs, 2017; Lee & Eng, 2011).

NONINSULIN VERSUS INSULIN AND ORAL VERSUS INJECTION

For T2DM, most guidelines recommend metformin often coupled with an insulin secretagogue such as sulfonyurea. Older adults are susceptible to drug-induced hypoglycemia. The side-effect profile must be carefully considered. For example, it is well known that, in a patient with severe renal insufficiency, metformin is contraindicated. Additionally, for persons with high risk for cardiovascular events, the following medications have been found to specifically reduce cardiovascular events: metformin, empagliflozin, and liraglutide (Department of Veterans Affairs, 2017). Harms related to social determinants of health must be considered in older homeless persons.

Noninsulin therapy is chosen based on the side-effect profile, kidney function, alcohol use, liver function, and/or whether weight loss or gain is desired. For example, DPP-4 inhibitors in a patient with known or suspected alcohol use disorder are dangerous. Also, GLP-1 inhibitors require refrigeration before opening. This may be impossible for some and difficult for others in homeless shelters (Kalinowski et al., 2013). Additionally, GLP-1 inhibitors may be dangerous if the patient has triglycerides greater than 500 or is struggling with alcohol use disorder due to secondaryrisk of pancreatitis (BYDUREON BCise [(exenatide extended-release) injectable suspension] full Prescribing Information, 2017; Handelsman & Jellinger, 2011).

ORAL NONINSULIN MEDICATIONS

Biguanides (Metformin)

Mechanism of action (MOA): Decrease hepatic glucose production
Metformin alone decreases HbA1 by 1.5% and is not associated with weight gain or risk of hypoglycemia. Adverse effects to warn patients to look out for include nausea, diarrhea, and lactic acidosis in those with renal failure,

although it is a rare complication. If the patient cannot tolerate the side effects, then other oral agents can be prescribed. Patients should be advised, if living in a shelter that limits bathroom privileges, to anticipate diarrheal episodes. Providers can write a letter to the shelter to explain their special need.

Meglitinides (Repaglinide, Nateglinide)

MOA: Stimulate insulin secretion
Meglitinides are short-acting insulin secretagogues that can decrease post-prandial hyperglycemia. This agent causes weight gain and risk of hypoglycemia.

Alpha glucosidase inhibitors (Acarbose, Miglitol)

MOA: Decrease intestinal carbohydrate absorption
Alpha glucosidase inhibitors are rarely used due to gastrointestinal side effects.

Thiazolidinediones (Pioglitazone, Rosiglitazone)

MOA: Increased peripheral insulin sensitivity
Thiazolidinediones also cause weight gain and may exacerbate heart failure and other cardiovascular (CV) events.

Incretin Modulators

GLP-1 agonists (Exenatide, Liraglutide)

MOA: Increase glucose-dependent insulin secretion
Adverse effects include weight loss, nausea, vomiting, diarrhea, and acute pancreatitis.

DPP-4 inhibitors (Sitagliptin, Saxagliptin, Linagliptin)

MOA: Accentuates GLP-1 activity and decreases glucagon
DPP-4 inhibitors are weight-neutral and do not increase risk of hypoglycemia, but do increase risk of acute pancreatitis.

Amylin Mimetic (Pramlintide)

MOA: Analogue of amylin
Released along with insulin by the pancreas after meals to aid in regulation of glucose via slowing gastric emptying, inhibiting secretion of glucagon, and

promoting satiety in the hypothalamus. Lastly, amylin mimetic (Pramlintide) is generally well tolerated, but cannot be mixed with insulin.

Insulin

T2DM may eventually require treatment with insulin. Treatment of T1DM requires insulin. Understanding the different preparations of insulin, especially lispro, regular, neutral protamine Hagedorn (NPH), glargine, and detemir insulin, is also key to appropriate management and effective education (Department of Veterans Affairs, 2017).

Caution with intensifying treatment to use of insulin is merited inhomeless persons. Long-acting basal insulins such as insulin glargine and insulin detemir are less likely to cause hypoglycemia than NPH insulin. Sliding-scale insulin should be avoided due to increased risk of hypoglycemia, without evidence that it can improve glycemic control (Williams et al., 2014).

The adverse effect of uncontrolled hyperglycemia in T2DM can lead to hyperglycemic hyperosmolar syndrome, landing a patient in the hospital. Classically, T1DM was more commonly associated with DKA, but increasing rates of DKA in T2DM patients are being studied. However, this is a less common cause of hospital admission. Diabetes will usually be secondary to another comorbidity, but hyperglycemia may be exacerbated by acute illness or infection (Wiener, Wiener, & Larson, 2008).

Inpatient Insulin Management

The following are some recommendations for patients in an inpatient setting supported by strong evidence as listed by the VA guideline:

- Patients receiving insulin in the hospital target blood glucose lesser than 110 mg/dL, 110 being the minimum. Previously, tight glycemic control was recommended, but risk of hypoglycemia outweighed the benefits.
- Adjust insulin to maintain blood glucose between 110 and 180 mg/dL for patients with type 2 diabetes, for patients who are critically ill, or for those with acute myocardial infarction (Department of Veterans Affairs, 2017; Malmberg, 1997).
- Strong evidence recommends against the use of split mixed regimen of all hospitalized T2DM patients. In other words, a twice-a-day insulin injection regimen with a fixed amount of mixed NPH insulin (intermediate-acting insulin) and regular insulin is recommended for patients who can receive consistent meal plans, which is difficult in the hospital.

- In an inpatient setting, basal bolus regimens can be replaced safely by noninsulin regimens with the use of dipeptidyl peptidase-4 inhibitors alone or in combination with basal bolus (Umpierrez, 2017).

Studies are unlikely to include older adults, but the guidelines may be helpful.

STRATEGIES TO REDUCE COMMON DIABETIC COMPLICATIONS

Cardiovascular

Adequate control of comorbid conditions should start with minimizing CV risk. Atherosclerosis is the most important cause of permanent disability and accounts for more hospital days than any other illness. Meanwhile, reducing CV risks will also reduce risk of microvascular dementia.

Cognitive Impairment

Patients who are homeless may have cognitive impairment due to various etiologies, such as intoxication or psychiatric, developmental, or neurologic deficits. Cognitive functioning may be impaired due to dementia, as such a work-up may help patients gain some clarity in condition and lapses in memory, especially if caught very early. Diabetics may need to enlist help from friends or shelter managers to ensure appropriate management of their medications. Inquire about head trauma, history of dementia in their family, and inability to carry out simple financial transactions; these may be some early-on clues to underlying dementia.

Infection

If a patient is not vigilant or is intoxicated, he or she may not be able to prevent a minor infection from becoming septic. Infections can cause blood glucose to become elevated, and providers should educate their patients who are monitoring their blood sugars during an infection.

Gastrointestinal Neuropathy

Patients may experience alternating constipation and diarrhea. A provider can choose to write to shelter administrators to allow for access to bathrooms.

Erectile Dysfunction

HbA1c is inversely proportional to erectile function (ED); cigarette smoking cessation can reduce the risk of CV and ED.

Renal Insufficiency

Signs and symptoms include polyuria, nocturia, increased frequency, foamy urine, hematuria, oliguria, and symptoms of anemia such as fatigue. Alternatively, physical exam findings consistent with anemia may be present, such as pale conjunctiva, fatigue, and so on. Appropriate work-up includes ordering a complete blood count and comprehensive metabolic panel, as well as calculation of creatinine clearance because glomerular filtration rate (GFR) and creatinine must be adjusted for by age and weight in addition to other factors.

Prophylaxis and Diabetes-Related Health Maintenance Recommendations

The conversation about the benefits of diet and exercise and the health benefits of a plant-based diet should be at least mentioned, although studies have shown this approach to be ineffective in environments lacking food security and high rates of venous stasis and neuropathy, ulcers, and other foot conditions, which preclude exercise. Soup kitchens do not usually follow diabetes-friendly menus. However, if the patient expresses interest, appropriate recommendations also include weight loss if he or she is obese. Obesity increases the risk of mortality at any age, and also increases hypertension, heart disease, coronary artery disease, insulin resistance, sleep apnea, DM, hypertriglyceridemia, osteoarthritis, thromboembolism, and varicose veins. Recall, however, that at the age of 80 patients are deficient of lean body mass. The following recommendations are suggested: If the patient has a body mass index (BMI) of greater than 30 kg/m², caloric restriction with the goal of weight loss, limiting saturated fat to less than 7% of total calories, minimizing trans fats, and limiting cholesterol intake to less than 200 mg/day. For patients with hypertension and diabetes, the "Mediterranean" diet, a plant-based diet; Dietary Approaches to Stop Hypertension (DASH) diet; and Bananas, Rice, Applesauce, Toast (BRAT) diet are some options. However, among frail homeless individuals, diabetic older adults' food restriction may increase risk of hypoglycemia. The "Mediterranean" diet consists of high intake of vegetables, fruits, nuts, unrefined grains, and olive oil; moderate intake of fish and poultry; low or moderate intake of wine; and low intake of red meat, processed meat, dairy, and sweets (Kalinowski et al., 2013). Furthermore, providers should be aware that medical nutritional therapy provided by a registered dietician is a covered Medicare benefit. Approach to exercise recommendations is to start slow and increase activity based on improved conditioning.

Clinicians should advocate for their homeless patients and visit with the director of nutrition services at the local soup kitchen to understand which healthy options are available and if more diabetic-friendly options can be made available. Other ways a provider can advocate for older diabetic patients is by securing a podiatrist for future referrals. Additionally, keeping a supply of padded socks available for providers to give to their patient during the visit is also helpful.

CONCLUSION

People without homes have a wide range of housing situations that may be temporary or permanent. In any case, their unique story and understanding of it without judgment and with ample empathy is the cornerstone of diabetic management in older homeless persons. In other words, only through genuine dialog strengthened by patience will a provider begin to facilitate trust and understanding. This is key to relationship building. Asking appropriate questions is a way that a provider can assure the survivor in front of him or her that he or she is not expected to be a passive recipient of services determined by the provider's professional expertise. The older adult is unlikely to respond or adhere, or even return for follow-up if subjected to the role of a passive recipient. Deliberate teaching about microvascular complications, such as retinopathy, neuropathy, and nephropathy, especially if HbA1c is greater than 9%, is necessary. Partner with the patient by using coaching techniques to remind the patient that focusing on and strengthening his or her internal locus of control is key. In other words, a provider's hope and encouragement can help replace the external locus of control that may be adding to the patient's complexities. The complications of diabetes develop over an extended period of time, which gives the provider serving this population ample time to be patient and resilient in caring for, educating, and goal-setting with the older, homeless person. Self-management is complex, and motivating a homeless patient to follow-up requires provider leadership; consistent, repetitive education (teachback method); and deep compassion.

CASE STUDY

Mr. X, a 68-year-old male with a past medical history of T2DM, hyperlipidemia, hypertension, psychosis, mood disorder, impulse control disorder, and major neurocognitive disorder, presented to the emergency department (ED) in a confused state and was unable to identify himself. He was wearing an arm band, identifying a local nursing and rehabilitation center. He was likely assisted to the ED by a good Samaritan.

On initial intake interview, although able to speak in full sentences, Mr. X was unable to recall his name. He was able to recognize it once it was stated. He perseverated on the fact that he was hungry and needed money to get home. The patient stated that he was in an airport and that he " is here for an eye exam." He was in no acute distress. Social work was immediately called to help piece-together his story. Meanwhile, the medical team began to work-up his confused state.

Six months prior to this admission, the patient was picked up at the airport while sitting in a wheelchair appearing confused. He presented to the ED awake and alert. The patient was unable to perform visual acuity assessment screening. On initial review of systems, he denied any chest pain, shortness of breath, nausea, vomiting, diarrhea, or constipation. He did not have any medications among his belongings. On initial exam, his physical exam was largely normal. His neurological exam was normal; he demonstrated equal strength bilaterally, and had a negative pronator drift. His mental status exam was grossly abnormal. His CT scan was notable for encephalomalacia without any acute findings; he was discharged back to the local nursing and rehabilitation center, which subsequently transferred him to a psychiatric unit.

Later, additional documentation helped confirm that Mr. X had been in and out of hospitals and nursing centers, but his records were incomplete.

On this admission, the patient was disheveled and dirty; he was oriented only to person. He was able to make his needs known such as food, water, and sleep, but was unable to state where he lived, his source of income, or his family or collateral contacts. He believed he lived in a big house in Arizona and had two ladies, and he also said that he was staying in a "nice new tent." A folder of documents included his past resume and other past employment-related documents. No collateral contact or identifying data was found in his belongings. He was recommended to stay in a unit within the hospital dedicated to care for older adults with psychiatric and medical needs. He remained in the unit while diagnostic work-up and further placement was arranged.

On review of systems, he only complained of difficulty hearing, double vision, and leg cramping. From ED records, six months prior, he has a history of T2DM. On admission, his glucose was 259 and he had an HbA1c of 10%. He began treatment with metformin 1000 twice a day. He was also hypertensive for which he received amlodipine, which immediately brought down his systolic blood pressure to 134 after being elevated in the ED, ranging from 147 to 170 mmHg. For his hyperlipidemia, he was previously prescribed atorvastatin 20 mg daily, but had not been taking any medications on arrival to the ED. His total cholesterol level was 180, HDL 61, LDL was 98, and triglycerides were 104.

Regarding his DM with a markedly elevated A1c, elevated blood sugars had been in the 300s. Weight-based calculations estimated that he would need approximately 34 units daily of insulin for coverage, but given his lability of blood sugars and advanced age, his team decided to err on the side of caution and prescribe low-dose long- and short-acting insulin, increasing the dose based on sliding-scale needs over a 24-hour period. He was also prescribed glargine 10 units daily, Lispro 3 units TID AC, and Lispro on a sliding scale. Endocrinology was consulted.

The patient's ocular symptoms and leg pain reports were concerning for diabetic retinopathy and neuropathy. Given his homeless situation, he had not had regular monitoring of his diabetes. He was appropriately arranged for outpatient follow-up, as well as optometry evaluation for a dilated fundoscopic exam. A urine microalbumin/creatinine ratio was checked and was found to be within normal limits.

Furthermore, his leg pain was most concerning for diabetic neuropathy, although the provider could not exclude peripheral vascular disease, given the patient's risk factors and comorbidities. His symptoms were reported as more claudication-like, especially given his vascular risk factors. Appropriate work-up included bilateral lower extremity venous ultrasound.

To make the picture complicated, his CT scan was notable for large encephalomalacia/gliosis of the left middle cerebral territory, left caudate head, and left lenticular nucleus. These findings were unchanged from a prior head CT. Moderate periventricular subcortical hypoattenuation was observed, which was likely due to chronic microvascular ischemia. There was no evidence of mass-effect or midline shift. The basal cisterns were patent. There was no evidence of an intracranial hemorrhage or mass lesion. It was observed that the patient had calcified intracranial vasculature.

The patient was diagnosed with a major neurocognitive disorder, with a vascular component, based on imaging. Laboratory assessment was performed to rule out organic contribution to disease. He received neurocognitive testing, and displayed evidence of a prior cerebral vascular accident on his head CT. No focal deficits were found on his neurologic exam, and he was managed with aspirin and atorvastatin to reduce the risk of future vascular accidents.

Given his multiple comorbidities, namely DM, HLD, hypertension (HTN), major neurocognitive disorder, and geropsychiatry, his primary provider co-managed his medications. Meanwhile, the unit social worker helped secure a safe aftercare plan.

His discharge plan entailed placement in a dementia unit, once medical management of his DM was optimized. Placement in a dementia memory care unit may help prevent future visits to the ED and help resolve his homeless status, ultimately providing a better environment for him with care, food, and boarding. The team set goals to optimize his medical management before discharge to the dementia unit.

REFERENCES

American Diabetes Association. (2013). Standards of medical care in diabetes—2013. *Diabetes Care, 36*(Suppl. 1), S11–S66. doi:10.2337/dc13-S011

Bernstein, R. S., Meurer, L. N., Plumb, E. J., & Jackson, J. L. (2015). Diabetes and hypertension prevalence in homeless adults in the United States: A systematic review and meta-analysis. *American Journal of Public Health, 105*(2), e46–e60. doi:10.2105/AJPH.2014.302330

BYDUREON BCise ([exenatide extended-release] injectable suspension) full Prescribing Information. (2017). Wilmington, DE: AstraZeneca Pharmaceuticals, LP.

California Healthcare Foundation/American Geriatrics Society Panel on Improving Care for Elders With Diabetes. (2003). Guidelines for improving the care of the older person with diabetes mellitus. *Journal of the American Geriatrics Society, 51*(5 Suppl Guidelines), S265–S280. doi:10.1046/j.1532-5415.51.5s.1.x

Department of Veterans Affairs. (2017). VA/DoD Clinical practice guideline for the management of type 2 diabetes mellitus in primary care (Vol. Version 5). Washington, DC: Author. Retrieved from https://www.healthquality.va.gov/guidelines/CD/diabetes/VADoDDMCPGFinal508.pdf

Egede, L. E. (2015). Diabetes and hypertension prevalence in homeless adults in the United States: A systematic review and meta-analysis. *Journal of General Internal Medicine, 105*(2), e46–e60. doi:10.1007/s11606-016-3786-z

English, E., Idris, I., Smith, G., Dhatariya, K., Kilpatrick, E. S., & John, W. G. (2015). The effect of anaemia and abnormalities of erythrocyte indices on HbA1c analysis: A systematic review. *Diabetologia, 58*(7), 1409–1421. doi:10.1007/s00125-015-3599-3

Handelsman, Y., & Jellinger, P. S. (2011). Overcoming obstacles in risk factor management in type 2 diabetes mellitus. *The Journal of Clinical Hypertension (Greenwich), 13*(8), 613–620. doi:10.1111/j.1751-7176.2011.00490.x

Kalinowski, A., Tinker, T., Wismer, B., & Meinbresse, M. (2013). *Adapting your practice: Treatment and recommendations for people who are homeless with diabetes mellitus.* Nashville, TN: Health Care for the Homeless Clinicians' Network. Retrieved from http://www.nhchc.org/wp-content/uploads/2013/06/2013DiabetesGuidelines_FINAL_20130612.pdf

Lee, S. J., & Eng, C. (2011). Goals of glycemic control in frail older patients with diabetes. *Journal of the American Medical Association, 305*(13), 1350–1351. doi:10.1001/jama.2011.404

Malmberg, K. (1997). Prospective randomised study of intensive insulin treatment on long term survival after acute myocardial infarction in patients with diabetes mellitus. DIGAMI (Diabetes Mellitus, Insulin Glucose Infusion in Acute Myocardial Infarction) Study Group. *British Medical Journal, 314*(7093), 1512–1515.

Maness, D. L., & Khan, M. (2014). Care of the homeless: An overview. *American Family Physician, 89*(8), 634–640.

Mehta, S. N., & Wolfsdorf, J. I. (2010). Contemporary management of patients with type 1 diabetes. *Endocrinology and Metabolism Clinics of North America, 39*(3), 573–593. doi:10.1016/j.ecl.2010.05.002

Mohamed, Q., Gillies, M. C., & Wong, T. Y. (2007). Management of diabetic retinopathy: A systematic review. *Journal of the American Medical Association, 298*(8), 902–916. doi:10.1001/jama.298.8.902

Reuben, D. B., Herr, K., Pacala, J. T., Potter, J. F., Semla, T. P., & Small, G. W. (2017). *Geriatrics at your fingertips: 2017*. Belle Mead, NJ: Excerpta Medica.

Umpierrez, G. E. (2017). Diabetes: SGLT2 inhibitors and diabetic ketoacidosis: A growing concern. *Nature Reviews Endocrinology, 13*(8), 441–442. doi:10.1038/nrendo.2017.77

Umpierrez, G. E., & Pasquel, F. J. (2017). Management of inpatient hyperglycemia and diabetes in older adults. *Diabetes Care, 40*(4), 509–517. doi:10.2337/dc16-0989

Vellanki, P., & Umpierrez, G. E. (2017). Diabetic ketoacidosis: A common debut of diabetes among African Americans with type 2 diabetes. *Endocrine Practice.* doi:10.4158/EP161679.RA

Viberti, G., Lachin, J., Holman, R., Zinman, B., Haffner, S., Kravitz, B., . . . Group, A. S. (2006). A Diabetes Outcome Progression Trial (ADOPT): Baseline characteristics of type 2 diabetic patients in North America and Europe. *Diabetic Medicine, 23*(12), 1289–1294. doi:10.1111/j.1464-5491.2006.02022.x

Wiener, R. S., Wiener, D. C., & Larson, R. J. (2008). Benefits and risks of tight glucose control in critically ill adults: A meta-analysis. *Journal of the American Medical Association, 300*(8), 933–944. doi:10.1001/jama.300.8.933

Williams, B., Chang, A., Landefeld, S., Ahalt, C., Conant, R., & Chen, H. (2014). *Current diagnosis & treatment: Geriatrics* (2nd ed.). New York, NY: McGraw-Hill.

11

Geriatric Nutrition and Homelessness

Victoria Clark and Elizabeth Lake

MALNUTRITION AND AGING

Malnutrition impacts an estimated 22.8% of elderly adults worldwide, with prevalence as high as 38.7% in hospitalized elderly patients (Kaiser et al., 2010). The American Society for Parenteral and Enteral Nutrition defines malnutrition as "An acute, subacute or chronic state of nutrition, in which a combination of varying degrees of overnutrition or undernutrition with or without inflammatory activity have led to a change in body composition and diminished function" (Definitions, n.d.). Malnutrition can result from acute disease/injury, chronic disease, or starvation. The costs associated with malnutrition are vast. Malnutrition is associated with increased healthcare costs and hospital length of stay, decreased quality of life, and poor outcomes with increased rates of morbidity and mortality (Kaiser et al., 2010). Physiological, psychosocial, and medical changes that occur with aging put the elderly at increased risk for developing malnutrition.

Food intake typically decreases with age, a phenomenon commonly referred to as "anorexia of aging" (Bernstein & Munoz, 2012). With decreased intake, the risk for undernutrition increases for elderly patients. To understand this phenomenon, one must first delve into the many physical, social, and psychological factors that influence the aging process. Body composition itself changes with age as muscle begins to decrease in both mass and strength, also known as sarcopenia (Mahan, Escott-Stump, & Raymond, 2012). Physical activity level also typically begins to decrease, and these two factors combined ultimately result in reduced energy needs; however, requirements for many other nutrients remain constant or even increase (Bernstein & Munoz, 2012). Older adults are more likely to experience early satiety and feel less hungry when compared with their younger counterparts, thus making achieving adequate intake more difficult (Bernstein & Munoz, 2012). Overall, disability and functional limitations may inhibit independent performance of activities of daily living such as their ability to prepare meals, grocery shop, and feed themselves (Bernstein & Munoz, 2012).

Sensory decline is also associated with aging. Older adults may experience decreased sense of taste, smell, and hearing. Decreased taste and smell not only deters food intake, but fails to stimulate important metabolic processes such as salivation and release of pancreatic and gastric secretions (Mahan et al., 2012). The immune function declines. Xerostomia, dry mouth, is a common side effect of medications and contributes to difficulty with chewing and swallowing foods (Mahan et al., 2012). Overall gastric acid secretion declines and results in decreased nutrient absorption, especially vitamin B_{12} (Mahan et al., 2012). Older adults may also experience delayed gastric emptying, which contributes to early satiety. They are also more likely to experience constipation. General decline in liver, kidney, and pancreatic function impacts efficiency of nutrient metabolism, digestion, and absorption (Mahan et al., 2012).

Presence of chronic diseases also has nutritional implications. In addition to the impact chronic conditions have on nutrient needs and the patient's appetite/intake, diet modification may be encouraged to help manage the disease process. Although aimed to improve health outcomes, a more restrictive diet may be unpalatable to the older adult and negatively impact intake and quality of life (Bernstein & Munoz, 2012). In 2015, the Centers for Disease Control (CDC) estimated that approximately 80% of older adults have at least one chronic condition and 50% have a minimum of two (CDC, 2015). In addition to the physiological impact of chronic disease, medications used to manage these conditions also often have nutritional side effects and interactions, leading to taste changes, anorexia, nausea, and vomiting. Many elderly adults experience varying levels of cognitive decline from either aging or a disease process such as dementia. Impaired memory and cognition may cause patients to forget to eat or drink adequately and can also negatively impact chewing and swallowing function. Depression, social isolation, living situation, and economic limitations can also negatively impact intake and nutritional status. This chapter will further explore the impact that homelessness and food insecurity has on the nutritional status of older adults.

NUTRITION AND HOMELESSNESS

The U.S. Department of Agriculture (USDA) defines food security as access by all people at all times to enough food for an active, healthy life. Food insecurity is a day-to-day reality for the elderly homeless population. Food security is basic to maintain the nutritional status of the elderly, as it addresses hunger and a consistent source of nutritionally adequate food, which will help with the management of chronic diseases (Kertesz, 2004; Wellman, Weddle, Kranz, & Brain, 1997).

It is predicted that homeless people greater than 65 years of age will double by 2050 from 44,000 to over 88,000 as the population ages (Goldberg, Lang, & Barrington, 2016). Homeless persons 65 years and older have previously been a lower percentage among the homeless population, as they become eligible for Medicare and Social Security. Older adults, aged 50 to 65 years of age, is an increasing homeless population (National Coalition for the Homeless, 2009). In 2012, the Department of Agriculture reported 49 million people, or 14.5% of the population, had inadequate access to food (Supplemental Nutrition Assistance Program). The 2016 U.S. Conference of Mayors' Report on Hunger and Homelessness (2016), which surveyed 32 cities in 24 states, found that of those requesting emergency food assistance, 63% were members of a family, 51% were employed, 18% were elderly, and 8% were homeless. In the U.S. Conference of Mayors' report, the surveyed cities estimated that 13.8% of the demand for emergency food assistance went unmet. Of those cities, 47% had emergency kitchen and food pantries decrease the amount of food offered per meals and the quantity of food received per visit. About 29% of the cities had to reduce the number of times a person could visit the food bank. Due to the lack of resources, 47% of the surveyed cities had facilities turn away individuals.

Homeless individuals are faced with difficult decisions to provide their basic needs for survival, often with limited financial resources. They have to choose between prioritizing shelter, food, and medical care, which may include medications (Supplemental Nutrition Assistance Program [SNAP], 2013; Wellman et al., 1997). The elderly homeless have additional barriers to accessing food resources. They may have limited mobility and/or weakness, lack of transportation, memory issues, and the absence of a permanent address. The elderly homeless may not be able to walk to a soup kitchen, food pantry, or agency to apply for benefits. Waiting in line for food or other services can be a challenge. They may not be strong enough when challenged by their younger counterparts for a place in line. Cognitive impairment of the elderly may make applying for programs difficult, or even being aware that they may be eligible for benefits that are available to the homeless (Goldberg et al., 2016).

Sources for food and/or meals for the homeless include shelters, soup kitchens, food banks, and government programs, such as the Supplemental Nutrition Assistance Program (SNAP). These resources help with reducing the food insecurity experienced by the elderly homeless. Some shelters serve meals; however, others just provide a bed for sleeping. Soup kitchens vary greatly in the number of meals they serve per day; often, it is only one instead of two or three (Sprake, Russell, & Barker, 2013; Strasser, Damrosch, & Gaines, 1991). The Holy Apostle Soup Kitchen in New York City serves one meal a day, about 1,200 meals. It costs about $2.2 million a year to run this kitchen. They survive on donated money for the most part. To serve more meals a day or include healthier food choices that are more expensive, more money would have to be raised as budgets are limited with little room to stretch (Bradfield, Greene, Watman, & Watman, 2014).

Traditionally, shelters and soup kitchens have relied on donations, food banks, and surplus commodity distributions (Homelessness, n.d.; Luder, Ceysens-Okada, Koren-Roth, & Martinez-Weber, 1990). Overall, foods provided to homeless individuals through shelter feeding facilities are high in fat, low in fiber, and inadequate in the provision of most nutrients (Johnson & McCool, 2003). This presents a real challenge for an elderly homeless person with a chronic disease, as well as decreased bowel motility, diverticulosis, and constipation. The choice is often eating or obtaining adequate food to prevent hunger or choosing the appropriate foods for their chronic disease, which most likely would limit the adequacy of their daily calorie, protein, and nutrient intake (Luder et al., 1990; Strasser, Damrosch, & Gaines, 1991).

Nutritional issues for the homeless individual include calorie deficiency or excess, as well as possible nutrient or vitamin deficiency (Kertesz, 2004). It has been reported through dietary questionnaires of homeless persons that their intake is deficient in thiamine, folic acid, calcium, magnesium, iron, vitamin A, and vitamin C (Homelessness, n.d.; Kertesz, 2004). The elderly homeless face additional nutritional challenges. The elderly often have chronic diseases, such as heart disease and diabetes mellitus, as well as high blood pressure. Obtaining medically appropriate foods that help with the management of these chronic diseases is particularly challenging. Foods that are lower in sodium, saturated fat, cholesterol, sugar, and refined carbohydrates are needed, but not always available.

Sisson and Lown (2011) collected survey and interview data about the local soup kitchens in Grand Rapids, Michigan. They found that a single meal did not provide two-thirds of the estimated average requirement for energy, vitamin C, magnesium, zinc, or two-thirds of the average intake for dietary fiber and calcium. However, the meal did exceed the recommendation for saturated fat. If two meals from the soup kitchen were consumed, they would meet the goals for all nutrients, except dietary fiber. But, the two meals also had an excess of energy, sodium, and saturated fat. The authors concluded this could potentially lead to overweight/obesity. Lyles, Drago-Ferguson, Lopez, and Seligman (2013) randomly analyzed meals served at six soup kitchens over a 10-week period in San Francisco. They found results similar to earlier studies. The meals provided were high in fat and sodium and inadequate in dietary fiber. The nutrients found in insufficient quantities were potassium, calcium, vitamin A, and vitamin C. The total calories would be insufficient for the day if two of the meals were consumed.

Food banks usually provide staples that are nonperishable. Food items include canned fruits, vegetables, beans, and meats. Boxed cereals and bags of dried beans or rice are other foods frequently included, whereas fresh foods are a minimal part of what is available. Homeless persons may not be able to utilize all the foods offered. The Hennepin County Medical Center (HCMC) in Minneapolis, Minnesota, has established a Food Shelf. This program was developed to address hunger and food insecurity among the patients they serve. HCMC found that half of their patients are food insecure. The food items provided are tailored to the specific population and are packaged in handled bags for easy transport (Hennepin County Medical Center, n.d.). Food banks in Grand Rapids are now providing more frequent access to fresh fruits and vegetables, as well as lower-sodium canned goods (Sisson & Lown, 2011). Surveyed cities in the 2016 U.S. Conference of Mayors' report noted some changes in the type of food purchased by their emergency food programs. In general, there was more purchasing of fresher, healthier, and more nutritious foods, particularly fresh produce and foods high in protein and low in sodium.

Other cities are taking the provision of food one step further. They are adding nutrition and health education in the form of a food prescription. The San Francisco General Hospital (SFGH) of the San Francisco Health Network developed a Therapeutic Food Pantry in order to improve health outcomes, promote healthy eating, provide nutrition education, and address food insecurity. This hospital-based program uses a prescription food program in which the provider writes a prescription for fresh fruits and vegetables and other healthy foods the patients will receive from the food pantry. These patients will also receive onsite nutrition education relevant to their health needs (SFGH Therapeutic Food Pantry, 2017). Another hospital, Boston Medical Center, runs a Prevention Food Pantry. This pantry was started to address illness and chronic diseases that are impacted by nutrition as well as undernutrition. It also connects the patient with a provider and nutritionist. As in San Francisco, the provider writes a prescription for the appropriate foods, which will include fresh fruits and vegetables, as well as meat (Boston Medical Center, 2017).

Some homeless persons scavenge for food, which increases the concern for food safety and adequacy (Supplemental Nutrition Assistance Program [SNAP], 2013). The homeless mentally ill are more likely to obtain food from garbage cans instead of soup kitchens or shelters (Wiecha, Dwyer, & Dunn-Strohecker, 1991). By scavenging places, the homeless are at risk for food-borne illnesses, as well as nutrient and caloric deficiencies (Supplemental Nutrition Assistance Program [SNAP], 2013).

Homeless persons are unable to follow the normal routine to purchase food. Lack of storage and cooking facilities limit the foods that can be bought, stored, and prepared. They often can only purchase food to eat immediately that requires minimal preparation and that does not require cooking or storage. Higher food costs may result in the need to buy smaller amounts of food that usually have a higher unit cost. There are foods available that do not need cooking or refrigeration for storage, but the lack of space and reduced ability to carry, and protect food from the heat present further barriers (Sprake et al., 2013; Wellman et al., 1997). For the elderly homeless persons, additional obstacles include decline in mobility, strength, and memory issues. They may not be able to walk to the discount grocery store, but rely on the local convenience store that has a limited selection at a higher cost (Goldberg et al., 2016). It is, therefore, difficult for the homeless elderly to meet their basic nutritional needs.

Obesity has become a growing health concern in the United States. There has been little research on the prevalence of obesity in the homeless population. Tsai and Rosenheck (2013) conducted a multivariate regression analysis using the data from the Collaborative Initiative by the U.S. Interagency Council on Homelessness. They found that 57.3 percent of the participants were overweight or obese. In a study by Koh, Hoy, O'Connell, and Montgomery (2012), the findings suggest that obesity is highly prevalent in the adult population. They found a 29% prevalence of obesity in those homeless who were greater than 60 years of age. They discovered potential reasons that were related to food and their altered metabolism. To avoid hunger, the homeless purchase inexpensive, energy dense but low-nutrient dense foods. These foods often taste good, leading to excessive intake of these low-nutrient and unhealthy foods. Obesity can produce an adaptive response to the inconsistent intake experienced by those with irregular meal intake. The homeless often eat more when there is food available. This inconsistent intake can also affect the metabolism by making it more efficient, thus producing weight gain with excessive meal intake. Other factors may include a sedentary lifestyle, sleep debit, and stress. Obesity adds other health risks such as high blood pressure, diabetes, and arthritis. Obese homeless can face additional challenges with facilities or shelters. They may not be able to accommodate a lower bunk or a large-enough bed, as well as any specialized medical equipment such as a CPAP machine.

NUTRITIONAL IMPACT OF SUBSTANCE ABUSE

Homeless individuals are faced with the difficult task of prioritizing their limited resources. Addiction to drugs and/or alcohol carries a big price tag, both financially and nutritionally. Substance abuse and addiction often divert financial resources away from securing healthy foods in adequate quantities. Excess substance intake and corresponding inadequate nutrition intake place the person at increased risk for developing malnutrition and nutrient deficiencies.

The National Coalition for the Homeless (2009) estimates that 38% of the homeless population is dependent on alcohol. Coppenrath (2001) found in a study on nutritional intake in the homeless population that, of the individuals who consumed alcohol, a majority of total calories for that day were derived from alcohol alone (53% average). While alcohol is calorically dense, providing approximately seven kilocalories per gram as opposed to four kilocalories per gram derived from protein and carbohydrate foods, it has little nutritional value to offer. Of the people included in this study, approximately 32% of their remaining caloric intake was obtained from carbohydrate food sources and only 6% from protein (Coppenrath, 2001). While calories consumed may numerically meet the person's estimated caloric needs, diets that are high in alcohol are ultimately lacking in necessary nutrients. Alcoholics who consume greater than 30% of daily calories from alcohol have increased risk for vitamin A, vitamin C, and thiamine deficiencies (Salz, 2014). Thiamine deficiency associated with alcohol consumption may lead to development of Wernicke-Korsakoff syndrome, which is characterized by encephalopathy and altered mental status ranging from confusion to coma (Mahan et al., 2012). Treatment involves cessation of alcohol, hydration, and thiamine supplementation. Although thiamine and vitamin C deficiencies are the most commonly reported, other nutrient deficiencies may also occur such as vitamins B_2, B_6, B_9, B_{12}, and vitamin E (Ijaz et al., 2017). Alcohol dependence also may result in weight changes, anorexia, decreased digestive enzymes, and liver disease, all of which have direct nutritional implications.

Alcohol is not the only substance with nutritional consequences. Opioids ultimately slow body processes, including digestion, often resulting in constipation. Withdrawal symptoms such as nausea, vomiting, and diarrhea may also result in inadequate intake and electrolyte imbalances. Methamphetamine use typically suppresses appetite and leads to weight loss. Additionally, methamphetamine abuse is associated with dental disease, which may contribute to chewing difficulties and decreased diet tolerance. Marijuana, on the other hand, is associated with increased appetite

(Salz, 2014). In addition to the direct nutritional implications of substance abuse, lifestyle factors associated with addiction, such as lack of exercise, altered sleep patterns, and altered eating habits, places people at increased risk for developing diabetes, hypertension, weight problems, and metabolic syndrome (Salz, 2014).

One may assume that homeless persons with substance addictions do not have financial means to procure housing or food; however, that is not always the case. Some homeless individuals have adequate funding from pensions, Social Security, and so on, but prioritize alcohol and drugs over their health and well-being. For example, a man in his sixties was admitted to the hospital with cardiomyopathy. The man had a history of meth abuse.He was underweight with a history of weight loss and subsequent decreased physical function and mobility, leaving him wheelchair-bound. This presentation is consistent with the typical nutrition implications of stimulant abuse. The man made approximately $1,500/month from Social Security; however, he chose not to spend the money on housing or food. Educating patients on the importance of prioritizing their health and optimizing food intake within their available resources is an important component of nutrition intervention for the homeless.

NUTRITION ASSESSMENT AND INTERVENTION

Nutrition assessment is a tool that can be used for prevention, diagnosis, and treatment of malnutrition. The Nutrition Care Process (NCP) incorporates assessment, diagnosis, interventions, monitoring, and evaluation to identify and address nutritional problems, including malnutrition. In order to evaluate a patient's nutritional status, the registered dietitian must collect and analyze the patient's nutritional data, including anthropometrics, biochemical/lab data, food and nutrition history, intake, medical history, and nutrition-focused physical exam (Academy of Nutrition and Dietetics, n.d.).

Nutrition assessment of the homeless patient focuses on obtaining diet and intake history and evaluating for adequacy, identification of existing nutrient deficiencies, and interpretation of weight trends. Obtaining essential information to conduct a full nutrition assessment may be difficult. Infrequent trips to the doctor may result in gaps in the patient's weight history, laboratory data, and so on. Patients also do not likely have access to scales regularly; thus, they may also be unable to fill in these gaps in their weight history. Oftentimes, patients are resistant to discuss their previous intake, and it may even be impossible to provide a recall of "typical" intake, given its sporadic nature. Patients are often vague when describing their intake and frequently use statements like "I eat sometimes," "I eat one to two times a day," "I eat what is available," thus making an accurate evaluation of their past diet difficult. The nutrition diagnosis is determined by the data collected in the nutrition assessment. Example nutrition diagnosis for the elderly homeless would include problems such as inadequate oral intake, unintentional weight loss, malnutrition, swallowing and chewing difficulties, and limited access to food or water. The nutrition diagnosis dictates the interventions.

Nutrition interventions are aimed at improving balance and adequacy of intake, correcting deficiencies, and managing disease processes. While homeless patients are hospitalized, the first priority is addressing the acute issue. After the major acute medical and nutritional problems are treated, interventions shift to connecting the patient to community resources in order to expand their access to adequate nutrition and overall improve their dietary profile. Nutrition education is one tool that can also be used to improve nutritional status. When providing nutrition education to homeless individuals, the focus is first on meeting the basic essential nutrition requirements to survive. Disease management is often a secondary priority, given food insecurity and inability to meet basic calorie and protein needs. Nutritional problems must be prioritized and addressed in order of health impact, but also importance to the patient. An interdisciplinary approach is essential to effectively implement nutrition interventions. Social work is integral in finding and connecting the patient to the best-suited resources for that patient. Collaboration with physicians and pharmacists can be useful to help simplify medication regimens to encourage compliance and manage disease processes such as diabetes. Psychological evaluation and intervention is also essential, especially with patients with substance abuse.

Nutrition interventions are much easier to control within the hospital setting. Patients typically eat well while institutionalized because the food is available and they continue to eat with a "feast or famine-type" pattern. Homeless elderly likely lack access to nutrition services such as one-on-one appointments with registered dietitians. Veterans have the advantage of having access to these services; however, they must also take initiative and seek them. In addition to obvious barriers to compliance with nutrition recommendations, such as limited financial resources, lack of food preparation, and storage amenities, it is important to remember some limitations are directly a result of the aging process, such as impaired cognition, forgetfulness, and decreased functional ability. All potential barriers must be carefully explored in order to develop a successful, feasible nutrition care plan that can be implemented by the patient. Individualization is essential (Coppenrath, 2001). Interventions must be tailored to accommodate the patient's financial resources, medical conditions, and ultimately his or her own personal goals in order to be effective. Patients may be completely disengaged from nutrition education and focused on other priorities, which are essential for survival, that is, shelter and safety, thus making nutrition education the least effective intervention for that patient at that moment in time. Ideally, the homeless geriatric person would be monitored and re-evaluated; however, follow-up may be unrealistic. What does nutrition assessment look like in action? See the following case.

NUTRITION ASSESSMENT PUT INTO PRACTICE—CASE STUDY

A homeless man aged 70 years was referred by an inpatient critical care dietitian to an outpatient nutrition clinic after discovering during a recent hospitalization that the patient was living in a storage unit with no facilities available to cook or store food. The man was underweight (89% of his ideal body weight for height) and had a history of gradual, progressive weight loss of 33 lb. in the past four years (17% body weight). His medical history was significant for tetraplegia secondary to cervical stenosis, neurogenic bowel and bladder, hyperlipidemia, gastroesophageal reflux disease, major depression, and chronic pain.

Due to limited income and no kitchen amenities, his diet was heavily dependent on processed, convenient, inexpensive food items. He reported he mostly bought food items from convenience stores and discount-type grocery stores. The patient's budget was approximately $10 per week at the grocery store plus additional funds he set aside to purchase burritos. Two weeks prior to his second assessment, all of his shower supplies were stolen, which he estimated would cost him just over $20 to replace. He prioritized replacing the supplies over purchasing burritos for the next weeks. The patient reported largely variable intake dependent on available resources. He stated he always ate breakfast, but that consumption of lunch and dinner meals was more sporadic. He had been prescribed nutrition supplements by the inpatient dietitian; however, he had not been drinking them due to an inability to transport and store large quantities of the supplement. He recently decreased his physical activity to help prevent further weight loss. The patient also reported some difficulty with chewing due to missing teeth and difficulty swallowing characterized with the sensation of foods getting stuck in his throat. He had previously been referred to a speech and language pathologist who deemed a regular diet with thin liquids safe for the patient to swallow.

Outpatient nutrition counseling was focused on problem-solving, with the first priority being achieving adequate intake to prevent further weight loss.

The dietitian focused on educating the patient on selecting nutrient-dense foods that provided more nutrition/calories for less money and reviewed how to read a nutrition label to help facilitate making the best food selections possible. The dietitian explained the basic process behind nutrition expenditure versus intake in relation to the patient's physical activity level and history of weight loss. The dietitian recommended the patient continue to receive liquid nutrition supplements and brainstormed ways with the patient that he could successfully transport and store the supplement. In collaboration with the pharmacist,, smaller, more manageable quantities of the supplement were ordered, which were provided more frequently. The dietitian also discussed the patient's case and provided the patient with a referral to social work to help connect the patient to more nutrition resources in the local community. At a follow-up appointment, the dietitian further investigated the patient's willingness to participate in community food programs, and the patient adamantly declined. He stated he desired to "maintain a low profile" and did not wish to participate in any programs that were supported by the government. Ultimately, the patient self-limited available nutrition resources. The patient also described transportation issues to go to shelters for meals. Three months post intervention, the patient was maintaining his weight without any further weight loss.

REFERENCES

Academy of Nutrition and Dietetics. (n.d.). Nutrition Terminology Reference Manual (eNCPT): Dietetics language for nutrition care. Retrieved from http://ncpt.web author.com

Bernstein, M., & Munoz, N. (2012). Position of the Academy of Nutrition and Dietetics: Food and nutrition for older adults: Promoting health and wellness. *Journal of the Academy of Nutrition and Dietetics, 112*(8), 1255–1277. doi:10.1016/j.jand.2012.06.015

Boston Medical Center. (2017, February 1). Preventive Food Pantry. Retrieved from https://www.bmc.org/programs/preventive-food-pantry

Bradfield, S., Greene, C., Watman, M., & Watman, D. (2014, May 15). Homeless population and soup kitchens. Retrieved from https://www.bing.com/cr?IG=D200DC775BFF49C29E 30250DA0999801&CID=34CB1D5F11086CBF0A2217EF100E6D17&rd=1&h=Is4BH qPcpOaIk9b9bKDnoEX9Yn3x0tpZIyJS_sinFKY&v=1&r=https%3a%2f%2fmacaulay .cuny.edu%2feportfolios%2fadiv14_magazine%2f2014%2f05%2f15%2fhomeless- population-and-soup-kitchens%2f&p=DevEx,5034.1

Centers for Disease Control and Prevention. (2015, September 14). Healthy aging at a glance, 2015: Helping people to live long and productive lives and enjoy a good quality of life. Retrieved from https://stacks.cdc.gov/view/cdc/43961

Coppenrath, W. (2001). Problems in nutritional status among homeless populations: An introduction. *Nutrition Bytes, 7*, 1–7. Retrieved from https://escholarship.org/uc/ item/5hm1p27p

Definitions. (n.d.). Malnutrition. Retrieved from https://www.nutritioncare.org/ Guidelines_and_Clinical_Resources/Toolkits/Malnutrition_Toolkit/Definitions

Goldberg, J., Lang, K., & Barrington, V. (2016, April). How to prevent and end homelessness among older adults. Retrieved from http://www.justiceinaging.org/wp-content/uploads/2016/04/Homelessness-Older-Adults.pdf

Hennepin County Medical Center. (n.d.). The FOOD SHELF at Hennepin County Medical Center. Retrieved from http://www.hcmc.org/foodshelf/index.htm

Homelessness. (n.d.). Retrieved from https://www.diet.com/g/homelessness?get=homelessness

Ijaz, S., Jackson, J., Thorley, H., Porter, K., Fleming, C., Richards, A., . . . Savović, J. (2017). Nutritional deficiencies in homeless persons with problematic drinking: A systematic review. *International Journal for Equity in Health, 16*, 71. doi:10.1186/s12939-017-0564-4

Johnson, L., & McCool, A. (2003). Dietary intake and nutritional status of older adult homeless women: A pilot study. *Journal of Nutrition for the Elderly, 23*(1), 1–21. doi:10.1300/J052v23n01_01

Kaiser, M. J., Bauer, J. M., Ramsch, C., Uter, W., Guigoz, Y., Cederholm, T., . . . Sieber, C. (2010). Frequency of malnutrition in older adults: A multinational perspective using the mini nutrition assessment. *Journal of the American Geriatrics Society, 58*(9), 1734–1738. doi:10.1111/j.1532-5415.2010.03016.x

Kertesz, S. G. (2004). Nutritional issues. In J. J. O'Connell (Ed.), *The health care of homeless persons*. Boston, MA: Boston Health Care for the Homeless Program. Retrieved from https://www.bhchp.org/sites/default/files/BHCHPManual/pdf_files/Part3_PDF/Nutritional_Issues.pdf

Koh, K. A., Hoy, J. S., O'Connell, J. J., & Montgomery, P. (2012). The hunger–obesity paradox: Obesity in the homeless. *Journal of Urban Health : Bulletin of the New York Academy of Medicine, 89*(6), 952–964. doi:10.1007/s11524-012-9708-4

Luder, E., Ceysens-Okada, E., Koren-Roth, A., & Martinez-Weber, C. (1990). Health and nutrition survey in a group of urban homeless adults. *Journal of the American Dietetics Association, 90*(10), 1387–1392. Retreived from https://www.ncbi.nlm.nih.gov/pubmed/2212420

Lyles, C. R., Drago-Ferguson, S., Lopez, A., & Seligman, H. K. (2013). Nutritional assessment of free meal programs in San Francisco. *Preventing Chronic Disease, 10*. doi:10.5888/pcd10.120301

Mahan, L. K., Escott Stump, S., & Raymond, J. L. (2012). *Krause's food and the nutrition care process* (13th ed). St. Louis, MO: Elsevier/Saunders.

National Coalition for the Homeless. (2009). Substance abuse and homelessness. Retrieved from http://www.nationalhomeless.org/factsheets/elderly.html

Salz, A. (2014). Substance abuse and nutrition. *Today's Dietitian, 16*(12), 44. Retrieved from http://www.todaysdietitian.com/newarchives/120914p44.shtml

SFGH Therapeutic Food Pantry. (2017). Retrieved from https://sfghf.org/funded-initiatives/prescription-healthy-food

Sisson, L. G., & Lown, D. A. (2011). Do soup kitchen meals contribute to suboptimal nutrient intake & obesity in the homeless population? *Journal of Hunger & Environmental Nutrition, 6*(3), 312–323. doi:10.1080/19320248.2011.597832

Sprake, E. F., Russell, J. M., & Barker, M. E. (2014). Food choice and nutrient intake amongst homeless people. *Journal of Human Nutrition and Dietetics, 27*, 242–250. doi:10.1111/jhn.12130

Strasser, J. A., Damrosch, S., & Gaines, J. (1991). Nutrition and the homeless person. *Journal of Community Health Nursing, 8*(2), 65–73. doi:10.1207/s15327655jchn0802_2

Supplemental Nutrition Assistance Program (SNAP). (2013). Health status, homelessness and hunger: A fact sheet. Retrieved from http://www.nhchc.org/wp-content/uploads/2013/12/nhchc-snap-fact-sheet-nov-2013.pdf

The U.S. Conference of Mayors. (2016, December 13). The U.S. Conference of Mayors' Report on Hunger and Homelessness. Retrieved from https://endhomelessness.atavist.com/mayorsreport2016

Tsai, K., & Rosenheck, R. A. (2013). Obesity among chronically homeless adults: Is it a problem? *Public Health Reports, 128*(1), 29–36. doi:10.1177/003335491312800105

Wellman, N. S., Weddle, D. O., Kranz, S., & Brain, C. T. (1997). Elderly insecurities: Poverty, hunger, and malnutrition. *Journal of the American Dietetics Association, 97*(10), S120–S122. doi:10.1016/S0002-8223(97)00744-X

Wiecha, J. L., Dwyer, J. T., & Dunn-Strohecker, M. (1991). Nutrition and health services needs among the homeless. *Public Health Reports, 106*(4), 364–374. Retrieved from https://www.ncbi.nlm.nih.gov/pmc/articles/PMC1580272

12

Barriers and Applications of Medication Therapy Management in the Homeless Population

Kevin M. Krcmarik

INTRODUCTION: MEDICATION THERAPY MANAGEMENT (MTM) IN THE HOMELESS POPULATION

Over the past three decades, a growing shortage of affordable rental housing with a concomitant rise in poverty has contributed significantly to an increased rate of homelessness in America. Individuals who are homeless face multiple challenges, which can prove to be both causes and subsequent effects of their lack of housing. Social isolation, unemployment, poverty, domestic abuse, drug addiction/substance abuse, mental illness, challenges to personal hygiene, food scarcity, the high cost of medications, and lack of health insurance are some examples of such, and they can all contribute to the financial hardship and de-stabilization of the individual in society. Regardless of the particular circumstances of a homeless person, his or her basic needs oftentimes cannot all be sufficiently met, and so sacrifices must be made. Because it frequently constitutes the largest portion of one's financial commitments, stable housing may be abdicated or compromised at the expense of obtaining other vital necessities such as food, clothing, healthcare, and even medication therapy. In the case of medication therapy management (MTM), homeless persons may face significant hardship in not only procuring and using effective drug therapy, but also in following-up with their providers and establishing provider–patient relationships that will help them to meet their target therapeutic goals. In this chapter, a review of the more common barriers to MTM in the homeless population will be enumerated, followed by a number of practical applications of MTM in optimizing the health of the homeless. In order to appreciate the value and role that stable MTM can offer the homeless, perspectives on homeless health and the concept of MTM will first be briefly discussed.

Perspectives on Health Matters

Despite popular mischaracterizations about the homeless being aloof about their health, various studies have shed light about how homeless people actually view their health risks and habits, as well as their health management. One recent survey analysis by Steward et al. (2016) attempted to identify concerns that the homeless have regarding aspects of their primary care. Ease of accessibility, provision of evidence-based care that can be easily understood, and coordination and cooperation with their providers all ranked as the highest priorities related by homeless participants. Another study by Asgary, Sckell, Alcabes, Naderi, and Ogedegbe (2015) reveals that the homeless may believe that their risk of cancer is higher than the general population and consider cancer screening as a high priority despite other health-related concerns. In this analysis, patients were eager to understand their health needs and issues and receive advice about preventive care. They requested interventions such as incentives, the use of mobile clinics, and using text messaging to receive reminders for appointments. In a focus group survey study by authors Salem and Ma-Pham (2015), middle-aged and older homeless women cited problems with taking medications and being able to safely store them to treat their chronic illnesses. An anthropological study conducted by Whitley (2013) found that rural homeless persons had a strong aversion to "professional healthcare" (services given by doctors, hospitals, clinics, and professional medical staff), as opposed to the nonprofit, mobile delivery of care more characteristic of community social volunteer services. Study participants cited previous "demeaning and disparaging" encounters with health professionals with frequent cases of misdiagnosis and iatrogenesis as the causes of their distrust. When considered in total, these aforementioned studies illustrate that the homeless are not detached from their healthcare, but rather seek high-quality professional care that they can actively be a part of.

The Field of Medication Therapy Management

The goal of MTM is to optimize the medication management of individuals to assist them in achieving therapeutic targets that have been established in professional health guidelines. In the wake of the Medicare Modernization

Act of 2003, the field of MTM has had a growing influence on the medical care of millions of Americans. The approach to chronic disease state management has been revitalized and strengthened as a result of this legislation, which requires Medicare Part D prescription drug plans to include MTM services by qualified healthcare professionals. As defined by the American Pharmacists Association under the description of "patient-centered" health, the core elements of the MTM practice include: assessing the health status of patients and comprehensively reviewing their medication (prescription and nonprescription) regimens; formulating a medication treatment plan after prioritizing either actual or potential medication-related problems; monitoring the efficacy and safety of medications; optimizing medication adherence through patient empowerment and education; and documenting and communicating findings and treatment suggestions to prescribers (Lemay, 2012). Authors Greysen, Allen, Rosenthal, Lucas, and Wang (2013) described patient-centered health provision as (one) that places a high emphasis on acknowledging and addressing patient concerns in *every* clinical interaction. Previous studies have demonstrated the effectiveness of this approach in optimizing both patient adherence to their medications (Roumie et al., 2011) and shared decision making in health management matters between physicians and underserved primary care patients (Cooper et al., 2011). In addition, authors Smith, Bates, Bodenheimer, and Cleary (2010) also describe a pharmacist's "personalized" medication care plan (as one that) addresses "medication errors, inappropriate medication selection, omissions, duplications, sub-therapeutic or excessive dosages, drug interactions, adverse events, adherence problems, cultural competency and health literacy challenges, and costly regimens." These clinical services are normally performed before a clinical visitation with a provider and can be employed in almost any context, ranging from conventional outpatient primary clinics to senior centers, community specialty pharmacist practices, and clinics for the uninsured. Having glimpsed a brief introduction into the elements of MTM, let us now examine more closely the barriers and challenges to optimizing MTM in the homeless.

BARRIERS TO MEDICATION THERAPY MANAGEMENT IN THE HOMELESS POPULATION

Barriers to Providing Pharmaceutical Care

For many impoverished individuals in the United States, especially within the minority and homeless demographic, community and migrant health centers receiving federal funding may serve as their only resource for obtaining primary healthcare. A 2003 survey of medical directors and pharmacists at over 1,000 of these sites across the nation helped identify several key common barriers to providing adequate pharmaceutical care to this population (Brown, Barner, & Shepherd, 2003): (a) structural issues, including lack of available clinic space, especially areas for private pharmaceutical counseling; (b) insufficient time allotted for pharmacists to address the pharmaceutical/health needs of patients; (c) equipment problems (chiefly inadequate or antiquated computer systems and software); (d) patient-related issues, including their lack of proficiency in English when bilingual or multilingual staff were not available, as well as their lack of educational background; and (e) personnel issues, including inadequate staffing (especially language translators and pharmacy technicians), incompetence of technicians, and lack of commitment/support from higher management to pharmaceutical care. Pharmacists in other community settings have also identified several of these same issues as barriers to providing acceptable pharmaceutical care (Bell, McElnay, Hughes, & Woods, 1998; McAuley, Mott, Schommer, Moore, & Reeves, 1999). In regard to these financial and logistical limitations that many clinics face in addressing the MTM needs of the homeless population, much experience has been documented in identifying solutions to many of these barriers. Authors Brown et al. (2003) have suggested several, including: cultural sensitivity training of pharmaceutical staff, recruitment and retention of culturally and language-competent staff to proportionally match the languages and cultural backgrounds of their patient populations, and expansion and modernization of pharmacy school curricula to educate trainees on the "health and illness behaviors of multicultural and indigent populations as well as their access to and use of health services." In the overall scheme of providing MTM to the homeless, the foundational issue of access to healthcare services should also be considered.

Barriers to Healthcare Access

Success with MTM in the homeless population cannot be extricated from larger policy issues, including the availability of health insurance. Without continuous, stable access to primary care and MTM services, efforts, such as health screening, drug therapy education, and medication reconciliation, may be compromised or nonexistent. Subsequently, MTM loses its intended purpose in optimizing patient health and helping homeless and indigent patients to reach their target therapeutic medication goals. Previous studies have already demonstrated the association between homelessness or low socioeconomic status and diminished access to healthcare (Duchon, Weitzman,

& Shinn, 1999; Kushel, Vittinghoff, & Haas, 2001; K. W. Reid, Vittinghoff, & Kushel, 2008; Wood & Valdez, 1991), as well as homelessness and a higher propensity for using acute care services (Han & Wells, 2003; Kushel et al. 2001; K. W. Reid et al., 2008). These associations point to the concept of "competing priorities," which authors K. W. Reid et al. (2008) have defined as a situation where people must choose between their "subsistence needs and their health-care needs" when confronted with other financial demands. Oftentimes, they will choose paying for the former over the latter, even potentially delaying seeking medical care and remaining without health insurance. This can ulti-mately translate into reduced primary care access and potentially poorer health outcomes (Chwastiak, Tsai, & Rosenheck, 2012; Institute of Medicine, 2009; White & Newman, 2015). A meta-regression using nationally represen-tative surveys by K. W. Reid et al. (2008) already demonstrates that housing instability should be considered as having a proportional risk for poor access to healthcare and higher rates of hospitalization. Other contributing factors have also been described as increasing the risk for diminished access to pri-mary care services or increased emergency room use:

- Food insecurity (Modrek, Stuckler, McKee, Cullen, & Basu, 2013)
- Economic downturns and recession resulting in individual unemploy-ment and acute losses in income and health insurance loss (Modrek et al., 2013; White, Jones, Moran, & Simpson, 2016)
- Racial minority status (Chang & Troyer, 2011; P. J. Johnson et al., 2012; O'Neil et al., 2010)
- Poor understanding of eligibility and enrollment for Medicaid services. In a 2014-based study by authors Fryling, Mazanec, and Rodriguez (2015), several barriers in accessing and maintaining Medicaid services were identified from an extensive survey of homeless subjects. Respond-ers highlighted "difficulty obtaining and providing required documen-tation, difficulty understanding the application, literacy barriers, lack of a constant phone number and address, lack of transportation, and not receiving notifications to renew Medicaid access"
- Uncertainty of where to seek care (Lewis, Andersen, & Gelberg, 2003; Rosenheck & Lam, 1997)
- Feelings of abandonment or being judged in professional healthcare set-tings (McCabe, Macnee, & Anderson, 2001; Whitley, 2013)
- Health policies influencing the allocation of funding for safety net resources. Government-appropriated funding for such is highly variable depending on the current political affiliation majority in state and federal legislatures (Navarro & Shi, 2001)

Various strategies for improving healthcare access have been proposed including: making patients aware of their eligibility for public assistance programs, finding ways to help them apply for and receive benefits, performing emergency room-based outreach and education regarding eligibility for Medicaid enrollment or renewal, and implementing the use of patient navigators to help the homeless better understand their health problems and management, apply for available resources, and partake in health screenings. In addition to issues with healthcare access and barriers to providing pharmaceutical care, the ability of each patient to adhere to a medication plan should also be considered, as successful adherence engenders multiple considerations as well.

Barriers to Adherence in the Homeless Population

The term *adherence* has been previously defined by the World Health Organization (WHO) as "the extent to which a person's behavior-taking medication, following a diet, and/or executing lifestyle changes correspond with agreed recommendations from a healthcare provider" (WHO, 2003). Medication adherence remains a major global challenge as more than half of the individuals with chronic diseases do not take any or all of their medications correctly (Haynes, McDonald, & Garg, 2002; WHO, 2003). In addition, multiple studies in patients with chronic diseases, such as HIV, TB, and bipolar disorder, have demonstrated an association between homelessness and decreased medication adherence. (Kidder, Wolitski, Campsmith, & Nakamura, 2007; Leaver, Bargh, Dunn, & Hwang, 2007; LoBue & Moser, 2003; Palepu, Milloy, Kerr, Zhang, & Wood, 2011; Parruti et al., 2006; Sajatovic, Valenstein, Blow, Ganoczy, & Ignacio, 2006; Sajatovic, Valenstein, Blow, Ganoczy, & Ignacio, 2007). As quoted from Chan, Patounas, Dornbusch, Tran, and Watson (2015), referencing studies from Moczygemba et al. (2011), Sleath et al. (2006), and Coe et al. (2015): "From a medication perspective, people suffering from homelessness are particularly vulnerable to medication-related problems, as well as exhibiting poor medication adherence and reporting more barriers to medication use."

So, what is at the root of medication nonadherence in the homeless population? The answer is quite complex, embodying a large spectrum of causes identified in several published investigations. It should be noted that any discussion of adherence *should first be considered broadly outside the context of the housing issue*, as both homeless persons and their housed counterparts may face many of the same common barriers to adherence. Multiple authors have attempted to organize the causes of nonadherence into different categories in order to identify solutions. Authors Bubalo et al. (2010) drew from a narrowed list of 55 publications containing information regarding pharmacists' perspectives on patient barriers to medication adherence, and utilized a classification system of treatment-related challenges, condition-related challenges, and patient characteristics. Another separate systematic review of the barriers affecting medication adherence in adults (regardless of housing status) by Yap, Thirumoorthy, and Kwan (2016) narrowed down a group of 65 articles from over 17,000, identifying 80 factors, which they subsequently grouped into five different categories: patient, physician, medication-related, systems-based, and all other factors—all of which contribute to poor medication adherence. One of the medication-related adherence barriers involves a lack of financial resources or insurance, which may be further exacerbated in the context of the high cost of medication therapy. Being characteristic of almost all homeless people, lacking insurance has been identified in several previous analyses and reviews identifying causes for nonadherence in housed and homeless persons (Briesacher, Gurwitz, & Soumerai, 2007; Kennedy, Tuleu, & Mackay, 2008; Kripalani, Henderson, Jacobson, & Vaccarino, 2008; M. D. Schoen, DiDomenico, Connor, Dischler, & Bauman, 2001; Sleath et al., 2006; Wheeler, Roberts, & Neiheisel, 2014). Authors C. Schoen et al. (2009) report that 58% of the U.S. primary care physicians they surveyed related that their patients have difficulties paying for medications and care. Restricting medications based on cost translates into suboptimal health management and has been previously associated with increased risks of subsequent decline in patient's self-reported health status (Heisler et al., 2004). In addition to lacking health insurance and the relatively high costs of healthcare and prescription medications, other factors have been identified as contributing to nonadherence:

- Isolation/lack of caregivers. Generally, patients with inadequate social support do poorly and have worse medication adherence (Catz, Kelley, Bogart, Benotsch, & McAuliffe, 2000; Scheurer, Choudhry, Swanton, Matlin, & Shrank, 2012; Zullig et al., 2015).
- Poor functional health literacy (Ad Hoc Committee on Health Literacy for the Council on Scientific Affairs, American Medical Association, 1999; Andrus & Roth, 2002). This problem is of special importance in elderly patients, taking into consideration other contributing contributions such as the level of education, cognitive impairment, and vision/hearing deficits (MacLaughlin et al., 2005; Murray et al., 2004).
- Cognitive impairment/Forgetfulness inclusive of memory and knowledge of medications (Campbell et al., 2016).

- Mental illness (especially depression) and/or higher levels of perceived stress (Nilsson-Schonnesson, Diamond, Ross, Williams, & Bratt, 2006; Royal et al., 2009; Starace et al., 2002; Vranceanu et al., 2008).
- Polypharmacy. One feasibility study of a systematic approach for discontinuation of multiple medications in 70 elderly adults reported an average use of 7.7 medications per adult (Garfinkel & Mangin, 2010). However, this issue of polypharmacy appears rather complicated. Although it has previously been stated that medication adherence may be negatively affected when the number of medications that one takes increases (Vlasnik, Aliotta, & DeLor, 2005), other studies demonstrate that the opposite relationship can also happen (Billups, Malone, & Carter, 2000; Sharkness & Snow, 1992).
- Frequent changes to the medication regimen and doubts as to a medication's therapeutic benefit (Hincapie, Taylor, Boesen, & Warholak, 2015; Vlasnik et al., 2005).
- Perceived adverse side effects (Hincapie et al., 2015; Lash, Fox, Westrup, Fink, & Silliman, 2006; MacLaughlin et al., 2005).
- Medications requiring multiple daily doses. Studies show that, when patients are required to take a medication more than once per day, their risk of nonadherence increases (Boyle et al., 2008; Claxton, Cramer, & Pierce, 2001).

If we add to these common adherence barriers several additional challenges that the homeless may cope with (such as personal safety, food insecurity, lack of resources for personal hygiene, and access to secure medication storage and transportation), it becomes evident that proper adherence to a healthy lifestyle and medications can be challenging tasks. Furthermore, an interdependent relationship between the causes and effects of homelessness can make it profoundly challenging for a homeless individual to improve his or her socioeconomic condition. If patients do not have stable access to healthcare and medication treatment, then they will potentially become more unhealthy and experience additional suffering that can further exacerbate their access issues. When examining the available research concerning barriers to medication adherence specifically identified in the homeless population, several notable examples have been described:

- Homelessness can present significant challenges to proper management of diabetes. Authors Hwang and Bugeja (2000) in their qualitative analysis of surveys from homeless adults in Toronto found that 72% of their survey participants identified poor availability of diabetic-friendly food offered at shelters, inability to obtain insulin and supplies when needed, and the inability to coordinate insulin with mealtimes as their most pressing challenges.

- Quoting from the National Alliance to End Homelessness, the NCH, in their 2009 report on HIV/AIDS, reports that "homelessness makes it more difficult to obtain and use antiretroviral treatments (ARTs). ARTs have complex regimens, and adherence is very difficult for people who don't' have access to stable housing, clean water, bathrooms, refrigeration, and food." Thus, these patients face potentially more complicated courses of disease, further complicating their efforts to overcome their homelessness.

- Sleath et al. (2006) concluded from their qualitative analysis of 164 homeless women in 18 homeless shelters across central North Carolina that "women with lower medical literacy were significantly more likely to report a barrier to giving their children a needed medication than women who read at the high school level." These authors further advised that, for homeless mothers taking care of their children, pharmacists should employ a strategy of providing both oral counseling and written materials/instructions about their children's medications. In total, 75% of those women surveyed actually preferred to have both forms of information.

- In their qualitative content analysis exploring factors for self-reported medication nonadherence in homeless persons in a behavioral health clinic, authors Coe et al. (2015) identified various patient-related factors (from documented pharmacist encounters) such as forgetting to take medications, losing medications or having them stolen, missing scheduled follow-up appointments, lacking sufficient knowledge and/or capacity in managing disease symptoms, and treatments, and having insufficient funding to afford medications.

- Homeless persons with bipolar disorder who were younger, nonwhite, and who had substance-abuse problems were more likely to be nonadherent to their psychiatric medications, as found in two separate studies by authors Sajatovic et al. (2006, 2007).

In addition to identifying adherence barriers, various study authors have emphasized provider- and pharmacist-driven strategies to optimize medication adherence. Several authors (mentioned in the following bulleted list) have offered pragmatic ideas that pharmacists and other health professionals can institute to address medication nonadherence for both homeless and low-income patients:

- Clarifying instructions and using uncomplicated language (especially for elderly patients or those who are cognitively challenged) to help patients better understand and see value in their medication regimen while enumerating potential side effects of medications
- Assessing patients' readiness to take more active roles in managing their medications responsibly via the use of formal screening tools. One of these tools is the "transtheoretical model" of Garfield and Caro (Ficke & Farris, 2005; Prochaska & Velicer, 1997; Willey et al., 2000), which offers a way for pharmacists to tailor interventions to improve adherence according to a patient's relative state of readiness to change
- Fostering transparent and open lines of communication with patients to both identify barriers to medication adherence and to collaboratively create tailored interventions to address those issues (Bubalo et al., 2010)
- Utilizing formal screening tools to evaluate patients' ability to manage their own medications. This includes assessing their capacity to know the dosing, function, and administration of their medications, as well as verifying that they are able to take their medications (Edelberg, Shallenberger, & Wei, 1999; Meyer & Schuna, 1989; Raehl, Bond, Woods, Patry, & Sleeper, 2002)
- Assisting with medication adherence monitoring via use of medication adherence technology (pillboxes, automated med organizers, etc.) and follow-up visitations. Authors Petersen et al. (2007) found that, when pharmacists provided a pillbox organizer to a group of HIV positive, urban poor (which included homeless patients) who demonstrated forgetfulness or missed doses, adherence rates improved
- Providing patients with wallet-sized cards containing a current medication list and health history in order to enhance communication between multiple providers and facilitate the medication reconciliation process (Blake, McMorris, Jacobson, Gazmararian, & Kripalani, 2010; Montauk, 2006)
- Establishing a trusting, continuous relationship with patients and initiating personalized follow-up visits. This includes setting aside adequate time for patient-centered interviews employing open-ended questions and education. Pharmacists and other providers should emphasize the importance of attendance at follow-up appointments and offer appointment reminder cards
- Advocating for regimens of medications that require less daily dosing that may be less expensive generic equivalents and that do not entail specialized administrative requirements to be effective (Claxton, Cramer, & Pierce, 2001; Kennedy, Tuleu, & Mackay, 2008; MacLaughlin et al., 2005).

- Considering the use of a 340B drug pricing program or other patient-assistance drug benefit program to help increase homeless patient access to medications (Robbins, Stillwell, Wilson, & Fitzgerald, 2012). A previous study has demonstrated that expanding access to medications via this route actually improves health outcomes and optimizes long-term healthcare spending and savings via decreasing unnecessary hospitalizations (M. D. Schoen et al., 2001). Alternatively, for those who have unstable housing and demonstrate poor management of their finances, the use of representative payee services (via the U.S. Social Security Administration) may help ensure that their needs are budgeted for. One recently published pilot study by authors Hawk, McLaughlin, Farmartino, King, and Davis (2016), investigating the impact of representative payee services on medication adherence among unstably housed HIV/AIDS patients, demonstrated improved adherence and decreased viral loads/improved rates of viral suppression.

PHARMACIST-DRIVEN MTM INTERVENTIONS TARGETING HOMELESS HEALTH

The Roles of Pharmacists in Optimizing Therapeutic Outcomes in the Underserved/Homeless Populations

Pharmacists are among the most important and skilled agents actively leading efforts to drive the implementation of MTM services for the homeless. In collaboration with other health professionals, they are reaching out to the homeless with targeted health interventions embracing educational, behavioral, and technical tools to address problems with their health management, especially that of their adherence. Their foundational knowledge and training in monitoring for adverse drug side effects, reconciling complicated or conflicting drug medication lists, identifying drug–drug interactions, preventing negative therapeutic outcomes, and offering medication counseling oftentimes equals or even surpasses that of providers. One study by Finley et al. (2002) comparing the management of depression by a psychiatric pharmacist to that of a primary care physician in a Health Maintenance Organization (HMO)-type setting demonstrated that the pharmacist-managed group experienced higher six-month adherence rates and less need for resources. The effectiveness of pharmacists in helping the homeless to meet their medication self-management goals is due in part to "pharmacists develop(ing) sustained partnerships with other healthcare providers, patients, families, and caregivers to focus on patient-specific prescribing options, medication use at home, and follow-up on the achievement of desired medication outcomes" (Smith, Bates, Bodenheimer, & Cleary, 2010). What then can be said about the effectiveness of pharmacists in helping the homeless to reach their therapeutic goals?

As an initial consideration, there is a substantial amount of data gathered from published studies that justifies the importance of clinical pharmacists in assisting *nonhomeless and nonunderserved* patients to significantly lower their % HbA1c, lipid levels, and blood pressure toward guideline-recommended target goals (Carter et al., 2009; Cioffi, Caron, Kalus, Hill, & Buckley, 2004; Cranor & Christensen, 2012; Cranor, Bunting, & Christensen, 2003; Hirsch et al., 2002; Kiel & McCord, 2005; Nkansah, Brewer, Connors, & Shermock, 2008; Ragucci, Fermo, Wessell, & Chumney, 2005; F. Reid, Murray, & Storrie, 2005; Till, Voris, & Horst, 2003). There is, however, relatively less data available to substantiate a similar role in the homeless population—but what is available is encouraging. To the best of this author's knowledge, most available studies examining pharmacist-driven therapeutic and clinical outcomes in homeless persons do not limit their inclusion criteria to homeless status. Although these studies generate data obtained from pharmacy services found in free clinics or community health centers, their patient populations engender wider descriptions of "underserved" or "uninsured" persons, many of whom have housing. Regardless, homeless persons fall within these descriptions even if their proportional contribution to the total studied population has not been established.

There are many published studies documenting the favorable outcomes of underserved patients at improving or attaining referenced target goals for diabetes, hypertension, and blood pressure with the assistance of pharmacist-led MTM efforts (N. Chung, Rascati, Lopez, Jokerst, & Garza, 2014; Enfinger, Campbell, & Taylor, 2009; Leal, Glover, Herrier, & Felix, 2004; Scott, Boyd, Stephan, Augustine, & Reardon, 2006; Shane-McWhorter & Oderda, 2005). However, most of these are mainly retrospective or descriptive in nature, and oftentimes do not include control groups against which to observe statistical significance in the effective outcomes. Two prospective studies, however, do show encouraging data that supports the role of pharmacists in helping the homeless and underserved to reach their therapeutic target goals. Authors Scott et al. (2006) conducted a nine-month unblinded, randomized, prospective trial comparing the effectiveness of a pharmacist-managed diabetes care program versus a control group (usual care without a fixed pharmacist collaboration) in helping largely underserved, indigent patients lower their serum HbA1c percentage values, blood pressures, and serum lipid concentrations toward guideline-recommended target levels. There were no significant demographic differences between the two groups of patients treated at the community health center. In total, 76 patients in the intervention group received more frequent follow-up appointments when necessary. Appointments with the clinical pharmacist were individually tailored to help patients focus on "disease management, lifestyle adjustments, and goal setting." An additional dietitian and nurse also reviewed diabetes management with the patient, provided reminders of upcoming appointments, and offered referrals for other health issues. At the conclusion of the study, mean HbA1c levels were significantly lowered by 1.7% points in the study group, and by 0.7% points in the control group ($p < .003$). A statistically significant 1.0 point difference between the mean of the two groups was seen ($p < .05$). Although the total change in blood pressure for each group over the nine-month duration was minimal from that of baseline, there was a significant difference in lowering between the two groups ($p = .023$). Mean LDL cholesterol levels were significantly decreased in both groups by an 11.2 mg/dL mean difference ($p = .012$). In addition, patients receiving the intervention along with pharmacy-guided follow-up reported a higher degree of satisfaction, less anxiety about their diabetes, and a higher perceived level of health.

Another prospective study by authors Shane-McWhorter and Oderda (2005) followed an intervention group of 176 underserved patients alongside a control group of 176 patients at a Salt Lake City Community Health Center over a one- to three-year time period. Significantly more patients were uninsured (88.1%) in the study group, while 67.6% of the control group patients were uninsured ($p < .001$). Both groups were closely matched, however, in sex, demographic identifiers, and diabetes type. The intervention group employed the use of a faculty pharmacist with multiple certifications in diabetes management. Working collaboratively alongside primary providers, this pharmacy specialist provided direct diabetes education, monitored glucose levels, and gave instructional feedback to patients at subsequent follow-up visits, and offered recommendations to providers. The control group did not have intentional access to this trained specialist, but rather were managed under the usual care of the primary provider unless, however, consultation with a certified diabetic pharmacist was personally requested by the provider. At the completion of the three-year study, serum HbA1c percentage values were significantly lowered to ADA target goals of lesser than 7% in both clinics, but significantly more in the intervention group (38.4% vs. 27.7% with $p < .042$). Lipid parameters improved in both groups without a statistically significant improvement in one over the other. Blood pressures were not improved from initial baseline in either group, however. Over 240 specific drug therapy recommendations were made by the pharmacist at the intervention clinic in addition to recommendations for laboratory tests, immunizations, and eye examinations. Although this study was not a tightly controlled randomized trial, it, nonetheless, offers value in describing the impact of employing a pharmacy diabetes specialist to optimize diabetes management for underserved diabetic patients.

In addressing the MTM needs of the homeless and assisting them with reaching their therapeutic goals, various healthcare delivery models embracing collaborative partnerships have been created. Academic–community partnerships between pharmacy colleges and homeless clinics, focusing on medication education and management, have resulted in improved health outcomes with fewer medication use problems (Connor, Snyder, Snyder, & Pater-Steinmetz, 2009; Gatewood et al., 2011; Moczygemba et al., 2011). The funding for such programs varies in different models, but is derived from a vested pharmacy college, a family practice group, or a university sponsoring resident education (Smith et al., 2010). Alternatively, clinical pharmacists have also been employed by private provider groups as part of pay-for-performance or quality improvement initiatives seeking to generate cost savings for the clinical practice, improve outcomes in medication therapy and chronic disease state management, personalize medication adherence programs for greater patient satisfaction, and curb the rate of medication-related hospital readmissions (Smith et al., 2010). Finally, under federal grant subsidizing, both "entrepreneurial groups" and state pharmacist associations have developed "independent networks of trained pharmacists to conduct comprehensive clinical services on a fee-for-service contractual basis with provider groups, payers, health plans, and employers" (Smith et al., 2010).

In light of these varied contractual partnerships, how can homeless patients benefit from the various unique and integrated roles of pharmacists?

Pharmacists in Medical Homes and Psychiatric Skid Row Clinics

In collaboration with primary providers and other secondary health professionals, including nutritionists and physical/occupational therapists, pharmacists have become a crucial factor in optimizing the healthcare of patients living in medical homes and transitional nursing facilities.

Although in these settings only some of these patients are considered homeless or impoverished, much has been learned regarding the valuable contributions contributed by pharmacists. Numerous studies already point to the importance of outpatient clinic pharmacists addressing medication adherence problems; assisting with health screening; optimizing therapeutic outcomes by identifying medication-related problems; educating patients on medication side effects, drug interactions, and safe medication use; and assisting providers with consultations (Bunting, Smith, & Sutherland, 2008; Carter et al., 2009; Cranor et al., 2003, 2012; Devine et al., 2009; Isetts et al., 2008; K. A. Johnson et al., 2010; F. Reid et al., 2005; Reilly & Cavanagh, 2003; Smith et al., 2010). Pharmacist interventions may help optimize how impoverished or homeless patients use their medications, as well as improve the cost-effectiveness of their treatment regimen (Lamsam et al., 1996).

As summarized by authors McKee, Lee, and Cobb (2013): "Patients with mental illness can especially benefit from psychiatric pharmacists' unique training in psychopharmacology and patient education about the risks and benefits of treatment. Psychiatric pharmacists embrace the concept of team-based care that involves the psychiatric and medical team and patient and family members; they also promote empowerment in the recovery process." And, it is not just patients who they are empowering. Primary care physicians have reported doubts regarding their ability to manage psychiatric illnesses or refill psychiatric regimens. This has translated into adverse drug reactions, accidental duplications of drug therapy, unaddressed/untreated psychiatric disorders, and patient noncompliance with his or her medications (Wang, Dopheide, & Gregerson, 2011). The high acceptance rate of recommendations offered by psychiatric clinical pharmacists providing MTM services for indigent patients suggests the willingness of physicians to embrace collaborative care in psychiatric settings (Caballero, Souffrant, & Heffernan, 2008).

Published experiences of psychiatric pharmacists in various Los Angeles skid row clinics have helped us to more fully understand the roles and breadth of expertise that a clinical pharmacist can offer in collaboration with psychiatrists and clinicians to optimize care for the mentally ill. Authors Wang et al. (2011), in their descriptive analysis of the roles of pharmacists in one such setting, detailed the primary routine tasks of psychiatric pharmacists: extensively reviewing patient histories (past psychiatric and medical problems, history of present illness, allergies, family psychiatric illness, social and medical history, and lab values) via chart exploration and patient interviews; evaluating refill histories to assess compliance; assessing for drug–drug interactions; counseling on illnesses and medications; and reviewing their personalized treatment plans with both the patient and the primary provider. The diverse roles of pharmacists in this clinic were appreciated, especially given their independence to make other referrals outside the clinic such as with dental care, psychotherapy, and social services.

Another study by authors B. Chung, Dopheide, and Gregerson (2011) describes a more expanded managerial role of psychiatric pharmacy specialists outside of traditional MTM responsibilities to also include initiating medications and laboratory monitoring, offering psychosocial support and education, making referrals to primary care physicians or social workers, and assisting underserved patients with completing mental health assessments necessary for housing and Social Security applications. This study highlighted the appreciation and overall satisfaction of primary care staff with the expertise and function of a clinical psychiatrist in their clinic, as several of the primary providers expressed low comfort with independently managing patients with mental illnesses. In particular, providers expressed satisfaction with the expertise and reliability of the pharmacist for consultation and medication management. In addition, patients related on their satisfaction questionnaires that their concerns were being addressed. They highly praised the initial hour-long visitation times that the psychiatric pharmacy resident was able to provide for both psychosocial support and education about their mental illnesses and medication use. Follow-up visits with the clinical pharmacist were 30 minutes in length, focusing on side-effect management. This study offers insight into the value of collaborative health management to help primary providers manage the time-intensive nature of visitations required for many homeless individuals who have complicated psychosocial issues and needs.

Academic–Community Partnerships Targeting Homeless Medication Management

Over the last few decades, mutually benefitting partnerships between academic institutions and various community health and free primary care clinics have provided invaluable experience and optimized care for pharmacy trainees and their homeless patients, respectively. Pharmacists in training reap pragmatic experience in MTM provision, including medication reconciliation and identification of medication-related problems. Confronting the barriers to medication adherence and the multitude of challenges that the homeless oftentimes must contend with has provided them with a valuable perspective and awareness. Conversely, the homeless have had opportunities to better understand their chronic disease states as well as the treatment strategies and medications employed to address these issues. They have been supported in accessing resources such as government assistance in finding stable health insurance and a means for obtaining their medications. Establishment of these partnerships has led to documented reductions in medication-related adverse events, as well as increased long-term cost savings for the respective clinic and financial contributors.

A descriptive study by authors Gatewood et al. (2011) chronicles the development and implementation of a university-sponsored pharmacy service in a federally sponsored Health Care for the Homeless (HCH) Clinic. Faculty and students from the Commonwealth University School of Pharmacy in Richmond, Virginia, have developed a comprehensive MTM (CMTM) model with the overall goal of addressing barriers to safe and effective medication use among homeless persons in both the behavioral health and the general medical clinics. Their roles and responsibilities have expanded over the years, from providing comprehensive medication education and reconciliation to collecting patient data engendering both medication adherence data and various patient lifestyle issues. They have pioneered "medication reconciliation campaigns" to support patient awareness of bringing their medications to their visits. The MTM services offered have also expanded to include personalized medication adherence counseling, education on disease, and provision of medication adherence devices and training in the general medical clinic. In their descriptive study, they report identifying over 600 medication-related problems over an observed interval of nearly one year. More than 85% of the treatment recommendations they subsequently offered to providers within the clinic were accepted, and the satisfaction of house staff was overall high, with a perceived improvement in the quality of care that was delivered.

Another published study by authors Connor et al. (2009) similarly describes the implementation of a pharmacy clinic within both a free clinic for primary care, as well as a community health center located in Pittsburgh, Pennsylvania. The Grace Lamsam Pharmacy Program for the Underserved (GLPPU) was founded in 1995 by faculty at the University of Pittsburgh School of Pharmacy and includes participation by both volunteer community pharmacists and pharmacy students throughout the Pittsburgh area. Approximately, 90% of the patients served within these safety-net settings had income 150% below the defined 2007 federal poverty level. The authors of this descriptive study described their patient population according to the frequency of pre-defined medication-related problems. They also demonstrated outcomes in the various pharmacy-led interventions targeting diabetes, hypertension, and serum cholesterol levels. Pharmacists actively assisted patients with filing 477 pharmaceutical manufacturer assistance program applications for 68 individual patients. As with the Richmond group previously mentioned, the pharmacist participants utilized an MTM-guided approach of comprehensive medication therapy review and reconciliation to assist patients in reaching therapeutic target goals. Over a 13-month period from 2007 to 2008, medication problems identified included noncompliance with medication therapy, incorrectly prescribed medication dosages, medical issues requiring drug therapy that was not being utilized, the presence of unnecessary medications and adverse drug reactions, and nonoptimal/poor choice of medication to treat a particular health problem. Of all of these issues, noncompliance was the most frequently observed medication-related problem within this population, occurring in 66% of all indexed problems. The pharmacy staff also recorded the type of interventions they recommended and performed, and an extrapolation of cost savings was performed based on patient survey and clinical data. This included pre- and end-point study values of HbA1c, blood pressure readings, and serum LDL-c concentration values for patients with diabetes, hypertension, and hyperlipidemia, respectively. Average blood pressure, HbA1c, and LDL-c readings improved in patients receiving care at both locations, although it could not be determined whether these reductions were actually clinically significant. Today, the GLPPU has extended its reach in caring for the homeless and low-income individuals at additional centers throughout the Pittsburgh area. As referenced from its website, the GLPPU continues to annually dispense over 6,000 prescriptions, serving approximately 3,000 patients at various clinics, shelters, and drop-in centers, and provide medications free of charge (valued at over 500,000 U.S. dollars), all while serving the educational and training needs of over 250 pharmacy students and residents each year (University of Pittsburgh, 2017).

Optimizing Medication Safety via a Quality Improvement Initiative

When patients such as the homeless are frequently transitioned between medical settings, they may accrue multiple medication lists and a growing collection of bottles. Oftentimes, these medication lists will have duplicated or conflicting classes of agents used to treat their ongoing health issues. Similar-looking medications or different strength dosages of the same medication may physically be mixed up in the same bottles in which they are found (Moczygemba et al., 2012). This confusing situation may unfortunately result in patients experiencing the unintended side effects of missed or excessive drug dosages, as well as drug–drug interactions. Ultimately, patients may become confused and distrustful, and their providers are left with the challenging and potentially time-intensive task of medication reconciliation. Reconciling drug regimens is a comprehensive process of carefully reviewing a patient's list(s) of medications between different settings. As detailed by authors Moczygemba et al. (2012), this involves a four-step process of: (a) verifying a current medication list by reviewing any available medical records or medication bottles that the patient may physically carry with him, (b) clarifying any dosage discrepancies or contradictions with both the patient and provider(s), (c) reconciling all discrepancies via written documentation of any new changes or corrections being made, and (d) educating the patient regarding all changes to the updated medication list with provision of a new list that reflects the changes made in the electronic medical record. This process of medication reconciliation serves a vital role in sustaining medication treatment continuity, supporting a patient's medication adherence, and preventing negative health outcomes.

A quality improvement project started in 2009 and detailed by Moczygemba et al. (2012) describes a "Pack Your Bag" campaign geared toward improving medication reconciliation in a central Virginia community of homeless and at-risk homeless patients. The goal of the endeavor was to "encourage patients to bring in all of their medications to clinic visits so that the best possible medication list (could be) created for them." In turn, the homeless healthcare clinic would have accurate and updated health records of their homeless patients, and thus be less likely to contribute to medication-related negative health outcomes. The project consisted of strategically placing large poster-type advertisement reminders around the clinic and distributing flyers, buttons, and individual carry bags that the homeless could use to store their medications in and remember to bring with them into their subsequent clinic follow-up visits. Eight months after initiation of the campaign, 40% (139 of 379) of those who were engaged by the promotional materials at earlier visits remembered to bring their medications into subsequent follow-up visits. Subsequently, they "received a personal medication record to share with other health care providers" (p. 561). From these successful patient encounters, 79% (157) of the 199 discrepancies identified were resolved by pharmacists.

CONCLUSION

Medication therapy management remains a challenging endeavor to optimally implement in the homeless population, which comprises a demographic with limited resources and significant challenges to sustaining their health. Working in various settings in collaboration with other health professionals, pharmacists are spearheading patient-centered efforts to optimize MTM and assist the homeless with attaining health insurance and continuity of care. Their evolving range of skills and knowledge allow them to better educate and equip homeless patients to reach acceptable therapeutic outcomes comparable with their housed and economically stable counterparts. Despite the persistent challenges to housing access and health maintenance, encouraging data from more recent studies over the last two decades demonstrates that their efforts are indeed achieving such.

REFERENCES

Ad Hoc Committee on Health Literacy for the Council on Scientific Affairs, American Medical Association. (1999). Health Literacy: Report of the Council on Scientific Affairs. *Journal of the American Medical Association, 10*, 281(6), 552–557.

Andrus, M. R., & Roth, M. T. (2002). Health literacy: A review. *Pharmacotherapy, 22*(3), 282–302.

Asgary, R., Sckell, B., Alcabes, A., Naderi, R., & Ogedegbe, G. (2015). Perspectives of cancer and cancer screening among homeless adults of New York City shelter-based clinics: A qualitative approach. *Cancer Causes Control, 26*(10), 1429–1438.

Bell, H. H., McElnay, J. C., Hughes, C. M., & Woods, A. (1998). Provision of pharmaceutical care by community pharmacists in Northern Ireland. *American Journal of Health-System Pharmacy, 55*(19), 2009–2013.

Billups, S. J., Malone, D. C., & Carter, B. L. (2000). The relationship between drug therapy noncompliance and patient characteristics, health-related quality of life, and health care costs. *Pharmacotherapy, 20*(8), 941–949.

Blake, S. C., McMorris, K., Jacobson, K. L., Gazmararian, J. A., & Kripalani, S. (2010). A qualitative evaluation of a health literacy intervention to improve medication adherence for underserved pharmacy patients. *Journal of Health Care for the Poor and Underserved, 21*(2), 559–567.

Boyle, B. A., Jayaweera, D., Witt, M. D., Grimm, K., Maa, J. F., & Seekins, D. W. (2008). Randomization to once-daily stavudine extended release/lamivudine, efavirenz versus a more frequent regimen improves adherence while maintaining viral suppression. *HIV Clinical Trials, 9*(3), 164–176.

Briesacher, B. A., Gurwitz, J. H., & Soumerai, S. B. (2007). Patients at risk for cost-related medication nonadherence: A review of the literature. *Journal of General Internal Medicine, 22*(6), 864–871.

Brown, C. M., Barner, J. C., & Shepherd, M. D. (2003). Issues and barriers related to the provision of pharmaceutical care in community health centers and migrant health centers. *Journal of the American Pharmaceutical Association (Wash), 43*(1), 75–77.

Bubalo, J., Clark, R. K. Jr., Jiing, S. S., Johnson, N. B., Miller, K. A., Clemens-Shipman, C. J., & Sweet, A. L. (2010). Medication adherence: Pharmacist perspective. *Journal of the American Pharmacists Association, 50*(3), 394–406.

Bunting, B. A., Smith, B. H., & Sutherland, S. E. (2008). The Asheville Project: Clinical and economic outcomes of a community-based long-term medication therapy management program for hypertension and dyslipidemia. *Journal of the American Pharmacists Association, 48*(1), 23–31.

Caballero, J., Souffrant, G., & Heffernan, E. (2008). Development and outcomes of a psychiatric pharmacy clinic for indigent patients. *American Journal of Health-System Pharmacy, 65*(3), 229–233.

Campbell, N. L., Zhan, J., Tu, W., Weber, Z., Ambeuhl, R., McKay, C., & McElwee, N. (2016). Self-reported medication adherence barriers among ambulatory older adults with mild cognitive impairment. *Pharmacotherapy, 36*(2), 196–202.

Carter, B. L., Ardery, G., Dawson, J. D., James, P. A., Bergus, G. R., Doucette, W. R., . . . Xu, Y. (2009). Physician and pharmacist collaboration to improve blood pressure control. *Archives of Internal Medicine, 169*(21), 1996–2002.

Catz, S. L., Kelly, J. A., Bogart, L. M., Benotsch, E. G., & McAuliffe, T. L. (2000). Patterns, correlates, and barriers to medication adherence among persons prescribed new treatments for HIV disease. *Health Psychology, 19*(2), 124–133.

Chan, V., Patounas, M., Dornbusch, D., Tran, H., & Watson, P. (2015). Is there a role for pharmacists in multidisciplinary health-care teams at community outreach events for the homeless? *Australian Journal of Primary Health, 21*(4), 379–383.

Chang, C. F., & Troyer, J. L. (2011). Trends in potentially avoidable hospitalizations among adults in Tennessee, 1998–2006. *Tennessee Medicine Journal, 104*(10), 35–38, 45.

Chung, B., Dopheide, J. A., & Gregerson, P. (2011). Psychiatric pharmacist and primary care collaboration at a skid-row safety-net clinic. *Journal of the National Medical Association, 103*(7), 567–574.

Chung, N., Rascati, K., Lopez, D., Jokerst, J., & Garza, A. (2014). Impact of a clinical pharmacy program on changes in hemoglobin A1c, diabetes-related hospitalizations, and diabetes-related emergency department visits for patients with diabetes in an underserved population. *Journal of Managed Care & Specialty Pharmacy, 20*(9), 914–919.

Chwastiak, L., Tsai, J., & Rosenheck, R. (2012). Impact of health insurance status and a diagnosis of serious mental illness on whether chronically homeless individuals engage in primary care. *American Journal of Public Health, 102*(12), e83–e89.

Cioffi, S. T., Caron, M. F., Kalus, J. S., Hill, P., & Buckley, T. E. (2004). Glycosylated hemoglobin, cardiovascular, and renal outcomes in a pharmacist-managed clinic. *The Annals of Pharmacotherapy, 38*(5), 771–775.

Claxton, A. J., Cramer, J., & Pierce, C. (2001). A systematic review of the associations between dose regimens and medication compliance. *Clinical Therapeutics, 23*(8), 1296–1310.

Coe, A. B., Moczygemba, L. R., Gatewood, S. B., Osborn, R. D., Matzke, G. R., & Goode, J. V. (2015). Medication adherence challenges among patients experiencing homelessness in a behavioral health clinic. *Research in Social and Administrative Pharmacy, 11*(3), e110–e120.

Connor, S. E., Snyder, M. E., Snyder, Z. J., & Pater Steinmetz, K. (2009). Provision of clinical pharmacy services in two safety net provider settings. *Pharmacy Practice, 7*(2), 94–99.

Cooper, L. A., Roter, D. L., Carson, K. A., Bone, L. R., Larson, S. M., Miller, E. R. 3rd., . . . Levine, D. M. (2011). A randomized trial to improve patient-centered care and hypertension control in underserved primary care patients. *Journal of General Internal Medicine, 26*(11), 1297–1304.

Cranor, C. W., Bunting, B. A., & Christensen, D. B. (2003). The Asheville Project: Long-term clinical and economic outcomes of a community pharmacy diabetes care program. *Journal of the American Pharmacists Association, 43*(2), 173–184.

Cranor, C. W., & Christensen, D. B. (2012). The Asheville Project: Short-term outcomes of a community pharmacy diabetes care program. *Journal of the American Pharmacists Association, 52*(6), 838–850.

Devine, E. B., Hoang, S., Fisk, A. W., Wilson-Norton, J. L., Lawless, N. M., & Louie, C. (2009). Strategies to optimize medication use in the physician group practice: The role of the clinical pharmacist. *Journal of the American Pharmacists Association, 49*(2), 181–191.

Duchon, L. M., Weitzman, B. C., & Shinn, M. (1999). The relationship of residential instability to medical care utilization among poor mothers in New York City. *Medical Care, 37*(12), 1282–1293.

Edelberg, H. K., Shallenberger, E., & Wei, J. Y. (1999). Medication management capacity in highly functioning community-living older adults: Detection of early deficits. *Journal of the American Geriatrics Society, 47*(5), 592–596.

Enfinger, F., Campbell, K., & Taylor, R. J. (2009). Collaboration with pharmacy services in a family practice for the medically underserved. *Pharmacy Practice, 7*(4), 248–253.

Ficke, D. L., & Farris, K. B. (2005). Use of the transtheoretical model in the medication use process. *The Annals of Pharmacotherapy, 39*(7–8), 1325–1330.

Finley, P. R., Rens, H. R., Pont, J. T., Gess, S. L., Louie, C., Bull, S. A., & Bero, L. A. (2002). Impact of a collaborative pharmacy practice model on the treatment of depression in primary care. *American Journal of Health-System Pharmacy, 59*(16), 1518–1526.

Fryling, L. R., Mazanec, P., & Rodriguez, R. M. (2015). Barriers to homeless persons acquiring health insurance through the Affordable Care Act. *Journal of Emergency Medicine, 49*(5), 755–762.

Garfinkel, D., & Mangin, D. (2010). Feasibility study of a systematic approach for discontinuation of multiple medications in older adults: Addressing polypharmacy. *Archives of Internal Medicine, 170*(18), 1648–1654.

Gatewood, S. B., Moczygemba, L. R., Alexander, A. J., Osborn, R. D., Reynolds-Cane, D. L., Matzke, G. R., & Goode, J. V. (2011). Development and implementation of an academic-community partnership to enhance care among homeless persons. *Innovations in Pharmacy, 2*(1), 1–7.

Greysen, S. R., Allen, R., Rosenthal, M. S., Lucas, G. I., & Wang, E. A. (2013). Improving the quality of discharge care for the homeless: A patient-centered approach. *Journal of Health Care for the Poor and Underserved, 24*(2), 444–455.

Han, B., & Wells, B. L. (2003). Inappropriate emergency department visits and use of the Health Care for the Homeless Program services by homeless adults in the northeastern United States. *Journal of Public Health Management Practice, 9*(6), 530–537.

Hawk, M., McLaughlin, J., Farmartino, C., King, M., & Davis, D. (2016). The impact of representative payee services on medication adherence among unstably housed people living with HIV/AIDS. *AIDS Care, 28*(3), 384–389.

Haynes, R. B., McDonald, H. P., & Garg, A. X. (2002). Helping patients follow prescribed treatment: Clinical applications. *Journal of the American Medical Association, 288*(22), 2880–2883.

Heisler, M., Langa, K. M., Eby, E. L., Fendrick, A. M., Kabeto, M. U., & Piette, J. D. (2004). The health effects of restricting prescription medication use because of cost. *Medical Care, 42*(7), 626–634.

Hincapie, A. L., Taylor, A. M., Boesen, K. P., & Warholak, T. (2015). Understanding reasons for nonadherence to medications in a Medicare Part D beneficiary sample. *Journal of Managed Care and Specialty Pharmacy, 21*(5), 391–399.

Hirsch, I. B., Goldberg, H. I., Ellsworth, A., Evans, T. C., Herter, C. D., Ramsey, S. D., Mullen, M., Neighbor, W. E., & Cheadle, A. D. (2002). A multifaceted intervention in support of diabetes treatment guidelines: A cont trial. *Diabetes Research and Clinical Practice, 58*(1), 27–36.

Hwang, S. W., & Bugeja, A. L. (2000). Barriers to appropriate diabetes management among homeless people in Toronto. *Canadian Medical Association Journal, 163*(2), 161–165.

Institute of Medicine. (2009). Committee on Health Insurance Status and Its Consequences, America's uninsured crisis: Consequences for health and health care. March 11, 2009. Retrieved from https://www.ncbi.nlm.nih.gov/books/NBK214966/pdf/Bookshelf_NBK214966.pdf

Isetts, B. J., Schondelmeyer, S. W., Artz, M. B., Lenarz, L. A., Heaton, A. H., Wadd, W. B., Brown, L. M., & Cipolle, R. J. (2008). Clinical and economic outcomes of medication therapy management services: The Minnesota experience. *Journal of the American Pharmacists Association, 48*(2), 203–211; 3 p following 211.

Johnson, K. A., Chen, S., Cheng, I. N., Lou, M., Gregerson, P., Blieden, C., Baron, C., & McCombs, J. (2010). The impact of clinical pharmacy services integrated into medical homes on diabetes-related clinical outcomes. *The Annals of Pharmacotherapy, 44*(12), 1877–1886.

Johnson, P. J., Ghildayal, N., Ward, A. C., Westgard, B. C., Boland, L. L., & Hokanson, J. S. (2012). Disparities in potentially avoidable emergency department (ED) care: ED visits for ambulatory care sensitive conditions. *Medical Care, 50*(12), 1020–1028.

Kennedy, J., Tuleu, I., & Mackay, K. (2008). Unfilled prescriptions of Medicare beneficiaries: Prevalence, reasons, and types of medicines prescribed. *Journal of Managed Care Pharmacy, 14*(6), 553–560.

Kidder, D. P., Wolitski, R. J., Campsmith, M. L., & Nakamura, G. V. (2007). Health status, health care use, medication use, and medication adherence among homeless and housed people living with HIV/AIDS. *American Journal of Public Health, 97*(12), 2238–2245.

Kiel, P. J., & McCord, A. D. (2005). Pharmacist impact on clinical outcomes in a diabetes disease management program via collaborative practice. *The Annals of Pharmacotherapy, 39*(11), 1828–1832.

Kripalani, S., Henderson, L. E., Jacobson, T. A., & Vaccarino, V. (2008). Medication use among inner-city patients after hospital discharge: Patient-reported barriers and solutions. *Mayo Clinic Proceedings, 83*(5), 529–535.

Kushel, M. B., Vittinghoff, E., & Haas, J. S. (2001). Factors associated with the health care utilization of homeless persons. *Journal of the American Medical Association, 285*(2), 200–206.

Lamsam, G. D., Stone, B. A., Rumsey, T., Shevlin, J. M., Scott, B. E., & Reif, C. J. (1996). Pharmaceutical services for a homeless population. *American Journal of Health-System Pharmacy, 53*(12), 1426–1430.

Lash, T. L., Fox, M. P., Westrup, J. L., Fink, A. K., & Silliman, R. A. (2006). Adherence to tamoxifen over the five year course. *Breast Cancer Research and Treatment, 99*(2), 215–220.

Leal, S., Glover, J. J., Herrier, R. N., & Felix, A. (2004). Improving quality of care in diabetes through a comprehensive pharmacist-based disease management program. *Diabetes Care, 27*(12), 2983–2984.

Leaver, C. A., Bargh, G., Dunn, J. R., & Hwang, S. W. (2007). The effects of housing status on health-related outcomes in people living with HIV: A systemic review of the literature. *AIDS and Behavior, 11*(6 Suppl), 85–100.

Lemay, G. (2012). Medication therapy management in community pharmacy practice. *Medicine and Health Rhode Island, 95*(9), 281–282.

Lewis, J. H., Andersen, R. M., & Gelberg, L. (2003). Health care for homeless women. *Journal of General Internal Medicine, 18*(11), 921–928.

LoBue, P. A., & Moser, K. S. (2003). Use of isoniazid for latent tuberculosis infection in a public health clinic. *American Journal of Respiratory and Critical Care Medicine, 168*(4), 443–447.

MacLaughlin, E. J., Raehl, C. L., Treadway, A. K., Sterling, T. L., Zoller, D. P., & Bond, C. A. (2005). Assessing medication adherence in the elderly: Which tools to use in clinical practice? *Drugs Aging, 22*(3), 231–255.

McAuley, J. W., Mott, D. A., Schommer, J. C., Moore, D. A., & Reeves, A. L. (1999). Assessing the needs of pharmacists and physicians in caring for patients with epilepsy. *Journal of the American Pharmacists Association, 39*(4), 499–504.

McCabe, S., Macnee, C. L., & Anderson, M. K. (2001). Homeless patients' experience of satisfaction with care. *Archives of Psychiatric Nursing, 15*(2), 78–85.

McKee, J. R., Lee, K. C., & Cobb, C. D. (2013). Psychiatric pharmacist integration into the medical home. *The Primary Care Companion for CNS Disorders, 15*(4).

Meyer, M. E., & Schuna, A. A. (1989). Assessment of geriatric patients' functional ability to take medication. *DICP, The Annals of Pharmacotherapy, 23*(2), 171–174.

Moczygemba, L. R., Gatewood, S. B., Kennedy, A. K., Osborn, R. D., Alexander, A. J., Matzke, G. R., & Goode, J. V. (2012). Medication reconciliation campaign in a clinic for homeless patients. *American Journal of Health-System Pharmacy, 69*(7), 558, 560–562.

Moczygemba, L. R., Goode, J. V., Gatewood, S. B., Osborn, R. D., Alexander, A. J., Kennedy, A. K., . . . Matzke, G. R. (2011). Integration of collaborative medication therapy management in a safety net patient-centered medical home. *Journal of the American Pharmacists Association, 51*(2), 167–172.

Modrek, S., Stuckler, D., McKee, M., Cullen, M. R., & Basu, S. (2013). A review of health consequences of recessions internationally and a synthesis of the US response during the great recession. *Public Health Reviews, 35*(7), 1–35.

Montauk, S. L. (2006). The homeless in America: Adapting your practice. *American Family Physician, 74*(7), 1132–1138.

Murray, M. D., Morrow, D. G., Weiner, M., Clark, D. O., Tu, W., Deer, M. M., . . . Weinberger, M. (2004). A conceptual framework to study medication adherence in older adults. *The American Journal of Geriatric Pharmacotherapy, 2*(1), 36–43.

National Coalition for the Homeless. (2009). HIV/AIDS and homelessness. Retrieved from http://www.nationalhomeless.org/factsheets/hiv.html

Navarro, V., & Shi, L. (2001). The political context of social inequalities and health. *Social Science & Medicine, 52*(3), 481–491.

Nilsson-Schonnesson, L., Diamond, P. M., Ross, M. W., Williams, M., & Bratt, G. (2006). Baseline predictors of three types of antiretroviral therapy (ART) adherence: A 2-year follow-up. *AIDS Care, 18*(3), 246–253.

Nkansah, N. T., Brewer, J. M., Connors, R., & Shermock, K. M. (2008). Clinical outcomes of patients with diabetes mellitus receiving medication management by pharmacists in an urban private physician practice. *American Journal of Health-System Pharmacy, 65*(2), 145–149.

O'Neil, S. S., Lake, T., Merrill, A., Wilson, A., Mann, D. A., & Bartnyska, L. M. (2010). Racial disparities in hospitalizations for ambulatory care-sensitive conditions. *American Journal of Preventive Medicine, 38*(4), 381–388.

Palepu, A., Milloy, M. J., Kerr, T., Zhang, R., & Wood, E. (2011). Homelessness and adherence to antiretroviral therapy among a cohort of HIV-infected injection drug users. *Journal of Urban Health, 88*(3), 545–555.

Parruti, G., Manzoli, L., Toro, P. M., D'Amico, G., Rotolo, S., Graziani, V., . . . Boyle, B. A. (2006). Long-term adherence to first-line highly active antiretroviral therapy in a hospital-based cohort: Predictors and impact on virologic response and relapse. *AIDS, Patient Care and STDs, 20*(1), 48–56.

Petersen, M. L., Wang, Y., van der Laan, M. J., Guzman, D., Riley, E., & Bangsberg, D. R. (2007). Pillbox organizers are associated with improved adherence to HIV antiretroviral therapy and viral suppression: A marginal structural model analysis. *Clinical Infectious Diseases, 45*(7), 908–915.

Prochaska, J. O., & Velicer, W. F. (1997). The transtheoretical model of health behavior change. *American Journal of Health Promotion, 12*(1), 38–48.

Raehl, C. L., Bond, C. A., Woods, T., Patry, R. A., & Sleeper, R. B. (2002). Individualized drug use assessment in the elderly. *Pharmacotherapy, 22*(10), 1239–1248.

Ragucci, K. R., Fermo, J. D., Wessell, A. M., & Chumney, E. C. (2005). Effectiveness of pharmacist-administered diabetes mellitus education and management services. *Pharmacotherapy, 25*(12), 1809–1816.

Reid, F., Murray, P., & Storrie, M. (2005). Implementation of a pharmacist-led clinic for hypertensive patients in primary care—a pilot study. *Pharmacy World & Science, 27*(3), 202–207.

Reid, K. W., Vittinghoff, E., & Kushel, M. B. (2008). Association between the level of housing instability, economic standing and health care access: A meta-regression. *Journal of Health Care for the Poor and Underserved, 19*(4), 1212–1228.

Reilly, V., & Cavanagh, M. (2003). The clinical and economic impact of a secondary heart disease prevention clinic jointly implemented by a practice nurse and pharmacist. *Pharmacy World & Science, 25*(6), 294–298.

Robbins, C., Stillwell, T., Wilson, S., & Fitzgerald, L. (2012). Formulary expansion to provide access to medications prescribed by a specialist in a low-income population. *Journal of Health Care for the Poor and Underserved, 23*(2), 834–841.

Rosenheck, R., & Lam, J. A. (1997). Client and site characteristics as barriers to service use by homeless persons with serious mental illness. *Psychiatric Services, 48*(3), 387–390.

Roumie, C. L., Greevy, R., Wallston, K. A., Elasy, T. A., Kaltenbach, L., Kotter, K., . . . Speroff, T. (2011). Patient centered primary care is associated with patient hypertension medication adherence. *Journal of Behavioral Medicine, 34*(4), 244–253.

Royal, S. W., Kidder, D. P., Patrabansh, S., Wolitski, R. J., Holtgrave, D. R., Aidala, A., . . . Stall, R. (2009). Factors associated with adherence to highly active retroviral therapy in homeless or unstably housed adults living with HIV. *AIDS Care, 21*(4), 448–455.

Sajatovic, M., Valenstein, M., Blow, F. C., Ganoczy, D., & Ignacio, R. V. (2006). Treatment adherence with antipsychotic medications in bipolar disorder. *Bipolar Disorders, 8*(3), 232–241.

Sajatovic, M., Valenstein, M., Blow, F. C., Ganoczy, D., & Ignacio, R. V. (2007). Treatment adherence with lithium and anticonvulsant medications among patients with bipolar disorder. *Psychiatric Services, 58*(6), 855–863.

Salem, B. E., & Ma-Pham, J. (2015). Understanding health needs and perspectives of middle-aged and older women experiencing homelessness. *Public Health Nursing, 32*(6), 634–644.

Scheurer, D., Choudhry, N., Swanton, K. A., Matlin, O., & Shrank, W. (2012). Association between different types of social support and medication adherence. *The American Journal of Managed Care, 18*(12), e461–e467.

Schoen, C., Osborne, R., Doty, M. M., Squires, D., Peugh, J., & Applebaum, S. (2009). A survey of primary care physicians in eleven countries, 2009: Perspectives on care, costs, and experiences. *Health Affairs (Millwood), 28*(6), w1171–w1183.

Schoen, M. D., DiDomenico, R. J., Connor, S. E., Dischler, J. E., & Bauman, J. L. (2001). Impact of the cost of prescription drugs on clinical outcomes in indigent patients with heart disease. *Pharmacotherapy, 21*(12), 1455–1463.

Scott, D. M., Boyd, S. T., Stephan, M., Augustine, S. C., & Reardon, T. P. (2006). Outcomes of pharmacist-managed diabetes care services in a community health center. *American Journal of Health-System Pharmacy, 63*(21), 2116–2122.

Shane-McWhorter, L., & Oderda, G. M. (2005). Providing diabetes education and care to underserved patients in a collaborative practice at a Utah community health center. *Pharmacotherapy, 25*(1), 96–109.

Sharkness, C. M., & Snow, D. A. (1992). The patient's view of hypertension and compliance. *American Journal of Preventive Medicine, 8*(3), 141–146.

Sleath, B. L., Jackson, E., Thomas, K. C., Galloway, J., Dumain, L., Thorpe, J., . . . Morrissey, J. (2006). Literacy and perceived barriers to medication taking among homeless mothers and their children. *American Journal of Health-System Pharmacy, 63*(4), 346–351.

Smith, M., Bates, D. W., Bodenheimer, T., & Cleary, P. D. (2010). Why pharmacists belong in the medical home. *Health Affairs (Millwood), 29*(5), 906–913.

Starace, F., Ammassari, A., Trotta, M. P., Murri, R., DeLongis, P., Izzo, C., . . . NeurolCoNA Study Group. (2002). Depression is a risk factor for suboptimal adherence to highly active antiretroviral therapy. *Journal of Acquired Immune Deficiency Syndromes, 31*(Suppl. 3), S136–S139.

Steward, J., Holt, C. L., Pollio, D. E., Austin, E. L., Johnson, N., Gordon, A. J., & Kertesz, S. G. (2016). Priorities in the primary care of persons experiencing homelessness: Convergence and divergence in the views of patients and provider/experts. *Patient Preference and Adherence, 10*, 153–158.

Till, L. T., Voris, J. C., & Horst, J. B. (2003). Assessment of clinical pharmacist management of lipid-lowering therapy in a primary care setting. *Journal of Managed Care Pharmacy, 9*(3), 269–273.

University of Pittsburgh. (2017). Grace Lamsam Pharmacy Program for the Uninsured. Retrieved from http://www.pharmacy.pitt.edu/programs/GraceLamsam/lamsam.php

Vlasnik, J. J., Aliotta, S. L., & DeLor, B. (2005). Medication adherence: Factors influencing compliance with prescribed medication plans. *The Case Manager, 16*(2), 47–51.

Vranceanu, A. M., Safren, S. A., Lu, M., Coady, W. M., Skolnik, P. R., Rogers, W. H., & Wilson, I. B. (2008). The relationship of post-traumatic stress disorder and depression to antiretroviral medication adherence in persons with HIV. *AIDS Patient Care and STDs, 22*(4), 313–321.

Wang, I., Dopheide, J. A., & Gregerson, P. (2011). Role of a psychiatric pharmacist in a Los Angeles "Skid-Row" safety-net clinic. *Journal of Urban Health, 88*(4), 718–723.

Wheeler, K. J., Roberts, M. E., & Neiheisel, M. B. (2014). Medication adherence part two: Predictors of nonadherence and adherence. *Journal of the American Association of Nurse Practitioners, 26*(4), 225–232.

White, B. M., Jones, W. J., Moran, W. P., & Simpson, K. N. (2016). Effect of the economic recession on primary care access for the homeless. *Journal of Health Care for the Poor and Underserved, 27*(3), 1577–1591.

White, B. M., & Newman, S. D. (2015). Access to primary care services among the homeless: A synthesis of the literature using the equity of access to medical care framework. *Journal of Primary Care & Community Health, 6*(2), 77–87.

Whitley, R. (2013). Fear and loathing in New England: Examining the health-care perspectives of homeless people in rural areas. *Anthropology and Medicine, 20*(3), 232–243.

Willey, C., Redding, C., Stafford, J., Garfield, F., Geletko, S., Flanigan, T., Melbourne, K., . . . Caro, J. J. (2000). Stages of change for adherence with medication regimens for chronic disease: Development and validation of a measure. *Clinical Therapeutics, 22*(7), 858–871.

Wood, D., & Valdez, R. B. (1991). Barriers to medical care for homeless families compared with housed poor families. *The American Journal of Diseases of Children, 145*(10), 1109–1115.

World Health Organization. (2003). Adherence to long term therapies: Evidence for action. Geneva, Switzerland: Author. Retrieved from http://www.who.int/chp/knowledge/publications/adherence_report/en

Yap, A. F., Thirumoorthy, T., & Kwan, Y. H. (2016). Systematic review of the barriers affecting medication adherence in older adults. *Geriatrics and Gerontology International,* *16*(10), 1093–1101.

Zullig, L. L., Stechuchak, K. M., Goldstein, K. M., Olsen, M. K., McCant, F. M., Danus, S., . . . Bosworth, H. B. (2015). Patient-reported medication adherence barriers among patients with cardiovascular risk factors. *Journal of Managed Care & Specialty Pharmacy,* *21*(6), 479–485.

13

Dermatologic Conditions in the Homeless Population

Laura S. Romero, Kevin Broder, Nicola Natsis, and Richard Bodor

Skin problems are one of the most common presenting complaints of home-less persons to emergency departments and community clinics, estimated at 20% of such visits. There is sparse data that specifically focuses on skin dis-ease in the elderly homeless; nevertheless, recent U.S. surveys estimate that 69% of the homeless persons are adults (over age of 24 years). Approximately one-third of this population is over the age of 50 years, and less than 6% are over 61 years (Henry, Watt, Rosenthal, & Shivji, 2016).

Adult homeless suffer the usual skin diseases common to nonhomeless adults, but in addition can suffer more frequent infections, dermatitis, and wounds related to their compromised living status. They may have inade-quate access to clean clothes and bedding, washing facilities, and properly fitting shoes. Furthermore they tend to delay seeking healthcare often due to limited financial means, lack of insurance, or other access problems. Many also have mental health or substance-abuse disorders that also delay their treatments until their medical problems become much more severe (Colburn, 1989; Raoult, 2001). This chapter will focus on the diagnosis, treatment, and triage of common skin complaints in homeless adults.

Given the limited scope of this section, the clinical final treatments depend on local personal clinical judgments. This rough guide and discussion is restricted to the most common, significant skin ailments with limited and brief treatment considerations, and triage. Treatments are based on adult patients no longer of childbearing potential, with normal renal function, treated on an outpatient basis. The understanding is that homeless patients often will return to their current poor living situation with ongoing challenges of homelessness, including difficult access to regular healthcare and limited ability to store supplies, and, in general, maintain optimal wound hygiene and health status. The majority of medication treatments listed are derived from UpToDate and other clinical resources and are not to be taken as a final prescription for any patients without first an examination and then a local provider formulating the best customized treatment plan for each patient. However, it does offer a framework of some common regimens, which can be considered as a component of the local clinician's overall suggested final treatment plan. Other local experts in infectious disease, dermatology, vascular surgery, or plastic surgery may suggest their own preferred treatment regimens. Hospital admission should be considered whenever fever, chills, tachycardia, hypotension, or severe or rapidly progressing infection or other admission criteria are present (UpToDate, n.d.). Additionally, if outpatient treatment is unrealistic given limited social or logistical challenges, admission may be appropriate even without the aforementioned standards, in order to ensure appropriate critical treatments and resolution. This section will be divided into infestations, bites and infections, wounds, neoplasms, and rashes.

INFESTATIONS, BITES, AND INFECTIONS

Sample Case One

A 68-year-old male, who was homeless for three months, presents with severe itching and excoriations, which he has been experiencing for two months (Figures 13.1 and 13.2).

Physical Exam: The patient was disrobed for a complete skin exam. Physical examination revealed a disheveled male, oriented, afebrile with stable vital signs. Mucosa are clear. Rash consists of diffuse excoriations,

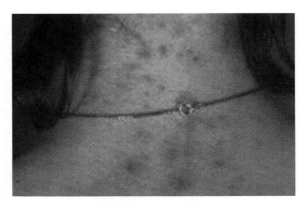

FIGURE 13.1   Body lice

Source: https://commons.wikimedia.org/wiki/File:Fig.4.Louse_bites.jpg

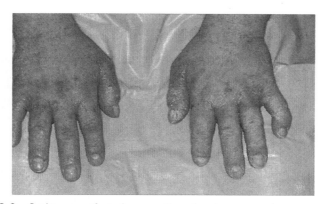

FIGURE 13.2 Scabies manifested as crusting of web spaces.

bleeding, eschars, and crust on the trunk and proximal extremities that spares the face, penis, palms, and soles. Web spaces and wrists are clear.

Differential Diagnosis: Scabies, body lice, atopic or xerotic dermatitis, drug eruption, and Grover's disease.

The most *common infestations* include body lice, and scabies, transmitted from other infested individuals or bedding in marginal living conditions. Both of these infestations are associated with moderate to severe pruritus, disturbing sleep, and typically spare the face. Body lice infestation presents with diffuse excoriations on the trunk (Figure 13.1), often to the point of bleeding. Lice and nits are detected in the clothing seams, rather than on the patient (Figure 13.2). Effective treatment also involves hot water detergent washing (or discarding) of affected clothing and bedding (Table 13.1). Scabies infestation manifests as excoriations, burrows (serpentine plaques with fine scale), and erythematous scaly papules, symmetrically involving the web spaces, wrists, anterior axillae, nipple, waistline, medial buttock, and penis (Figure 13.2). Symptoms are typically of sudden onset. For practical reasons, scabies in the homeless is often best treated with oral Ivermectin 200 mcg/kg for two treatments, one week apart. Ideally, with both type infestations, the patient would also bathe in hot, soapy water. Low to medium strength topical steroid creams for one to two weeks post treatment can relieve itch and promote skin healing. Often, there is a *secondary infection* from extensive scratching in both processes, and empiric treatment that covers gram-positive organisms, including methicillin-resistant *Staphylococcus aureus* (MRSA), is often indicated (see cellulitis treatment in Table 13.1). Homeless persons are at increased risk of MRSA, and it may be prudent to always cover for this organism in the case of soft-tissue infection (Health Care for the Homeless Clinician's Network, 2006; Stevens et al., 2014).

TABLE 13.1 *Infestations, Bites, and Infections Table Summary*

	Common Infestations and Bites	
Disease	**Medication(s)**	**Some Treatment Options**
Scabies	Ivermectin	200 Ug/kg single dose with second dose 7–10 days later
Pediculosis corporis	Low-potency topical steroid can be given for symptom relief	Wash clothing and bedding in greater than 149°F followed by drying in hot dryer or seal in airtight bag for two weeks; have patient bathe in hot soapy water.
	Common Infections	
Tinea (pedis, limited corporis, cruris)	Allylamines, imidazoles* and pyridines in cream, lotion, or gel form Note that nystatin is not appropriate treatment	Topical 1–2 times/day for 1 month
Widespread or multifocal tinea corporis	Terbinafine Other oral agents may be used, but have more potential drug interactions. Simultaneous topical therapy as for limited tinea corporis is often recommended Note that nystatin is not appropriate treatment	Oral terbinafine 250 mg daily for 7–14 days along with topical therapy as described for limited tinea corporis as stated earlier Or Oral Itraconazole 200 mg daily for 7 days Or Oral fluconazole 150–200 mg once weekly x 2–4 weeks
Intertrigo (Candidiasis)	Topical anti-candidal creams, lotions, or gels (nystatin, imidazoles*, ciclopirox) and topical hydrocortisone Severe or refractory disease may require oral antifungals (prescribe cautiously in unique cases only)	Anticandidal creams: 1–2 times/day for 2–4 weeks Hydrocortisone for short-term initial use at two times/day for 7–10 days to hasten symptom relief (use with caution as steroids can thin the skin in these sensitive areas) Fluconazole 150 mg once weekly or 50–100 mg daily x 2–6 weeks Or Itraconazole 200 mg twice daily x 2–6 weeks

(continued)

TABLE 13.1   *Infestations, Bites, and Infections Table Summary (continued)*

	Common Infections	
Disease	**Medication(s)**	**Some Treatment Options**
Onychomycosis	Topical ciclopirox, efinaconazole, or tavaparole for 48 weeks; if high risk recurrent cellulitis and an alcohol abstainer, consider oral terbinafine	Nail lacquer daily for up to 48 weeks Oral terbinafine 250 mg once daily for six weeks for fingernail and three months for toenail involvement (check LFTs, CBC at baseline and at six weeks in those on three-month regimen) Consider: pulsed Itraconazole therapy (200 mg twice a day) for one week per month. Duration: × two months for fingernail disease, and x three months for toenail disease
Dermatophytosis complex	Topical antifungals, topical antibiotics covering for staphylococcus and gram-negatives such as levofloxacin or based on culture results	Ciclopirox gel .77% twice daily for 28 days, topical tolnaftate, naftitine, or imidazole* combined with either 1% Neomycin ointment twice daily, or oral antibiotic based on culture results such as levofloxacin: 500 mg twice daily for 7–10 days
Pitted keratolysis	Topical erythromycin, clindamycin, fusidic acid	Twice daily erythromycin for 10 days
Cellulitis nonpurulent, no abscess, secondary skin infection from bites, tinea, infestations, etc.	Recommend empiric coverage of MRSA and beta-hemolytic until culture results indicate more narrow coverage Oral clindamycin, or amoxicillin + trimethoprim-sulfamethoxazole, or amoxicillin + doxycycline	Oral clindamycin: 300 mg–450 mg four times a day for 10–14 days Oral amoxicillin 500 mg three times a day + trimethoprim-sulfamethoxazole: 1 DS tab two times a day, respectively, for 10–14 days Oral amoxicillin 500 mg two times a day + doxycycline: 100 mg two times a day, respectively, for 10–14 days
Cellulitis purulent, no abscess	Empiric coverage for MRSA until culture results indicate otherwise Oral clindamycin, doxycycline, or minocycline, TMP-SMX	Oral clindamycin: 300–600 mg TID for 10–14 days Doxycycline, minocycline: 100 mg two times a day for 10–14 days TMP-SMX: 1 DS tab two times a day for 14 days
Cellulitis purulent, with abscess	Above antibiotics for purulent cellulitis plus incision, drainage; dressings	

(continued)

TABLE 13.1   *Infestations, Bites, and Infections Table Summary (continued)*

Common Infections		
Disease	**Medication(s)**	**Some Treatment Options**
Folliculitis	Topical clindamycin, oral dicloxacillin, or cephalexin	Clindamycin: topical for two weeks
		Oral dicloxacillin, cephalexin: four times daily for 7–10 days
		If severe or recurrent, treat for MRSA as listed under aforementioned "cellulitis, purulent"
Verruca vulgaris (nonfacial, nonfiliform)	Cryotherapy	Cryotherapy applied twice allowing for a thaw period in between, with duration of freezing as necessary such that the entire lesion is fully whitened as well as a 2 mm rim of normal skin
	Salicylic acid solution or impregnated bandages daily is an alternative, but would be difficult for homeless individuals	

*Imidazole agents include ketoconazole, clotrimazole, econazole, and miconazole.
CBC, complete blood count; DS, double strength; LFTs, liver function tests; MRSA, methicillin-resistant staphylococcus aureus; TMP-SMX, trimethoprim-sulfamethoxazole.

Arthropod bites or stings are also particularly common in homeless persons due to their dwelling outdoors or in temporary shelters. Bites appear as solitary or clustered erythematous papules or nodules on exposed skin of the extremities and face. Lesions may be pruritic, tender, or asymptomatic. Arthropods can include fleas, spiders, ants, and mosquitos. Treatment is with mild- to mid-potency topical steroids (triamcinolone 0.1%) and/or antipruritic lotions such as calamine or camphor/menthol. If concern exists for secondary infection, treatment with antibiotics that cover gram-positive organisms may be appropriate such as topical bacitracin or mupirocin and oral cephalexin. Rapid onset and short duration are features that help distinguish bites from infections and *neoplasms* such as lymphoma. Follow-up remains important for all of these problems. Note that bites can sometimes transmit other diseases secondarily (e.g., mosquitos can transmit West Nile and Zika virus), and so comprehensive patient evaluation, taking into account the specific geographic location, patient signs, and symptoms, will ensure that no secondary infections are missed.

Case One Final Diagnosis: Body lice. Clothing seams revealed nits and lice (Figure 13.3), and scabies preparation was found to be negative.

Sample Case Two

Thumbnail: A homeless 36-year-old male, active IV drug abuser, reports four days of swelling and pain in his left anterior forearm.

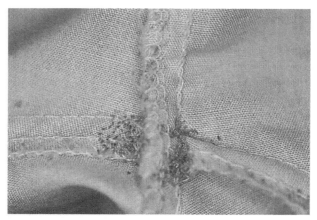

FIGURE 13.3 Lice in seams.

Source: Burkhart, C. N., Burkhart, C. G., & Morrell, D. S. (2012). Infestations. In J. L. Bolognia, J. L. Jorizzo, & J.V. Schaeffer (Eds.), *Dermatology* (3rd ed., pp. 1423–1432). Philadephia, PA: Elsevier.

Physical Exam: Vital signs show a temperature of 101°F, BP 140/82, and HR of 100. Left arm shows a 4-cm hot, fluctuant nodule, extremely tender, with patch-like erythema extending several centimeters up the arm.

Differential Diagnosis: Abscess, infected cyst or neoplasm, cellulitis. Skin and soft-tissue infections are frequent in the homeless, and treatment is challenging, given inadequate social support and concerns with access, compliance, and follow-up. Risks for infections are particularly concerning with HIV positive and other immunocompromised individuals. Fever, elevated white count, constitutional symptoms, and HIV positivity are all features whose presence may favor more proactive inpatient treatment. Again, while some of our listed treatment considerations are primarily obtained from UpToDate, the final treatment regimen should be customized for the individual patient's need. The most common skin infections occur on the lower extremity and include tinea pedis, onychomycosis, pitted keratolysis, and cellulitis (Contag, Lowenstein, Jain, & Amerson, 2017; Stratigos et al., 1999). *Tinea pedis* is a dermatophyte infection that presents characteristically as macerated, erythematous plaques, and occasionally pustules, in the web spaces (Figure 13.4). There is associated itching and burning. It is treated with topical antifungal creams or gels twice daily for approximately one month. Occasionally, this infection develops a secondary bacterial infection with Staphylococcus or gram-negative organisms (dermatophytosis complex). This secondary infection presents with more erosive, edematous, and draining plaques that can be quite painful (Figure 13.5). A bacterial culture swab should be performed, and the patient should be started on oral antibiotics, such as fluoroquinolones or other empiric options, until the results are

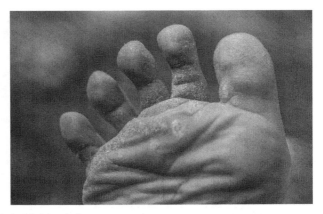

FIGURE 13.4 Athlete's foot.

Source: Russaquarius (Photographer). (2017). *Athlete's foot* (Photograph). Retrieved from https://www.istockphoto.com/photo/athletes-foot-gm823679170-133382463

finalized to further refine treatment. Topical antifungals should be used concomitantly as for uncomplicated tinea pedis. Oral antifungals may be used in extensive cases, for one to two weeks of duration; however, there are drug interactions, as well as liver toxicity considerations. *Pitted keratolysis* presents as asymptomatic, albeit malodorous, pits and superficial erosions on the plantar foot, especially in weight-bearing areas. This infection is caused most commonly by Corynebacterium species and is best treated with topical antibiotics. All the aforementioned foot infections should ideally be treated with the following additional daily measures: washing of feet, including web spaces, followed by thorough drying, exposing feet to air, changing socks whenever wet, and avoiding occlusive footwear such as boots. Topical

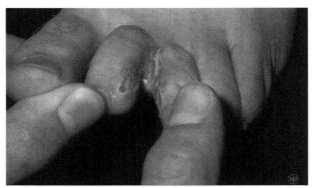

FIGURE 13.5 Dermatophytosis complex.

antifungal powders can minimize recurrence, but are insufficient to treat active infections. *Onychomycosis* presents as nail thickening, yellow or white discoloration, and subungual debris and is typically caused by a dermatophyte infection, less commonly by yeasts such as Candida species or nondermatophyte molds. Treatment is generally not recommended unless there is significant pain, recurrent secondary infection, or fingernail involvement. Topical treatment alone is curative in well under 50% of cases, although it generally results in partial improvement and may reduce the chance of progression. Oral therapy is indicated for six weeks to three months or longer for finger and toenail disease, respectively, and achieves 70% response rates. Screening for liver toxicity and drug interactions is prudent.

Bacterial cellulitis can develop whenever skin integrity is broken. Causes include untreated tinea infection, wounds created by ill-fitting footwear, untreated stasis dermatitis, and from traumatic injury. Diagnosis is made by clinical features of local or progressing erythema, heat, pain, edema, drainage, or tenderness, more so than elevated white count or fever, which can be a later finding. *Nonpurulent infections*, or mild infections lacking indicators for hospitalization, should receive a careful examination and close follow-up to ensure improvement to therapy. Initial outpatient treatment should begin with oral antibiotics (many suggest starting with regimens that cover MRSA and beta-hemolytic streptococcus) typically for 10 to 14 days. If the aforementioned signs of cellulitis are associated with frank pus or *abscess* (discrete area of tender, fluctuant intact skin), treatment for MRSA is appropriate (Figure 13.6). Abscesses should be incised, drained, and loosely packed with gauze. Reassessment (if admission is not indicated) should occur in 24 to 72 hours. If an area of concern for abscess demonstrated no purulence on aspirations or incision, or if no clinical improvement, then return for reassessment in 24 to 48 hours. Poor response to antibiotics may indicate that the abscess was not mature at the earlier visit, or inadequately drained, and at times radiographic guidance may even be needed. Affected limbs should be elevated and movement limited, if at all possible. Pain control with oral nonsteroidals, acetaminophen, or opiates may be indicated, but underlying causes must be aggressively resolved to avoid *complications* from untreated infections, such as necrotizing cellulitis, compartment syndrome, or sepsis.

The following infections occur most commonly on the trunk and are often related to occlusion, sweating, and poor hygiene. Symptoms of itching and burning may be present. *Folliculitis* is a bacterial infection manifested as pustules and red papules restricted to hair follicles. Local infection can be treated topically, although more extensive treatment requires oral antibiotics covering Staphylococcus for 7 to 10 days. *Tinea corporis* is a dermatophyte infection

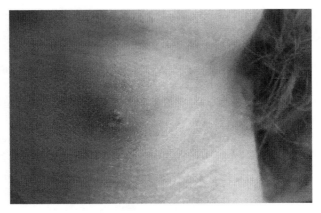

FIGURE 13.6 Abscess under chin.

Source: MementoImage (Photographer). (2015). *Abscess under chin* (Photograph). Retrieved from https://www.istockphoto.com/photo/abscess-under-the-chin-gm492372260-76267849

that presents as large, annular plaques with a scaly border. Potassium hydroxide (KOH) of the active scaly border may reveal branching hyphae. Limited involvement can be treated with topical antifungals, whereas more extensive involvement requires oral antifungal therapy. Baseline or recent (within three months) normal liver function tests are recommended prior to treatment.

Tinea cruris, or "jock itch," presents as scaly, pruritic, or burning plaques in the medial thighs and inguinal folds. It is usually treated with topical antifungal therapy, although severe or recurrent infections may warrant oral therapy. This infection is distinguished from *candidiasis*, which can also present in the inguinal crease and groin, by the presence of maceration, bright red erythema, and satellite pustules. Candida commonly also involves the flexural folds underneath breasts and abdominal pannus, and may involve the scrotum and penis. Topical antifungal therapy is indicated for two to four weeks. Note that topical nystatin is appropriate for limited candidal infection, but is ineffective for tinea cruris or corporis (dermatophyte infections). If symptoms of pain or itching are prominent, concomitant mild topical steroids may be used initially. Oral ketoconazole is no longer indicated for any cutaneous fungal infections, given the risk of liver toxicity, but many effective options remain and should be evaluated on a case-by-case basis.

Common *viral skin infections* include verruca vulgaris, which appear as filiform papules on the face and as more keratotic, verrucous plaques on the body. Treatment with liquid nitrogen, preceded by paring down of the lesion for particularly thick lesions, is the most efficient way to treat.

While *sexually transmitted diseases (STDs)* occur in this patient population, they have not been found to be a common presenting complaint in multiple studies (Oyerinde, 2014; Raoult, 2001; Stratigos et al., 1999) and will not be detailed here. Nevertheless, STD screening in this population is often indicated, and if detected, patients and their partners should be treated appropriately. Certain diseases require reporting to local county health departments. Universal precautions should also be used during all examinations and procedures. Treatment as per CDC (www.cdc.gov/std) guidelines with treatment counseling is recommended.

Case Two Diagnosis: Abscess with cellulitis, with systemic symptoms of significant pain, tachycardia and fever, and elevated blood pressure. Admit for incision and drainage (I&D) in the operating room (OR), labs, IV antibiotics, local wound care, and pain control.

LACERATIONS AND WOUNDS

See Table 13.1.

Sample Case Three

Thumbnail: A 70-year-old female with history of chronic lower extremity bilateral edema and darker surrounding skin above both ankles recently presents with an open wound at the medial mid-shin for the past several months. No history of trauma.

Physical Exam: Large 4-cm diameter irregular, shallow ulcer with surrounding chronic, nonwarm erythema, hemosiderin, and varicose veins; bilateral chronic edema.

Differential Diagnosis: Diabetic ulcer, trauma, stasis or other chronic ulcer, malignancy.

Homeless persons are prone to *lacerations and wounds* from poorly fitting shoes, falls, and physical or other environmental assaults. Persons who suffer puncture or other penetrating wounds should be assessed whether they have indications to be vaccinated with tetanus. Lacerations and wounds should all be irrigated copiously with sterile saline, preferably under pressure, to cleanse and remove all foreign or frankly necrotic material. Intralesional anesthesia is generally required first, typically 0.5% or 1% lidocaine with epinephrine.

Lacerations that are less than 24 hours old, or those that are on the scalp and face for longer duration, may occasionally be closed, primarily with sutures after thorough cleansing. Irregular edges may need sharp debridement, for best approximation with repair. Lesions in highly cosmetic areas such as the vermilion lip, deep or complex wounds, wounds near neurovascular structures, on the hands are typically treated by plastic surgeons or hand surgery referral for sub-specialty care. After vigorous irrigation and confirmation of hemostasis, anatomic suture repair is then the mainstay of treatment. Dressing regimen should include topical nonadherent dressings followed by padded protective dressings. Exudative, open wound areas may not be able to be repaired primarily and may require dressing change regimens that also maintain a moist wound environment while avoiding local skin maceration. Wrapping wounds with gentle padded gauze compression (along with elevation) helps control edema and offers healing tissues support. Various nonstick wound surface dressings (held in place with padded supportive overwrap dressings) may prevent or support healing of skin tears to fragile, compromised aging skin.

Ulcer wounds may be venous, arterial, diabetic, lymphatic, malignant, or mixed in origin and often appear on characteristic locations (Figure 13.7).

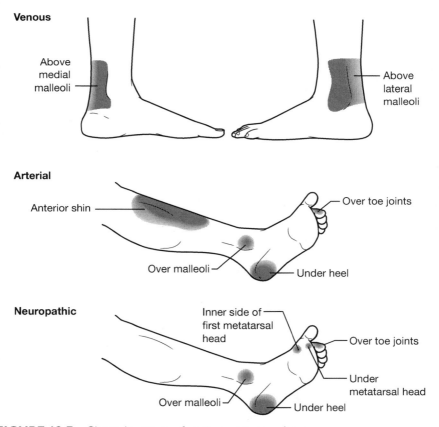

FIGURE 13.7   Classic locations of various common ulcers.

Source: Explore Nursing Diagnosis, Nursing Assessment, and more! (n.d.). Retrieved from https://www.pinterest.com/pin/553942822899116573

Ulcer wounds in the lower extremity are important for clinicians to understand, especially in the lower third of the leg where deep wounds can become limb threatening if neglected. With the underlying tendons or bone having little soft tissue covering, complex reconstructions may be required if such distal ulcers fail to heal. *Venous stasis ulcers* occur most commonly around the medial ankle and appear as irregular, shallow ulcers that are moderately painful (Figure 13.8). Risk factors include chronic prolonged standing, age greater than 64 years, venous hypertension (mostly due to valvular venous incompetence), lower leg trauma, and obesity. There are common clinical signs of venous stasis (hemosiderin deposition, edema, and varicose veins). Arterial perfusion should also always be assessed to determine whether adequate for compression bandages to be safely placed, and whether conservative treatment (elevation, local wound care, padded compression garments, etc.) will be sufficient to heal the venous ulcer. Peripheral arterial disease (PAD) can also cause distal limb ulcers. Such *arterial ulcers* may appear distally in the extremities and are not pressure related, perhaps appearing deep and punched out, and often are quite painful. They may occur on nonplantar pressure points, such as over the toe joints, on the anterior shin, and occasionally also on the heel. Clinical signs suggesting inadequate arterial perfusion include: absent foot pulses, claudication, leg pain with leg elevation, cold and hairless feet, discoloration or wounding of toes, persistent nonhealing distal ulcers despite good local care and no infection. An ankle-brachial index (ABI) can readily be performed bedside in minutes to also help diagnose arterial disease for planning care, triage, and referral for vascular specialists. *Diabetic ulcers* primarily have a neuropathic component and often occur in similar areas as arterial ulcers, but also classically occur on the pressure points of

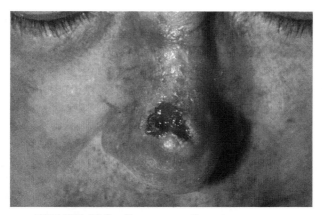

FIGURE 13.8   Squamous cell carcinoma.

Source: https://commons.wikimedia.org/wiki/File:Squamous_Cell_Carcinoma.jpg

the plantar foot (e.g., such as a painless ulcer over the metatarsal head level). They are often surrounded by thick callus and are typically anesthetic.

All such nonhealing chronic ulcers may require some level of *surgical* intervention for biopsy and debridement, to stimulate healing, or to rule out underlying causes such as squamous cell carcinoma (Marjoin's ulcer) for chronic nonhealing. Pathology or microbiology specimens or stains may be indicated. Postoperative management of such wound ulcers may include local dressings, with physiologic normal saline (or occasionally with 0.25 strength Dakin's or similar antimicrobial wound dressing solution). This may be followed by moist wound dressings with topical antibiotics, hydrogels, honey, calcium algenates, or some of the many other moist wound environment dressings. Wound matrix interventions and biological dressings, as well as negative pressure therapy type dressing can also be helpful in healing many such cases. If procedures are performed on extremities, patients should elevate the affected part to reduce edema as much as possible. Surgeons of lower extremity wounds may allow toe flexion/extension exercises to activate the calf muscle to assist in leg venous circulation, and reduce complications from immobilization. Close postoperative follow-up for such complex wounds helps ensure progressive improvement. Referral to a wound care clinic or plastic surgeon may also be helpful. Serial wound measurements and photographs help to follow progress especially in critical anatomic regions and help with continuity of care. Nutrition should be optimized, and smoking should be stopped. Laboratory results from culture and pathology results should be followed, with appropriate treatments initiated. Wounds should be followed until healed, and more closely if local signs of significant erythema, swelling, and pain exist.

For further details of presentation and management of diabetic foot ulcers, please refer to the section later in this chapter on "Foot and Nail Diseases."

Case Three Final Diagnosis: Venous Stasis ulcer

Patient had complete work-up, demonstrated adequate arterial perfusion, and was treated with local debridement, padded compression, leg elevation, daily moist dressings, medical and nutritional optimization, and weekly assessment.

NEOPLASMS

Sample Case Four

Thumbnail: A 68-year-old male presents with new, brown facial discoloration at the left upper cheek. He reports chronic sun exposure starting at age 10.

Physical Exam: Light brown irregular patch superficial to the left zygomatic arch measuring 1.4 cm in largest diameter.

Differential Diagnosis: Cafe-au-lait macule, solar lentigo, early seborrheic keratosis, lentigo maligna melanoma.

Pigmented lesions are fraught with fears of misdiagnosis. History should include duration, growth, history of pain or bleeding, and family or personal history of skin cancer/melanoma. Long-standing stable lesions without changing or symptoms are reassuring. Lesions that are discrete, symmetric, homogenous in color, and small (less than 6 mm) are more likely to be benign. If several atypical features exist, it is helpful to examine the patient to look for other growths that appear similar. This finding can be reassuring as some people simply produce atypical-appearing nevi (moles) and lentigos (liver spots). Dark black new lesions can occasionally represent nodular melanoma and should be biopsied or referred to dermatology. Lentigo maligna melanoma often presents as a tan or pink patch, greater than 1 cm, on sun-damaged skin with irregular coloration. They are typically long-standing, although the patient often notes that they may have grown darker or larger over time. Dermoscopy, using a device that utilizes a magnifier and polarized light, can help identify specific clinical features for malignancy such as an atypical pigment network or blue–gray veil. Generally, dermatopathologists prefer either a well-performed scoop shave biopsy or an excisional biopsy, rather than smaller punch biopsies, when evaluating pigmented lesions. A long scoop shave biopsy provides a larger area of epidermis to evaluate for malignant features, including asymmetry, while also excising the full lesion without transecting it, to the complete depth down to fat. For suspicious or questionable lesions, including borderline lesions located on the back or other areas where history of duration of change is not available, the provider should act conservatively and perform a limited biopsy that preserves depth and architectural pathology, or refer for biopsy from surgeons able to process a rapid effective diagnosis and trigger treatment without delays.

BENIGN LESIONS

Seborrheic keratoses (SKs) are waxy, stuck-on plaques, typically tan, pink, or brown in color, concentrated in the truncal area, that show verrucous or small pore-like surface change. They can occasionally look erythematous or atypical after trauma or irritation.

Solar lentigos are light-brown flat patches on sun-exposed skin and the trunk, which appear uniformly colored, are long-standing, and typically exist with many similar appearing lesions. Darker, larger, or more irregularly shaped lesions, or those that have changed per patient history, should be biopsied. Similarly, if the lesion is an isolated one that shows large size or asymmetry, biopsy is often indicated.

LESIONS WITH PREMALIGNANT POTENTIAL

Actinic keratoses (AKs) are premalignant growths located on sun-exposed skin caused by ultraviolet damage. If left untreated, AKs can occasionally progress to squamous cell carcinoma. AKs and nonmelanoma skin cancers are a significant risk for elderly homeless persons, particularly given their regular sun exposure, lack of sunscreen use, and low levels of skin cancer screening (Wilde, Jones, Lewis, & Hull, 2013). These risks are particularly high for homeless populations in states with high sun exposure—for example, California, where approximately one-fifth of the U.S. homeless persons live, with 10% specifically in Los Angeles (Henry et al., 2016). AKs present as scaly, erythematous, sometimes tender papules, and plaques on sun-exposed areas of the face, alopeciac scalp, forearms, and dorsal hands. The risk of transformation to skin cancer is low (less than 1% per lesion-year) (Werner et al., 2013), although the overall patient risk increases with multiple lesions if left untreated. Larger, more indurated lesions, or those that have not responded to standard therapy, should be biopsied or referred for biopsy. Cryotherapy of thicker lesions and of those located in higher risk sites (ears, nose, lips, and periocular skin) is appropriate. Use of *topical* creams, such as 5-fluorouracil, ingenol mebutate, diclofenac, and imiquimod, is ideal for field treatment of diffuse sun damage, although they are generally more expensive and run the risk of noncompliance.

Atypical nevi present as irregular or large pigmented or erythematous macules or papules. The presence of multiple nevi, including atypical nevi, are a marker of increased risk of melanoma. About 20% of the melanomas show an associated nevus. If two or more features are found on a clinical ABCDE lesion evaluation—A: asymmetry, B: border (sharp or blurred), C: color (presence of multiple colors or shades), D: diameter (greater than 6 mm), and E: evolution (history of change, growth, or bleeding)—biopsy may be appropriate. Another reasonable practice is to biopsy the most atypical nevus or nevi present ("ugly duckling").

MALIGNANT LESIONS

Squamous cell carcinoma and basal cell carcinoma account for approximately 90% of all skin malignancies, with the lifetime risk of development one in five in the United States. Both are directly related to sun exposure, although genetic and environmental factors play a lesser role (Hosler & Patterson, 2016). Treatment recommendation details will be restricted to those who are most realistic for homeless persons facing great logistical and access challenges, and therefore serial sessions of radiation therapy and photodynamic therapy, occasional options for these cancers, are not further discussed here.

Squamous cell cardinoma (SCC) is a skin cancer that presents typically as a keratotic or ulcerated erythematous plaque (Figure 13.8). It appears most commonly on the scalp, face, dorsal upper extremities, and lower vermilion lip and accounts for 20% of all nonmelanoma skin cancers. Although ultraviolet B with its subsequent induction of p53 tumor suppression gene is a common risk factor, other risks include immunosuppression, actinic keratosis sites, and human papilloma virus infection. Squamous cell carcinoma may also occur in skin that is not sun exposed, including sites of chronic ulceration, burns, scars, and chronic inflammatory processes, such as lichen planus. These SSC cancers are somewhat more aggressive than basal cell carcinoma, with a metastatic rate of 0.5% to 2% for the low-risk lesions (less than 2 cm, well differentiated, less than 4–5 mm in thickness histologically, sun-exposed skin, nonimmunosuppressed states) (Hosler & Patterson, 2016). High-risk SSC features include size greater than 2 cm, poor differentiation histologically, acantholysis, rapid growth, location on lip or ear or scars, perineural invasion, and depth greater than 6 mm. Treatment includes excision (with 4–5 mm clear margins) and, in anatomically critical areas, performing Mohs micrographic surgery. Tumor recurrence, if likely, is generally in the first five years post removal.

Basal cell carcinoma (BCC) is the most common skin cancer (80% of all nonmelanoma skin cancers) and presents classically as a pearly papule or plaque, often with central ulceration, rolled border, and overlying telangiectasia. Shave biopsy or referral for biopsy to confirm the diagnosis is recommended for any nonhealing, suspicious lesions. BCCs are characteristically located on sun-exposed skin, such as the upper face, upper trunk, and upper extremity, in the setting of chronic actinic skin damage. Ultraviolet B-induced mutations in the p53 tumor-suppressor gene are present in 50% of BCCs, although other risk factors also include radiotherapy, HPV infection, tar and asphalt exposure, and arsenical intoxication (Hosler & Patterson, 2016). This tumor grows slowly, but can be locally destructive and invasive. There are multiple histologic subtypes with nodular, superficial, and cystic being some of the most frequent. High-risk features include: size greater than 6 mm on the central face in the T zone and ears; size greater than 2 cm on the body; immunosuppression; histologic subtypes, including infiltrating, micronodular, sclerosing, or metatypical; histologic evidence of perineural invasion; and recurrent tumors. The metastatic rate is 0.05%, and regional lymph nodes are the most common metastatic site (Hosler & Patterson, 2016). The following are several treatment options to consider for these cancers, depending somewhat on lesion thickness, location and histologic depth, and differentiation: electrodessication and curettage, excision (with 3–4 mm margins), Mohs micrographic surgery, and topical imiquimod. Recurrence is very low, but generally occurs in the first three years post removal.

Malignant melanoma is the most serious of the malignant skin lesions. There is a 1/40 chance of developing melanoma in Caucasians, a 1/200 chance in Hispanics, and a 1/1000 chance in African Americans. While the risk of developing melanoma increases with age, it remains a common diagnosis even in individuals younger than 30 years. Some of the most prominent risk factors include multiple dysplastic nevi (greater than 5), previous melanoma, numerous nevi (greater than 100), red hair, genetic mutations (particularly Xeroderma pigmentosum and *RB1* gene), and excessive sun/ UV exposure (Hosler & Patterson, 2016). As mentioned in the atypical nevus section, melanomas are characteristically pigmented lesions with more than one atypical feature on the clinical ABCDE criteria. Patients may also report symptoms of itching or bleeding. The most common melanoma locations include the upper back in males and lower extremities in women (Hosler & Patterson, 2016). Prognosis is based on clinical and pathologic stage, so the goal is early detection and excision. The pathologic stage is particularly based on the microscopic depth of invasion (Breslow depth) and, when appropriate, sentinel lymph node status. *Favorable* conditions such as Breslow depth less than 1 mm in depth, presenting without ulceration, confers a five-year survival rate upon treatment of 97%. Besides depth of skin invasion, the clinical features that are *unfavorable* include increasing age, immunosuppression, and male sex, to name a few.

Melanoma can be divided into four major subtypes: lentigo maligna, acral lentiginous, superficial spreading, and nodular. Lentigo maligna presents as a tannish brown patch on chronically sun-exposed areas in older patients. Acral lentiginous melanoma is overall less common than lentigo maligna (Figure 13.9), but is over-represented in individuals with darker complexions—for example, African American and Asian people. They may or may not follow the usual ABCDE criteria. In the case of *nail melanoma*, pigmentation often presents as a pigmented linear nail streak, greater than 3 mm in width, irregular or dark brown in pigmentation, with extension of pigment onto the proximal nail fold (Hutchinson sign). The great toe is the most common location, and for any apparent pigmentation changes in the nailbed, it is important to exclude post-traumatic trapped hemorrhage that can clinically mimic a subungual melanoma. *Superficial spreading* melanoma accounts for the greatest proportion of melanomas (30% to 60%). These melanomas occasionally arise from a preexisting nevus (20% of time) and are more likely to be identified using the ABCDE criteria. Namely, these are pigmented lesions

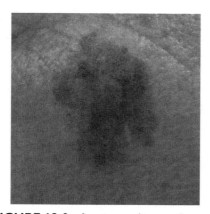

FIGURE 13.9 Lentigo maligna melanoma.
Source: https://en.wikipedia.org/wiki/File:Lentigo_maligna.JPG

that are irregular in border; asymmetric in color, shape, or size; large in size; and/or possess a history of growth or change. *Nodular* melanoma are typically blue or black nodules, though occasionally they may be flesh colored. They present with a more vertical growth phase, and so tend to have a greater depth of invasion upon biopsy diagnosis, with consequent poorer prognosis.

Melanomas, once diagnosed from a biopsy, typically are definitively treated by a pathologically driven wide surgical re-excision. The recommended *clear surgical margins* for treatment are as follows: 5-mm clear skin margins for an in-situ depth melanoma lesion, 1-cm clear skin margin for invasive lesion with depth less than 1 mm, 1- to 2-cm margin for invasive lesion with depth 1 to 2 mm (with clinical consideration of a *sentinel lymph node* biopsy for such intermediate depth lesions), and a 2-cm clear margin to be excised for lesion invasion depth greater than 2 cm. *Sentinel lymph node* biopsy (i.e., sampling of the main draining node) should be considered in melanomas greater than 1 mm in depth (or greater than 0.75 mm depth if additional high-risk features are present histologically, such as ulceration). This procedure should be performed at the same time as the re-excision, so as not to disrupt the lymphatic drainage. Patients after surgical treatment should *follow up* every three months for two years for invasive tumors; they should follow up at month 3, 6, 12, 18, and 24 months for in-situ melanomas. Melanoma can recur 10 or more years after initial diagnosis, and so annual long-term follow up for melanoma patients is appropriate. There are new therapies for advanced disease that target specific cytogenetic features of melanoma; however, these therapies are very expensive, and experimental regimens may likely be logistically difficult for homeless persons to access, so for homeless individuals (and all patients, actually), the goal for best effective treatment is early detection. Therapy for early melanoma (stage I or II) is highly successful with localized surgical treatment, and so outreach skin screening and education of patients are particularly effective measures.

Case Four Final Diagnosis: Lentigo maligna melanoma lesion on the left cheek of an elderly lady who had noticed it there for years. The patient's physician noted increasing thickness of certain regions in the pigmented, otherwise flat lesion.

RASHES, IRRITATIONS, AND MISCELLANEOUS

Sample Case Five

Thumbnail: An 80-year-old male with congestive heart failure and hepatitis C-associated cirrhosis presents with bilateral lower extremity redness, pain, and swelling.

Physical Exam: Bright red weepy *superficial* plaques on bilateral lower extremities.

Differential Diagnosis: Stasis dermatitis, cellulitis, deep venous thrombosis.

Dermatitis, denoting dry scaly skin, increases in frequency with age due to a decreased skin barrier. Homeless persons have increased exposures to irritants such as sun, cold, wet or rough clothing, ill-fitting shoes, and so on. Also, they may need to stand and sit for long periods, increasing stasis pressure on their venous system. Integral to the diagnosis of dermatitis is pruritus, which is why dermatitis is known as the "itch that rashes." Therefore, despite different causes, all the following various specific dermatitis entities may benefit from similar treatments, to resolve episodic clinical flares and prevent recurrences. Treatment for dermatitis includes the use of daily moisturizers and mild soaps, avoidance of irritants, restraint from scratching, and improved patient education (as to the underlying role of scratching and the need for long-term dry skin management). Diffuse dermatitis such as *atopic dermatitis* typically occurs in individuals with an atopic diathesis, including personal or family history of seasonal allergies, asthma, and dermatitis. Dry, ill-defined scaly, symmetric plaques can appear on the palms, antecubital and popliteal fossae, lateral neck, and eyelids. Pruritus is moderate to severe, and disease waxes and wanes in severity. Diagnosis is made by characteristic location, long-standing disease duration, and presence of personal and family atopic diathesis features. Treatment involves the aforementioned skin measures, and also mid-potency topical steroids, oral antihistamines, and, if appropriate, use of oral antibiotics covering staphylococcus, such as cephalexin, dicloxacillin, or doxycycline. Rarely, a short oral systemic steroid taper is given for severe flares to allow time for the more conservative topical therapy to take effect. Any type of *atypical dermatitis* that appears atypical in distribution or remains refractory to therapy should be referred for biopsy to confirm the diagnosis. Biopsy would also be prudent in the small subset of patients who require *systemic immunosuppressive* therapy for disease control such as methotrexate, azathioprine, or CellCept: This would be very challenging to manage in a homeless setting.

Xerotic dermatitis, also known as asteatotic eczema, presents most commonly in winter as diffusely dry skin with fine flakes, most severe on the extremities. Occasionally, the eczematous plaques show fine cracks running through them (eczema craquele), resembling the cracks seen in old porcelain dishes (James, Berger, & Elston, 2006). Treatment is similar to atopic dermatitis, with mid-potency topical steroids and antihistamines.

Lichen simplex chronicus presents as thickened plaques with overlying increased skin tension lines (lichenification) that appear on easily reached sites: These include the dorsal arms, legs, hands, and feet, as well as the scrotum, gluteal crease, and scalp. There is, sometimes, associated hyperpigmentation. These lesions are extremely pruritic and require use of potent topical steroids, sometimes with occlusion, to prevent perpetual scratching. Atypical appearing lesions might require biopsy for diagnosis, sometimes being mistaken for other neoplasms such as *squamous cell carcinoma* or *arthropod reaction*. Any lesions in the groin area should be studied with potassium hydroxide preparation for fungus.

Seborrheic dermatitis (a.k.a., "dandruff") presents as yellow, greasy scale in the scalp, hair-bearing facial skin (including eyebrow, beard, and moustache area), and nasal and nasolabial creases (Table 13.2). There is associated burning and itching, and severity and frequency are increased in HIV and spinal cord injury patients, likely from immune dysregulation. Treatment includes daily washing of involved areas with medicated or antifungal shampoo, topical steroid creams or solutions of mild to mid-potency, and/or antifungal creams to decrease Malassezia yeast levels on the skin, which appears to have a role in this disease (Hosler & Patterson, 2016). Seborrheic dermatitis arises in adolescence or young adulthood, flares with stress, and appears to be lifelong in duration.

Venous stasis dermatitis manifests as hyperpigmented thin plaques on the lower one-third of the leg, with variable associated varicose veins, hemosiderin deposits, pitting edema, and/or woody induration. Overlying skin dermatitis changes are present, and vary from dry and scaly to more

TABLE 13.2 *Irritations, Rashes, and Miscellaneous Summary*

Irritations and Rashes	
Disease	**Treatment Options**
Atopic dermatitis, xerotic eczema	Triamcinolone 0.1% or other mid-potency steroid ointment twice daily for two weeks, then as needed for persistent plaques, oral hydroxyzine 10–20 mg qhs, daily moisturizing cream 1 to 2 times daily. No skin scratching. Consider treatment with antibiotic against *Staphylococcus aureus*, such as cephalexin, dicloxacillin, or doxycycline.
Lichen simplex chronicus	Potent topical steroid such as clobetasol or diprolene ointment or cream twice daily for two weeks, or coverage with medicated tape such as cordran tape and change daily or every other day and wash with mild soap/dry in between, no scratching. Treatment is generally for two weeks, then treat for 7 days on / 7 days off cycle as needed for residual/recurrent lesions.
Seborrheic dermatitis	Scalp: ketoconazole or Selsun lotion or tar-, zinc-, or salicylic acid–containing shampoos once daily—leave on 5 to 10 minutes, then rinse out (twice in a row if flaring badly), followed by mid-potency topical steroid such as triamcinolone lotion or fluocinolone once nightly for two weeks, then three times weekly at night; wash out in the morning. Face: clotrimazole or ketoconazole cream, hydrocortisone, or triamcinolone 0.025% cream individually or mix antifungal with steroid and use twice daily for two weeks, then decrease to three times weekly; use sparingly as needed for chronic rash.

erythematous and weepy; the latter are often cool in temperature, but misdiagnosed as *acute cellulitis*. Treatment is with graduated compression stockings or wraps (check first for adequate arterial perfusion; see first part of chapter on venous ulcer), mid-potency topical steroid ointments, and cool water soaks.

Case Five Final Diagnosis: Venous stasis dermatitis. The patient's condition improved with elevation, local wound care, padded compression.

FOOT AND NAIL DISEASES

Sample Case Six

Thumbnail: An elderly homeless male presents with worsening pain at the great toe. He does not recall recent acute trauma to the toe, but wears ill-fitting shoes.

Physical Exam: Dystrophic nail from onychomycosis, with possible darkly pigmented nailbed.

Differential Diagnosis: Nailbed melanoma, ingrown toenail, subungual hematoma.

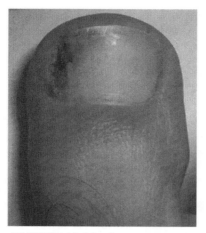

FIGURE 13.10   Ingrown toenail.

Ingrown toenails (Figure 13.10) are common problems in the homeless, with improperly fitting shoes present in approximately one-third of all the persons in one study (To, Brothers, & Van Zoost, 2016). Improper toenail trimming may contribute, and patients need educating to trim nails square and not too short. Shoes that compress the toes, augmented by prolonged standing, and poor hygiene cause the lateral "ingrown toenail" to pierce the adjacent nailfold skin, with resultant *foreign body reaction* or even acute secondary *infection*. The great toe is most commonly affected and may manifest as erythema, swelling, and sometimes purulent or sanguineous drainage. Treatment involves topical or local anesthesia, sterile skin preparation, and meticulous removal of the ingrown lateral portion of the nail. Dental floss or a small amount of cotton from cotton from a cotton swab can be placed between the nail plate and nailbed to help prevent further ingrown reaction, and some use phenol or cauterization of the nail growth plate laterally to reduce recurrence. After the healing wound stabilizes, careful washing with regular soap is ideal. Shoes need to be loose or more appropriately fitting: sandals would be ideal. Empiric antibiotics covering gram-positive organisms, including MRSA, as listed in the table for cellulitis, are recommended for patients with such an infectious component. Post-procedure follow-up is essential to confirm stable healing

Case Six Final Diagnosis: Ingrown toenail. Improved with removal, cauterization of the nail growth plate, and improved fitting of shoes and local nail care (Table 13.3).

TABLE 13.3 *Foot and Nails*

Ailment	Prevention and Treatment Options
Ingrown toenails	Avoidance of tight shoes, avoid close trimming of nails, or trauma to feet. Use warm Epsom salt soaks; use cotton or dental floss in-between nail plate and lateral nail fold to prevent recurrence
Diabetic foot ailments	Wear diabetic shoes, never go barefoot, always pare down all callosities. Examine feet daily.
Nailbed atypia	Evaluate any pigmented lesions by serial photos, measurement, and history Dystrophic lesions should be sent for fungal culture; nailbed lesions may need nail removal to evaluate for subungual warts or neoplasm; consider nail matrix or nailbed biopsy for persistent or growing neoplasms (especially if pigmented).

REFERENCES

Burkhart, C. N., Burkhart, C. G., & Morrell, D. S. (2012). Infestations. In J. L. Bolognia, J. L. Jorizzo, & J. V. Schaeffer (Eds.), *Dermatology* (3rd ed., pp. 1423–1432). Philadephia, PA: Elsevier.

Colburn, D. (1989). Homeless people suffer more serious skin diseases. *The Washington Post*, pp. 9–10. Retrieved from https://www.washingtonpost.com/archive/lifestyle/wellness/1989/11/28/homeless-people-suffer-more-serious-skin-diseases/c94e357f-9b7f-4db2-bdb7-72484377803e/?utm_term=.114732fa107f

Contag, C., Lowenstein, S. E., Jain, S., & Amerson, E. (2017). Survey of symptomatic dermatologic disease in homeless patients at a shelter-based clinic. *Our Dermatology Online, 8*(2), 133–137. doi:10.7241/ourd.20172.37

Explore Nursing Diagnosis, Nursing Assessment, and More! (n.d.). Retrieved from https://www.pinterest.com/pin/553942822899116573

Health Care for the Homeless Clinician's Network. (2006).Homeless people at higher risk for CA-MRSA, HIV and TB. *Healing Hands, 10*(5). Retrieved from http://www.nhchc.org/wp-content/uploads/2012/02/Dec2006HealingHands.pdf

Henry, M., Watt, R., Rosenthal, L., & Shivji, A.. (2016). *The 2016 Annual Homeless Assessment Report (AHAR) to Congress November 2016: Part 1-Point in Time estimates of homelessness*: The U.S. Department of Housing and Urban Development. Retrieved from https://www.hudexchange.info/resources/document/2016-AHAR-Part-1.pdf

Hosler, G. A., & Patterson, J. W. (2016). Lentigines, nevi and melanomas. In J. W. Patterson (Ed.), *Weedon's skin pathology* (4th ed., pp. 837–902). Philadephia, PA: Churchill Livingston Elsevier.

James, W. D., Berger, T. G., & Elston, D. M. (2006). *Andrews' diseases of the skin clinical dermatology* (pp. 51–90). Philadelphia, PA: Saunders Elsevier.

Oyerinde, O. M. D. (2014). The effect of hygiene on dermatological concerns in homeless patients GE-National Medical Fellowship: Primary care leadership *program*. Retrieved from https://nmfonline.org/wp-content/uploads/2016/02/Oyerinde-Oyetewa-Paper.pdf

Raoult, D. (2001). Infections in the homeless. *Lancet Infectious Diseases, 1*(2), 77–84. doi:10.1016/S1473-3099(01)00062-7

Red Book. (n.d.). Retrieved from https://redbook.solutions.aap.org

Stevens, D. L., Bisno, A. L., Chambers, H. F., Dellinger, E. P., Goldstein, E. J., Gorbach, S. L., . . . Wade, J. C. (2014). Practice guidelines for the diagnosis and management of skin and soft tissue infections: 2014 update by the Infectious Diseases Society of America. *Clinical Infectious Diseases, 59*(2), 147. doi:10.1093/cid/ciu444

Stratigos, A. J., Stern, R., Gonzalez, E., Johnson, R. A., O'Connell, J., & Dover, J. S. (1999). Prevalence of skin disease in a cohort of shelter-based homeless men. *Journal of the American Academy of Dermatology, 41*(2I), 197–202. doi:10.1016/S0190-9622(99)70048-4

To, M. J., Brothers, T. D., & Van Zoost, C. (2016). Foot conditions among homeless persons: A systematic review. *PLoS One, 11*(12), 1–14. doi:10.1371/journal.pone.0167463

UpToDate. (n.d.). Retrieved from https://www.uptodate.com

WebMD. (n.d.). Skin problems & treatments guide. Retrieved from http://www.webmd.boots.com/skin-problems-and-treatments/guide/abcess

Werner, R. N., Sammain, A., Erdmann, R., Hartmann, V., Stockfleth, E., & Nast, A. (2013). The natural history of actinic keratosis: A systematic review. *British Journal of Dermatology, 169*(3), 502–518. doi:10.1111/bjd.12420

Wilde, M., Jones, B., Lewis, B. K., & Hull, C. M. (2013). Skin cancer screening in homeless Salt Lake City 2013. *Dermatology Online Journal, 19*(1), 14.

14

End-of-Life Considerations in Homelessness and Aging

Kelly Conright, Ruth Simonis, Muhammad Atif Waqar, and Diane Chau

Perhaps end-of-life considerations for homeless elderly could be considered a topic of fictional creation, a sociomedical unicorn. Because, depending on one's perspective, the curse or blessing of homelessness is the failure to even reach an age that is generally acknowledged as "geriatric."

So, to begin the discussion for end-of-life considerations for homeless elderly, a revised definition of elderly relative to the realities of being homeless must be examined. Traditionally, geriatric medicine and gerontology have had a focus for populations aged 65 years and older. However, the average age of death of homeless people is 48 years (Claudia, 2016), with the average range being 42 to 56 years, far from the "typical" age profile considered geriatric. With challenges of premature aging and mortality, the growing consensus is that homeless individuals age 50 years and up be considered as "older homeless."

The harsh realities of homelessness and the associated poverty lend to a premature physiologic aging or "weathering." The homeless experience involves exposure to inclement weather, poor sanitary conditions with high prevalence of infections, and the stress of deprivation and hunger. Additionally, homeless are often afflicted with mental health issues, both organic in nature and resulting from factors such as exposure to violence, rape, and robbery. Of paramount significance to the compromised health of the homeless elderly are poor and inadequate sleeping conditions, which directly impact health and well-";being. For the homeless, sleep often becomes a matter of "where you can, when you can" it is often interrupted with noise, plagued with the insecurity of one's person and property, and can be limited to less than six hours of sleep in a day. With chronic sleep deprivation, the homeless suffer increased medical consequences, such as heart disease, diabetes, obesity, impaired immune function, and mental health illnesses, such as depression and anxiety, making the incumbent suffering abundantly clear. These are among the multitude of conditions that contribute to the higher incidence of chronic health conditions (Table 14.1), which when untreated and undertreated, as is common for the homeless, all lead to premature morbidity and mortality. The standardized mortality ratios reported vary between studies and countries but are typically two to five times the age-standardized general population (Fazel, Geddes, & Kushel, 2014).

In addition to the increased prevalence and severity of chronic health conditions in the homeless elderly population, there is the added burden of geriatric syndromes, such as functional decline, cognitive impairment, frailty, and incontinence. These syndromes are commonly associated with aging and result in a compromised independence and quality of life and are more prevalent for the homeless than sheltered cohorts (Brown, Kiely, Bharel, & Mitchell, 2012).

Access barriers to healthcare, along with distrust of the modern healthcare system, also accelerate and exacerbate chronic health conditions. All of these factors combined lead down a steeper, slipperier path to end-stage or terminal conditions, thus compounding the hardship of the elderly homeless experience.

Perhaps the most astonishing conclusion that could be drawn from the wealth of medical literature about modifiable risk factors for mortality in public health is homelessness. Many medical conditions have well-established

TABLE 14.1 *Prevalence of Specific Health Conditions Among the Homeless Population in Comparison to the General U.S. Population*

Health Condition	Estimate in the Homeless Population	Estimate in the United States
Hypertension	50%	29%
Diabetes	Up to 18%	9.3%
Myocardial infarction	35%	Up to 17%
HIV	Up to 21%	0.6%
Hepatitis C	Up to 36%	0.7%
Depression	Up to 49%	8%
Substance dependence	Up to 58%	Up to 16%

Source: Adapted and modified from Claudia, D. (2016). Advance care planning for individuals experiencing homelessness. *InFocus*, 4(2). Retrieved from https://www.nhchc.org/wp-content/uploads/2016/06/in-focus-advance-care-planning-final-for-posting.pdf

effects on mortality; with a variety of modifiable risk factors such as smoking (life reduction of 10 years), obesity (life reduction eight years), or diabetes that impact life expectancy often present in homeless individuals, one could easily conclude that one of the single greatest risk factors for early mortality is being homeless!

Indeed, even the end-of-life experience for homeless elders differs compared to sheltered cohorts. In the modern age of medicine, elderly people commonly experience changes of health, leading to gradual loss of independence, with health decline trajectories that typically play out over years, often with a waxing and waning course. For the homeless, death not only is premature, it is also more commonly sudden—from unintentional causes such as alcohol or drug overdoses, injuries due to falls, being struck by a motor vehicle, hypothermia or heatstroke from exposure to the elements, violence, and even suicide (Figure 14.1).

Adding the proverbial insult to injury of higher disease prevalence and earlier death, particular to homeless elderly, is a double jeopardy for the end-of-life journey: a disproportionate burden of suffering. This is seen through higher reports of pain and psychological distress found among the homeless nearing the end of life (Tobey et al., 2017). Adding fire to this fuel of suffering is the fact that homeless elders have experience with death, having had a

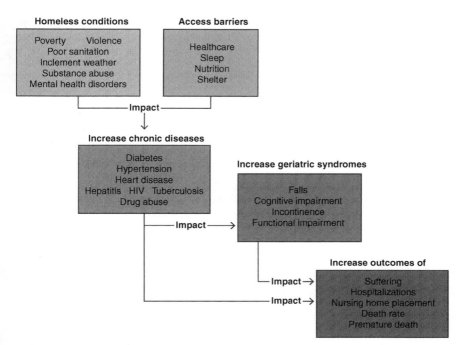

FIGURE 14.1 Homeless elderly premature death cascade.

disproportionately high, and almost universal, personal contact with death through family members and/or peers.

This constellation of challenges of homeless elders nearing end of life presents questions such as "What are the possibilities for a person-centered approach to prepare for this difficult reality?" and "How would care and services be created and delivered to best meet these unique needs?"

ADVANCE CARE PLANNING WITH AGING HOMELESS AT END OF LIFE

If you were to ask a young person what it would look like for an elderly individual to contemplate a life-limiting illness and end-of-life care, some might talk about someone having difficulty navigating around his or her home, requiring assistance to prepare a meal, use the toilet, take a shower, or get in and out of a vehicle due to increasing functional limitations. They may describe a general loss of strength and independence with an increasing need for family or other caregivers to step in to take over tasks such as shopping, cleaning, transportation to medical appointments, and paying bills.

But what happens when you do not have a home that shelters you from the freezing temperatures or the relentless heat; a place that provides a warm and safe place to sleep, shower, get undressed, and know that your clothes will be there in the morning; or a place to rest your weary and painful body in the comfort of a soft bed and nestle down into clean sheets that are not crawling with lice or soiled with layers of dirt and grime? What if there is no refrigerator to keep food from spoiling and you have to walk long distance just to have any food at all—assuming you have any money to purchase and prepare food, a way to haul it, and a place to keep it safe from the elements and natural predators (man and animal). Imagine looking into store-glass windows and seeing the face of someone who looks at least 70 years old when in truth you are in your late forties, but with crippling symptoms that make you feel 100. You have not been to a doctor, perhaps for decades. You may not be able to afford regular medical care or treatment because it takes everything you have just to survive being homeless.

Challenges in Accessing Healthcare for Homeless Aging at End of Life

In addition to typical challenges one faces when dealing with a decline in functional abilities and independence, the homeless elder encounters unique challenges. These challenges come in the form of a general mistrust of medical professionals, perceived or actual discrimination, or something as simple as a lack of identification, fixed address, or telephone number to establish contact or follow-up with medical providers (Dubbert, Garner, Lensing, White, & Sullivan, 2017). Given the competing interests of day-to-day survival, preventative care is simply not a high priority (Hubbell, 2017). Therefore, by the time elderly homeless individuals encounter a life-threatening illness, these specialty services are even more elusive (Hudson, Flemming, Shulman, & Candy, 2016). Assuming services were attainable, the delay in treatment can transform what may have been a preventable disease into a terminal illness. Ideally, conversations around preferences for medical care and treatment are ongoing within the context of long-term health management. However, statistically, the homeless use emergency room services four times as much as their nonhomeless cohort, contributing not only to the lack of continuity of care, but also to lost opportunities to engage the aging homeless in long-term advance care planning (Hudson, Flemming, Shulman, & Candy, 2016).

Perceptions of Dying of the Aging Homeless at End of Life

A qualitative study by Song and Ratner (2007) concluded that homeless individuals have significant exposure to death and dying, whether from trauma and losses sustained in childhood or the risks associated with being homeless and living on the streets (Claudia, 2016). The frequency of their exposure made the concepts of death and dying a constant companion, causing some to conclude that death could be "'right around the corner'" for any of them (Song & Ratner, 2007). The participants of the study voiced a number of fears, ranging from being subjected to unwanted invasive life-sustaining treatments, to dying alone and unacknowledged, to having no control regarding the disposition of their remains (Song & Bartels, 2007). The frequency of exposure to death and dying caused some to adopt a fatalistic attitude of seeming to accept the inevitable, while others would emotionally pull back and isolate as a means of coping with future loss (Song, 2010). Some used their experiences to justify continued participation in high-risk behaviors, while others used these experiences to pull together to improve their sense of safety and their chances for survival (Sumalinog, Harrington, Dosani, & Hwang, 2017). Interestingly, the homeless participants in this study placed significant importance on engaging in advance care planning and documenting their treatment preferences, given their prevalent experience with death and dying (Tarzian, 2005). Engaging in advance care planning empowered otherwise alienated and marginalized individuals to give voice to their treatment preferences and provided a sense of control for their future (Tobey et al., 2017).

Spiritual and Religious Consideration at End of Life

For many caught in addictions or experiencing the stress of loss or homelessness, a strong connection to God or a higher power can provide meaning and purpose for living and enable individuals to cope with or rise above their circumstances (Wikipedia, 2017). In a study by Tarzian, Neal, and O'Neil (2005) with the inner-city homeless, religious beliefs and spiritual experiences played an important role in how they approached end-of-life treatment decisions. Some held that, while individual preferences were important, there was equal—if not greater—importance attached to the individual's view of God's will as to the timing and circumstances of his or her death (Tobey et al., 2017). Some found comfort in an afterlife where they would be free from pain and suffering; determining that present circumstances could be managed in light of their hope for the future. Some sought guidance for local church leaders or through personal communion with God. In addition to their cognitive religious beliefs about God, the participants placed significant importance on their spiritual experiences of God, attributing their ability to overcome addiction and cope with loss to God's interventions in their lives. Participants described these spiritual experiences in terms of "feeling" God's presence and power, a kind of "spiritual knowing." In reviewing the comments made by the participants of this study, the process of making end-of-life treatment decisions may, among other factors, be significantly influenced by a complex and uniquely personal blend of an individual's spiritual and personal experiences and religious or doctrinal beliefs.

Advance Care Planning

Advance care planning is the process by which one decides what types of treatment one prefers at the end of life, but also who can speak on his or her behalf should the person become unable to speak for himself or herself. Individuals often know what they want or do not want with regard to life-sustaining treatments either through personal life experiences, general observations, or media education, but unless these decisions are documented and made part of the medical record, they will not be effective should the individual encounter a medical crisis.

The difficulty for homeless individuals engaging in advance care planning is complex and multi-factorial. The lack of access to primary care settings where these types of discussions predominantly take place presents few opportunities to engage in extended conversations about end-of-life care. In addition, the homeless individuals may be nomadic with a lack of consistent social environment or alienated from family and loved ones, making the selection of a healthcare surrogate challenging. The experiences of prejudice, discrimination, or general mistrust of healthcare institutions or governmental bodies may cause homeless individuals to be reluctant to document or sign anything because they do not believe they will receive quality medical care and treatment to reverse an acute illness or injury.

Engaging homeless individuals in advance care planning can be as simple as carrying a statement of medical preference or the name and contact information of a person in their wallet they want to serve as a surrogate decision-maker in the event of a medical emergency. Ideally, clinical providers and agency personnel in medical outpatient settings or connected to outreach programs for the homeless population will assist individuals to complete an advance directive to formalize their preferences and to file that document with the local hospital or agencies where the individuals are likely to receive medical care. In addition, many states have a general registry to hold electronic copies of an individual's advance directive and/or state-authorized portable order to be retrieved by medical care providers; in which case, the homeless individual need only carry a card in their wallet to reference the location.

This is not an exhaustive list, but does demonstrate that concerted effort needs to be made to actively engage homeless individuals in conversations about end-of-life care in a way that is meaningful, respectful, and mindful of their circumstances and their desire to have a voice in their future medical care and treatment.

Care Coverage

When discussing advance directive in the setting of palliative care, it is prudent to consider coverage for care and what options are available to homeless individuals to cover cost of care. Standard healthcare options include Medicare, Medicaid, and Veterans Affairs and each of these eligibility criteria should be considered. Publications are available to educate providers on how to use different resources to help homeless persons fund their palliative care needs. As regulations and criteria frequently change based on congressional budgets, only some of these will be referenced. For instance, A Primer on How to use Medicaid is available on the Internet at https://www.hhs.gov/programs/social-services/homelessness/research/how-to-use-medicaid-to-assist-homeless-persons/index.html. Each state is allowed to supplement their benefits with optional and mandated services, such as palliative care. These optional and mandated services are available on websites for each state-operated Medicaid program and vary greatly from state to state, i.e., California Medicaid covers palliative care costs in 2018.

PALLIATIVE AND HOSPICE CARE DELIVERY FOR THE GERIATRIC HOMELESS

Homeless elders express a surprising resilience and assign personal meaning to the suffering and afterlife as a balance against the burden of inordinate suffering. Perhaps as part of a disenfranchised, marginalized, and even invisible group, the homeless most desperately need a radically different model of care and delivery to meet the almost inconceivable challenges and suffering, which is the life of these elders. If we are judged as a society by how we care for the least of us, then we must heed the clarion call and rise to the moral imperative to serve the homeless elders where they are and where they go.

Often, the terminally ill subset of this population receive end-of-life care in shelters, hostels, or homes for the homeless (Hudson et al., 2016). This is in part due to the preference and wishes of homeless individuals to remain in the shelter during the course of their deteriorating health, rather than transferring to a healthcare facility (Håkanson et al., 2016). Usually, this stems from a mistrust and dislike of the healthcare system, familiarity of the shelter environment, and relationships that they have developed with the staff operating said facilities.

Unfortunately, this presents numerous challenges in trying to provide optimal end-of-life care in shelters and homes for the homeless that are cash strapped, have very limited resources, and were not designed to provide care to the terminally ill (Hudson et al., 2016; McNeil, Guirguis-Younger, & Dilley, 2012). Resources at such shelters need to be distributed equally among residents, and this may not be sustainable for individuals with very advanced and terminal conditions (Webb, 2015). Additionally, lack of necessary medical equipment and devices, essential medications required for palliation of symptoms, inadequate staffing, and lack of trained clinical expertise have all been noted as important factors why provision of end-of-life care in hostels and shelters is so challenging (McNeil, Guirguis-Younger, Dilley, Aubry, et al., 2012).

Despite the numerous barriers and challenges, sparks of hope in models of palliative and hospice care have sprouted across the United States. Models of housing and homes, for a few or for many, in cities big and small offer the guidance and inspiration of safety nets that speak to improve quality of life and relief of suffering for these at risk and most vulnerable elders.

INNOVATIVE PALLIATIVE CARE DELIVERY MODELS

Shelter-Based Palliative Care

One such model is the "Hospice for the Homeless" program at the Alpha Project, a nonprofit organization based out of San Diego, California (The

Alpha Project, 2009). Since the program began in 2007, they have supported efforts to empower over 3,000 homeless individuals. Their program initially focused on a "Dying With Dignity" aspect of care for homeless veterans and indigent people with serious and life-threatening diagnosis who had an estimated prognosis of six months or less to live. In addition to assistance with housing, case management, and support services, they also facilitated procuring medical care from local home hospice agencies in the community. Not surprisingly, with palliation from a supported safe living environment, some homeless receiving this comprehensive service led to improvement, stabilization, and an increased life span. Understanding that is occasionally an expected outcome with best supportive care, The Alpha Project included the "Living With Dignity" component as an extension of this program to cater to homeless people fortunate enough to come off of hospice care and continue to receive support as the project's funding permits.

A similar nonprofit hospice program for the homeless is "The INN Between" located in Salt Lake City, Utah (The INN Between, 2015). Since its inception in 2015, The INN Between has catered to many homeless patients with serious and life-threatening illnesses by providing over 8,000 housing nights to date. The facility is unique, in that they offer a 15-bed temporary housing option with comprehensive care and support services intended to serve homeless who may need care after serious illness or surgery, or while undergoing chemotherapy, or for palliative and even hospice care. The staff and volunteers cater beyond the basic needs to provide companionship; emotional and spiritual support; complementary and alternative care such as music therapy, pet therapy, activities, acupuncture, reiki, massage, salon services, and other services; and therapies that improve the quality of life while relieving pain and anxiety. Additionally, they attempt to reconnect the homeless with their family by reaching out to any known family members and relatives before the person passes away. Posthumously, many services are rendered that are unique yet inspirational at the same time. These include the posting of an obituary on their website, conduction of a memorial service in the homeless patient's honor, and placing the patient's name on a plaque in the memorial garden.

In Washington, DC, the Joseph House, which originally opened in response to the AIDS crisis in the early 1990s, offers a home and medical care to the homeless with advanced-stage AIDS and terminal cancers (Joseph House, 2017). The Joseph House offers a practice of compassionate relationship-centered care with dedicated nursing and personal care services around the clock. Understanding that many homeless patients continue to struggle with addiction and drug abuse, including toward the end of life, the Joseph House also supports their residents with addiction recovery and offers grief counseling. Impressively, through a network of trained volunteers from the community, the facility is also able to keep vigil with actively dying patients so that no resident dies alone. In addition to end-of-life care, the facility also supports residential respite care for patients with advanced HIV, with the goal to optimize them so that they can safely return to independent living. Along these same lines, they have begun a pilot project of supportive housing for residents discharged from the Joseph House, but who require ongoing medical case management, sobriety support, assistance with education, and employment. They have observed that many of their former residents continue to maintain a strong bond and relationship with the Joseph House and its staff members even after discharge, which speaks volumes about the quality of compassionate care that is provided at the facility.

REFERENCES

The Alpha Project. (2009). Hospice for the Homeless. Retrieved from https://www.alphaproject.org/programs/hospice-for-the-homeless

Brown, R. T., Kiely, D. K., Bharel, M., & Mitchell, S. L. (2012). Geriatric syndromes in older homeless adults. *Journal of General Internal Medicine, 27*(1), 16–22. doi:10.1007/s11606-011-1848-9

Claudia, D. (2016). Advance care planning for individuals experiencing homelessness. *InFocus, 4*, 2. Retrieved from https://www.nhchc.org/wp-content/uploads/2016/06/in-focus-advance-care-planning-final-for-posting.pdf

Dubbert, P. M., Garner, K. K., Lensing, S., White, J. G., & Sullivan, D. H. (2017). Engagement in steps of advance health care planning by homeless veterans. *Psychological Services, 14*(2), 214–220. doi:10.1037/ser0000147

Fazel, S., Geddes, J. R., & Kushel, M. (2014). The health of homeless people in high-income countries: Descriptive epidemiology, health consequences, and clinical and policy recommendations. *Lancet (London, England), 384*(9953), 1529–1540. doi:10.1016/S0140-6736(14)61132-6

Håkanson, C., Sandberg, J., Ekstedt, M., Kenne Sarenmalm, E., Christiansen, M., & Öhlén, J. (2016). Providing palliative care in a Swedish support home for people who are homeless. *Qualitative Health Research, 26*(9), 1252–1262. doi:10.1177/1049732315588500.

Hubbell, S. A. (2017). Advance care planning with individuals experiencing homelessness: Literature review and recommendations for public health practice. *Public Health Nursing, 34*(5), 1–7. doi:10.1111/phn.12333

Hudson, B. F., Flemming, K., Shulman, C., & Candy, B. (2016). Challenges to access and provision of palliative care for people who are homeless: A systematic review of qualitative research. *BMC Palliative Care, 15*(1), 96. doi:10.1186/s12904-016-0168-6

The INN Between. (2015). Hospice for the Homeless. Retrieved from https://www.theinnbetweenslc.org

Joseph House. (2017). End-of-life care. Retrieved from http://josephshouse.org/programs/residential-care

McNeil, R., Guirguis-Younger, M., & Dilley, L. B. (2012). Recommendations for improving the end-of-life care system for homeless populations: A qualitative study of the views of Canadian health and social services professionals. *BMC Palliative Care, 11*, 14.

McNeil, R., Guirguis-Younger, M., Dilley, L. B., Aubry, T. D., Turnbull, J., & Hwang, S. W. (2012). Harm reduction services as a point-of-entry to and source of end-of-life care and support for homeless and marginally housed persons who use alcohol and/or illicit drugs: A qualitative analysis. *BMC Public Health, 12*, 312. doi:10.1186/1471-2458-12-312

Song, J. (2010). Effect of an end-of-life planning intervention on the completion of advance directives in homeless persons. *Annals of Internal Medicine, 153*, 76–84.

Song, J., & Bartels, D. M. (2007). Dying on the streets: Homeless person's concerns and desires about end of life care. *Society of General Internal Medicine, 22*, 435–441.

Song, J., & Ratner, E. R. (2007). Experiences with and attitudes toward death and dying among homeless persons. *Society of General Internal Medicine, 22*, 427–434.

Sumalinog, R., Harrington, K., Dosani, N., & Hwang, S. W. (2017). Advance care planning, palliative care, and end-of-life are interventions for homeless people: A systematic review. *Palliative Medicine, 31*(2), 109–119.

Tarzian, A. J., Neal, M. T., O'Neil, J. A. (2005) Attitudes, experiences, and beliefs affecting end-of-life decision-making among homeless individuals. *Journal of Palliative Medicine, 8*(1), 36–48.

Tobey, M., Manasson, J., Decarlo, K., Ciraldo-Maryniuk, K., Gaeta, J. M., & Wilson, E. (2017). Homeless individuals approaching the end of life: Symptoms and attitudes. *Journal of Pain and Symptom Management, 53*(4), 738–744. doi:10.1016/j.jpainsymman.2016.10.364

Webb, W. A (2015). When dying at home is not an option: Exploration of hostel staff views on palliative care for homeless people. *International Journal of Palliative Nursing, 21*(5), 236–244. doi:10.12968/ijpn.2015.21.5.236

Wikipedia. (2017). Spirituality and homelessness [Updated 2017-02-06-t23:54Z]. Retrieved from http://en.wikipedia.org/wiki/Spirituality_and_homelessness

Index

Made in the USA
Middletown, DE
21 July 2022

69815528R00170